PREHOSPITAL EMERGENCY CARE SECRETS

PREHOSPITAL EMERGENCY CARE SECRETS

PETER T. PONS, MD, FACEP
Associate Professor of Emergency Medicine
Department of Surgery
University of Colorado Health Sciences Center
Senior Physician
Denver Health Medical Center
Denver, Colorado

VINCENT J. MARKOVCHICK, MD, FACEP
Director, Emergency Medical Services
Director, Denver Health Paramedics
Denver Health Medical Center
Professor of Emergency Medicine
Department of Surgery
University of Colorado Health Sciences Center
Denver, Colorado

HANLEY & BELFUS, INC./ Philadelphia

Publisher: HANLEY & BELFUS, INC.
                    Medical Publishers
                    210 South 13th Street
                    Philadelphia, PA 19107
                    (215) 546-7293; 800-962-1892
                    FAX (215) 790-9330
                    Web site: http://www.hanleyandbelfus.com

Note to the reader: Although the information in this book has been carefully reviewed for correctness of dosage and indications, neither the authors nor the editors nor the publisher can accept any legal responsibility for any errors or omissions that may be made. Neither the publisher nor the editors make any warranty, expressed or implied, with respect to the material contained herein. Before prescribing any drug, the reader must review the manufacturer's current product information (package inserts) for accepted indications, absolute dosage recommendations, and other information pertinent to the safe and effective use of the product described. This is especially important when drugs are given in combination or as an adjunct to other forms of therapy.

Library of Congress Cataloging-in-Publication Data

Prehospital emergency care secrets : questions you will be asked—at the scene,
    in the ED, on oral exams / [edited by] Peter T. Pons, Vincent J. Markovchick.
        p.   c.—(The Secrets Series®)
    Includes bibliographical references and index.
    ISBN 1-56053-250-5 (alk. paper)
    1. Emergency medical services—Miscellanea.   2. Emergency medicine—
Miscellanea.   I. Pons, Peter T.   II. Markovchick, V.   III. Series.
    [DNLM: 1. Emergency Medical Services—examination questions.
2. Emergencies—examination questions.   WX 18.2 P923 1998]
RA645.5.P736   1998
362.18'076—dc21
DNLM/DLC
for Library of Congress   97-51462
                                                                        CIP

PREHOSPITAL EMERGENCY CARE SECRETS   ISBN 1-56053-250-5

Last digit is the print number: 9   8   7   6   5   4   3   2   1

CONTENTS

CONTRIBUTORS

Jean T. Abbott, M.D., FACEP
Associate Professor, Division of Emergency Medicine, University of Colorado School of Medicine; Attending Emergency Department Physician, University Hospital, Denver, Colorado

Jonathan D. Apfelbaum, M.D.
Department of Emergency Medicine, Denver Health Medical Center Affiliated Residency in Emergency Medicine, Denver, Colorado

F. Keith Battan, M.D., FAAP
Associate Professor of Pediatrics, University of Colorado School of Medicine; Associate Director, Emergency Services, Children's Hospital, Denver, Colorado

David Bobes, EMT-P
Paramedic Division, Denver General Hospital, Denver, Colorado

Susan Elaine Bobes, M.D.
Staff Physician, Emergency Department, Davis Memorial Hospital, Elkins, West Virginia

Scott Bolleter, EMT-P, I/C
Flight Paramedic and Educator, San Antonio AirLife, San Antonio, Texas

Joan Bothner, M.D.
Associate Professor, Department of Pediatrics, University of Colorado School of Medicine; Medical Director, Emergency Department, Children's Hospital, Denver, Colorado

Marilyn K. Bourn, R.N., M.S.N., EMT-P
Emergency Medical Services Educator and Senior Instructor, Division of Emergency Medicine, University of Colorado School of Medicine, Denver, Colorado

Scott Wesley Branney, M.D.
Chief Resident, Denver Health Medical Center Affiliated Residency in Emergency Medicine, Denver, Colorado

Michael W. Brunko, M.D.
Associate Medical Director, Flight for Life, Centura St. Anthony Hospital, Denver, Colorado

Richard Frederick Buchanan, B.A., EMT-P
Emergency Medical Services Director and Education Program Director, Emergency Medical Services Department, Western State College (Continuing Education); Gunnison Valley Hospital, Gunnison, Colorado

Thomas G. Burke, M.D.
Attending Physician, Department of Emergency Medicine, Lutheran Medical Center, Denver, Colorado

Kevin H. Chu, M.B., B.S.
Fellow and Staff Emergency Physician, Department of Emergency Medicine, William Beaumont Hospital, Royal Oak, Michigan

Anne E. Clouatre, B.A., EMT-P
Department Coordinator, Porter Adventist Prehospital Services, Centura Health-Porter/Littleton Adventist Hospitals, Denver, Colorado

Pam Copeland, EMT-B
Paramedic Division, Denver Health Medical Center, Denver, Colorado

Tom Cribley, M.S.H.A., EMT-P
Paramedic Division, Denver Health Medical Center, Denver, Colorado

Kevin L. Crumpton, M.D.
Senior Resident, Department of Emergency Medicine, Denver Health Medical Center Affiliated
Residency in Emergency Medicine, Denver, Colorado

Catherine B. Custalow, M.D., Ph.D.
Resident Physician, Department of Emergency Medicine, Denver Health Medical Center, Denver,
Colorado

Paul Davidson, M.D.
Assistant Professor, Department of Surgery, University of Colorado School of Medicine; University
Hospital, Denver, Colorado

Robert M. Domeier, M.D.
Clinical Instructor, Department of Emergency Medicine, University of Michigan Medical School;
Emergency Medicine Residency Program, St. Joseph Mercy Hospital, Ann Arbor, Michigan

Susan A. Egaas, M.D.
Department of Emergency Medicine, Denver Health Medical Center, Denver, Colorado

Kim M. Feldhaus, M.D., FACEP
Associate Program Director, Denver Health Medical Center Affiliated Residency in Emergency
Medicine, Denver, Colorado

Herbert G. Garrison, M.D., M.P.H.
Associate Professor of Emergency Medicine, East Carolina University School of Medicine; Attending
Physician, University Health Systems of Eastern Carolina, Greenville, North Carolina

Marilyn J. Gifford, M.D., FACEP
Director, Emergency Services, Memorial Hospital, Colorado Springs, Colorado; Assistant Clinical
Professor, Department of Surgery, Division of Emergency Medicine, University of Colorado Health
Sciences Center, Denver, Colorado

Stewart L. Greisman, D.O., FACEP
Medical Director, United Healthcare of Colorado, Englewood, Colorado; Assistant Clinical Professor,
Department of Surgery, Division of Emergency Medicine, University of Colorado School of Medicine,
University of Colorado Health Sciences Center; Swedish Medical Center; Denver, Colorado

S. Scott Henderson, J.D., EMT-P
Emergency Medical Services Law Instructor, American College of Prehospital Medicine, New
Orleans, Louisiana; Private Practice, Lakewood, Colorado

Michael Hunt, M.D.
Emergency Medical Services Department, Columbia Health One, Englewood, Colorado

Lance W. Jobe, M.D.
Department of Emergency Medicine, Denver Health Medical Center, Denver, Colorado

Christina Johnson, M.D.
Attending Physician, Emergency Department; Associate Medical Director, Paramedic Division,
Denver Health Medical Center, Denver, Colorado

Jon R. Krohmer, M.D., FACEP
Associate Professor, Section of Emergency Medicine, Michigan State University College of Human
Medicine; Medical Director, Kent County Emergency Medical Services; EMS Director, Emergency
Medicine Residency, Butterworth Hospital, Grand Rapids, Michigan

Preston Love, R.N., B.S.N., CFRN, CEN, EMT-P
Flight Nurse, San Antonio AirLife, San Antonio, Texas

Ronald F. Maio, D.O.
Associate Professor, Department of Emergency Medicine, University of Michigan Medical School;
Attending Physician, University of Michigan Medical Center, Ann Arbor, Michigan

Vincent J. Markovchick, M.D., FACEP
Director, Emergency Medical Services, and Medical Director, Paramedics, Denver Health Medical Center; Professor of Surgery, Division of Emergency Medicine, University of Colorado School of Medicine, Denver, Colorado

John P. Marshall, M.D.
Department of Emergency Medicine, Denver Health Medical Center, Denver, Colorado

Robert F. McCormack, M.D.
Clinical Assistant Professor, Department of Emergency Medicine, State University of New York at Buffalo; Attending Physician, Buffalo General Hospital; Attending Physician, Erie County Medical Center, Buffalo, New York

William R. Metcalf, EMT
Publisher and General Manager, Jems Communications, Carlsbad, California

John Lawrence Mottley, M.D., MHSA, FACEP
Associate Clinical Professor, Department of Emergency Medicine, Boston University School of Medicine; Executive Director and Chief Medical Officer, Boston Emergency Medical Services; Attending Physician, Boston Medical Center, Boston, Massachusetts

Paul Murphy, EMT-P
Emergency Medical Technician-Paramedic, Chapel Hill, North Carolina

Peter T. Pons, M.D.
Associate Professor of Emergency Medicine, Department of Surgery, University of Colorado Health Sciences Center; Senior Physician, Denver Health Medical Center, Denver, Colorado

John C. Riccio, M.D., FACEP
Medical Director, Emergency Department and Prehospital Services, Centura Health-Porter Adventist Hospital, Denver, Colorado

Jedd Roe, M.D., FACEP
Assistant Professor, Division of Emergency Medicine, Department of Surgery, University of Colorado School of Medicine; Attending Faculty, Emergency Medical Services, Denver Health Medical Center, Denver, Colorado

Randolph N. Royal, B.S., NREMT-P, EMT-T
Lieutenant, Colorado Springs Fire Department; Instructor and Coordinator, EMT-B Program, Department of Health Sciences, Pikes Peak Community College, Colorado Springs, Colorado

Julie Seaman, M.D.
Department of Emergency Medicine, Denver Health and Hospital, Denver, Colorado

Lee W. Shockley, M.D., FACEP
Assistant Professor of Surgery, Division of Emergency Medicine, University of Colorado School of Medicine; Residency Program Director, Denver Health Medical Center Residency in Emergency Medicine, Denver, Colorado

Mike Smith, MICP
Vice President, Emergency Medical Training Associates, Olympia, Washington

Michael J. Stackpool, M.D.
Department of Emergency Medicine, Denver Health Medical Center, Denver, Colorado

Robert E. Suter, D.O., M.H.A., FACEP
Chief, Emergency Services, Medical City-Dallas Hospital, Dallas, Texas; Assistant Professor, Department of Emergency Medicine, Medical College of Georgia, Augusta, Georgia

Robert Swor, D.O.
Emergency Medical Services Director and Staff Physician, Department of Emergency Medicine, William Beaumont Hospital, Royal Oak, Michigan

Michael Taigman, EMT-P
Emergency Medical Technician-Paramedic, Denver, Colorado

John Stockman Tarr, Jr., M.D.
Associate Clinical Professor, Department of Family Medicine, University of Colorado School of Medicine, Denver, Colorado; Gunnison Valley Hospital, Gunnison, Colorado

Mitchell E. Tilstra, EMD-P, EMD I/C
Vice President, AMR of Colorado, Aurora, Colorado; Emergency Medical Technician and Emergency Medic Dispatcher and Instructor, Ambulance Service Co., Denver, Colorado

Tom Tkach, NREMT-P
Director, Emergency Medical Services Education, Denver Health Paramedic Division, Denver Health Medical Center, Denver, Colorado

Patricia L. Tritt, R.N., M.A.
Director of Emergency Medical Services and Trauma, Columbia Health One, Denver, Colorado

W. Peter Vellman, M.D., FACEP
Director, Emergency Medical Services, St. Anthony Hospital, Denver, Colorado

Vincent P. Verdile, M.D.
Associate Professor and Chair, Department of Emergency Medicine, Albany Medical College; Emergency Physician, Albany Medical Center Hospital, Albany, New York

PREFACE

The past twenty-five years have seen a virtual revolution in the area of prehospital emergency care. Where once the only therapy for an out-of-hospital emergency medical situation was a ride to the hospital at a speed limited only by the vehicle you were in and the driving conditions at the time, now virtually the full interventional capability of the Emergency Department has been moved into the ambulance, and sophisticated medical care is brought to the patient to begin the process of providing medical care at the point of first contact.

Today's prehospital emergency care provider will be faced with a wide variety of medical and traumatic emergencies, will need a strong foundation of medical knowledge, and will be using a large armamentarium of interventions and treatment. It is with this in mind that we have prepared this book. We hope that it will, in its own unique way, provide practical information applicable to the prehospital setting and help the prehospital emergency care provider be prepared to manage the emergencies he or she will be called upon to assist.

Peter T. Pons, M.D.
Vincent J. Markovchick, M.D.

DEDICATION

To my parents, John and Cecelia, whose love always guided me and whose support helps me achieve, and to my wife, Kathy, whose love and support see me through each day.

PTP

To Leslie, Nicole, Tasha, and Nadia, and to the EMTs and Paramedics at the Denver Health Paramedic Division and the Denver Fire Department.

VMJ

I. EMS Overview

1. HISTORY OF EMERGENCY MEDICAL SERVICES

Michael Hunt, M.D.

1. When did emergency medical services (EMS) originate?

The answer lies not in any single event but in the *record* that defines circumstances making a particular form of care unique. Biblical scholars may point to the parable of the Good Samaritan, who cared for a man found beaten at the side of a road and transported him to an inn, as the seminal recorded event in EMS history. But, it is only a parable.

2. What are the earliest recorded EMS events?

Aside from the forced removal of lepers and venereal disease victims from their homes to isolate them from the rest of the community, the earliest organized efforts at the care and transport of the ill and injured originated centuries ago. Art historians suggest that Caesar employed battlefield medics before 100 AD. The first wagon for transporting patients, the Anglo-Saxon hammock, was developed about 900 AD. Literally a hammock on wheels, its brakes were chains held by attendants who endeavored to keep downhill runaway to a minimum. The Norman conquest of England brought many changes, including a covered horse litter for moving patients. Consisting of a bed on poles extending to horses on either end, this device, invented about 1100 AD, improved riding comfort.

3. Who was responsible for the first ambulances?

Actually, "ambulances" (or *ambulancias* in Spanish) were field hospitals initially introduced by Queen Isabella of Spain at the siege of Malaga in 1487. Both Ferdinand and Isabella insisted on staying with their troops during their conflict with the Moors and took exceptional interest in the comfort and welfare of their troops. This interest was manifest in the accumulation of medical and surgical supplies and battlefield tents *(ambulancias)* for the wounded.

4. Did Napoleon's surgeons use ambulances?

Dominique-Jean Larrey, distressed over the observation that, during a battle with the Prussians, the wounded were left in the field until fighting ceased, developed the concept of mobile *ambulancias* for the Army of the Rhine in 1793. Because of Larrey's reputation of concern for wounded soldiers, he was ordered to join Napoleon's Army of Italy, where he worked in conjunction with his senior partner, Baron Percy. Together, they are credited with the development of light, two-wheeled ambulances, which could stay in the battlefield—allowing surgeons to work there—or be used to transport wounded soldiers to the hospital. These vehicles were known as "flying ambulances" because they accompanied the "flying artillery" into war.

5. When did EMS get its start in the United States?

EMS in the United States evolved under parallel but separate military and civilian lines. The Civil War produced several refinements of Larrey's original plans. Jonathan Letterman organized the field medical service of the Union Army, helping to create a system of field evacuation and treatment of wounded soldiers and establish a uniform army ambulance system. Under Letterman, dangerous two-wheeled Finleys gave way to the Rucker ambulance. Steamships and railcars were modified to accommodate patients and provide care during transport to tertiary facilities.

The first civilian ambulances were hospital-based and included those of Cincinnati's Commercial Hospital prior to 1865 and Bellevue's ambulance, initiated in 1869. The latter service was staffed by a driver and a surgeon and could be dispatched with supplies and equipment, including bandages, splints, sponges, brandy, handcuffs, and a strait jacket. Ambulances of that era might be staffed with a nurse but only rarely operated without medically trained personnel. Horse-drawn wagons gave way to motorized vehicles, including streetcars and automobiles by the turn of the century. While advances in transportation were progressive, the training of personnel did not necessarily keep pace. Private ambulance companies developed as business offshoots and were most frequently operated by funeral homes.

6. When did aeromedical services first develop?

As with ground ambulances, the first services were rudimentary transportation efforts that later incorporated medical care during patient movement. The first reported air transport is thought to have occurred by hot air balloon when 160 injured soldiers were removed from Paris during a siege by Prussians in 1870. French and American forces used modified airplanes to move injured soldiers during World War I, but it was not until 1929 that airplanes were designed for ambulance service. The use of helicopters to transport patients had its origins in the Korean War, and their subsequent use in Vietnam firmly established the role of rotor-wing aircraft in prehospital transportation. Largely due to the advances of prehospital care, some authorities claimed that a soldier wounded by enemy fire in Vietnam had a better chance of survival than a patient of a domestic motor vehicle accident.

7. What is the history of modern EMS?

There are two events to which the development of modern EMS can be attributed. The first is the creation of the first mobile coronary care units by J. F. Pantridge in Belfast in 1964. After reporting to the American College of Cardiology that prehospital care of acute myocardial infarction patients could reduce mortality, Pantridge found that several Americans attempted to duplicate his efforts. While the results were reproducible, the cost of putting doctors in the field was restrictive. Prehospital care became the domain of public safety and ambulance personnel who were trained to provide initial care in the form of EKG interpretation, intubation, defibrillation, medication, and safe transportation—the first paramedics.

The second is the publication of a position paper by the National Academy of Sciences in 1967 that found that emergency health care techniques and equipment were sorely inadequate. This study prompted the creation of the National Highway Traffic Safety Administration (NHTSA) within the Department of Transportation (DOT). NHTSA has been responsible for establishing the standard training curricula for all levels of prehospital providers, including dispatchers. Additionally, this organization has provided funds for program development and system improvement.

8. Who were Roy and Johnny of Rescue 51 out of Rampart General?

If you did not grow up in the 1970s or do not watch old reruns, these two characters will not ring a bell as the paramedics of the hit series "Emergency!" This program, much as "Rescue 911" of the 1990s, showcased the abilities of a prehospital system and fostered tremendous public acceptance and support. The American public saw what they could have in their own communities and demanded it.

9. How was this demand realized?

In 1973, Congress enacted the Emergency Medical Services System Act, which authorized the Department of Health, Education, and Welfare to fund more than 300 regional EMS systems across the country. Over 8 years, programs and standards were developed to promote a systems approach to prehospital care. Funds also were used to cover administrative expenses, purchase equipment, and create training centers. Once federal monies were exhausted, entities that did not disappear adapted their services and obtained other funding sources to continue the mission of advancing the cause of prehospital care.

10. Physicians used to ride in ambulances. How has their role changed?

The physician's role in prehospital care, especially in the civilian sector, while moving from "on-scene" to "behind the scenes," has remained intimate. The specialty of emergency medicine has grown in parallel with the development of EMS. While a few medical directors continue to respond to selected calls, it is unaffordable for the agency or individual physicians to spend most of their time in the field. The most important physician contribution is that of the extension of their license to prehospital care providers in the field. All prehospital providers are aware that their ability to function depends on this relationship. Additionally, medical directors participate in the development of protocols and quality assurance systems, education, and on-line medical control. The National Association of Emergency Physicians was organized in 1985 to address the concerns of medical directors and help direct the future course of EMS.

11. What is the more recent history of EMS?

No discussion of history can be considered truly current. The DOT recently revised the curricula for EMT-Basic training and is doing the same for paramedics. Of ongoing interest is the potential for expanding the scope of a paramedic's function beyond traditional boundaries. The base for prehospital functions continues to fluctuate among private, third-service, public utility and firebased operations. The value of a medical director's time and input is being increasingly recognized and the days of free service to agencies are rapidly dwindling. Almost certainly, financial considerations will be a major driving force in the future of EMS.

BIBLIOGRAPHY

1. Barkley JT: The Ambulance. Kiamesha Lake, NY, Load N Go Press, 1990.
2. Mustalish AC: Emergency medical services: Twenty years of growth and development. N Y State J Med Aug:414–420, 1986.
3. Page JO: Historical perspectives on EMS systems. In Roush WR (ed): Principles of EMS Systems, 2nd ed. Dallas, American College of Emergency Physicians, 1994, pp 1–10.
4. Smiley DR: Overview of the EMS system. In Pons P, Cason D (eds): Paramedic Field Care. St. Louis, Mosby, 1997, pp 4–16.
5. Stewart RD: The history of emergency medical services. In Kuehl A (ed): EMS Medical Directors' Handbook. St. Louis, Mosby, 1989, pp 3–6.

II. Medical Direction

2. MEDICAL DIRECTION—OVERVIEW

Marilyn J. Gifford, M.D.

1. Why do paramedics, who are licensed by the state, need a medical director or physician advisor?

Because the practice of medicine in most states is restricted to physicians, the extension of medical care into the field requires a physician to accept responsibility for the acts of each paramedic and, in many states, each basic emergency medical technician (EMT).

2. What is the difference between physician advisors and medical directors?

Although the terms are used interchangeably, *medical director* more accurately describes the role of providing the medical supervision necessary to assure a quality prehospital care program.

3. What is the difference between on-line and off-line medical direction?

On-line (or concurrent) medical direction is the direction given to the paramedic by the physician (usually an emergency physician) on the radio or phone while the paramedic is on the scene or en route to a hospital with a patient. Off-line medical direction is the direction provided by a medical director who plans and evaluates the prehospital care by reviewing and recommending equipment and medications to be used, protocols to be followed, and continuing education to maintain skills.

4. What is CECBEMS?

The Continuing Education Coordinating Board for EMS. CECBEMS reviews continuing education programs for EMTs and paramedics. They award national accreditation to programs that provide quality educational experiences.

5. What is NREMT?

The National Registry of EMTs. NREMT examines EMTs and paramedics who have completed approved training programs. An EMT who meets entry requirements and passes written and practical exams is "registered" by the NREMT. Reregistration is contingent on satisfying reregistration requirements. NREMT is the only organization to provide national testing and recognition to prehospital care providers.

6. What are the requirements to become an EMS medical director?

Although there are no nationally recognized requirements, the American College of Emergency Physicians recommends both *essential* and *desirable* selection criteria.

Essential criteria include:

1. License to practice medicine or osteopathy.
2. Familiarity with the design and operation of prehospital emergency medical services (EMS) systems.
3. Experience or training in the prehospital emergency care of acutely ill or injured patients.
4. Experience or training in medical direction of prehospital emergency units.
5. Active participation in the management of the acutely ill or injured patient.
6. Experience or training in the instruction of prehospital personnel.
7. Experience or training in the EMS quality improvement process.
8. Knowledge of EMS laws and regulations.

9. Knowledge or EMS dispatch and communications.
10. Knowledge of local mass casualty and disaster plans.
A **desirable** criterion is board certification in emergency medicine.

7. List six levels of prehospital care providers.

Emergency medical dispatch, first responder, emergency medical technician–basic, emergency medical technician–intermediate, paramedic, and advanced paramedic.

8. List the skills of a basic EMT that are not skills of a first responder.

1. Administration of oxygen
2. Use of oxygen-powered ventilation
3. Assistance with administration of medication
4. Use of automatic defibrillation
5. Application of pneumatic anti-shock garments
6. Immobilization for transport

9. What is an EMD program?

Emergency medical dispatchers (EMDs) are trained through a standard program that includes utilization of pre-arrival interrogation and instruction cards or computer programs designed to aid emergency victims before the arrival of first responders, EMTs, or paramedics. The second portion of their job is dispatching, which often requires knowledge of available units, geography, proximity, and whether first responders, EMTs, or paramedic units are required. Many of these decisions can be predetermined by dispatch protocols formulated by the medical director in coordination with the responding agencies.

10. What is the difference between QA, QI, CQI and TQM?

Quality assurance (QA) was an old term applied to searching for problems and trying to correct them. It did not "assure" quality and was eventually replaced by *quality improvement* (QI) activities, which were recognized to be ongoing activities. Thus, *continuous quality improvement* (CQI) was recognized as a process that was essential for a quality product. The shift in emphasis from "problem finding" to "system improvement" has created a more positive work environment. The concept of *total quality management* (TQM) refers to the overview of CQI activities on the total program.

11. What are treatment protocols?

Specific written guidelines that describe a general approach to common presenting conditions.

12. How do treatment protocols differ from standing orders?

Standing orders are specific authorizations to perform procedures or administer medications in clearly defined circumstances. Standing orders should be signed by the medical director who is ordering the procedure or medication.

13. Describe destination policies.

In any EMS system the medical director should determine, according to the resources available, where certain critical or high-risk patients should be transported. The lay public is not expected to know, for instance, which hospital has the pediatric critical care capabilities or which has the highest level trauma capabilities.

14. Are all paramedic training programs the same?

No. Paramedic programs have varied tremendously in the number of hours they require of their students. There has been increased adherence to standards, however, since accreditation has become available through the Joint Review Committee for EMT–Paramedic Educational Programs.

BIBLIOGRAPHY

1. Kuehl AE (ed): National Association of EMS Physicians EMS Medical Directors' Handbook. St. Louis, Mosby, 1989.
2. Werman HA (ed): American College of Emergency Physicians Medical Direction of Emergency Medical Services. Dallas, ACEP, 1993.

3. ON-LINE MEDICAL DIRECTION

Vincent P. Verdile, M.D.

1. What is meant by on-line medical direction?

On-line medical direction (OLMD), which is also referred to as direct medical control, on-line medical command, or real-time medical control, is the process by which advanced life support emergency medical services (EMS) providers receive physician directives contemporaneously for the care of patients encountered in the out-of-hospital venue. Treatment protocols are usually initiated based on a patient's symptoms or complaints, such as shortness of breath or chest pain. After assessment has been completed, the initiation of treatment is discussed with a physician. The physician and EMS providers decide on the best treatment plan given the patient's complaints, physical assessment findings, and treatment modalities available. OLMD is accomplished by radio, traditional telephone (landline), or cellular telephone.

2. Is there an alternative to OLMD?

Absolutely! Some EMS systems, whether because of topography, high patient volume, or unavailability of OLMD physicians, use a standing-order protocol system for patient care. This type of patient treatment procedure allows the EMS providers to initiate treatment based on either the patient's complaint or symptoms without contemporaneous contact with a physician. Implicit in this type of EMS patient care paradigm is a vigorous quality management program that ensures the timely review of the patient care record (PCR) to determine if the patient care is timely and appropriate given the presenting complaints or symptoms.

3. Does OLMD always involve contact with a physician?

In most instances, yes; however, there are some medical direction systems that allow nurses or other advanced life support EMS providers to provide OLMD in a delegated fashion. A physician needs to be in close proximity in the event of the need to change treatment protocols or if the patient does not fit neatly into one specific treatment protocol.

4. Why are most EMS systems designed around the OLMD model?

Currently, in most states, advanced life support EMS providers function under the medical licensure of a physician when they are caring for patients. Although certified and appropriately credentialed, EMS providers are not licensed to practice medicine. The EMS system medical director and the OLMD physician delegate certain functions to the EMS providers to effect patient care in the out-of-hospital arena. This stems from the recognition that for some medical and surgical conditions, such as acute myocardial infarction and multisystem injuries, early medical care may improve patient outcome.

5. Do only advanced life support EMS personnel require OLMD?

While there may be some variability from state to state, currently, because of the nature of the treatment modalities and pharmacotherapy, only advanced life support EMS providers are required to contact OLMD for patient care issues. In some parts of the country, basic emergency medical technicians who are performing automatic or semiautomatic external defibrillation on patients in cardiac arrest are required either to have a system medical director or to contact OLMD after defibrillation.

6. Does contacting OLMD delay treatment?

There will always be unavoidable delays encountered in out-of-hospital medicine. For instance, the time between receiving a call for assistance and dispatching an ambulance, the time to respond, and the time to access OLMD are all unavoidable. Most EMS systems, however, do not require OLMD for those therapies such as defibrillation and intubation that are life saving, time critical, and routinely done by advanced life support providers. Administration of other treatments beyond those that are immediately life saving will require contact with a physician. It is not uncommon for EMS systems that require OLMD to have built in a standing-order treatment plan in the event of communication failure for those life-saving interventions previously described or in order to begin routine advanced life support therapy such as oxygen administration, establishment of intravenous access, or provision of first-line ACLS drugs.

7. What is the configuration of successful OLMD?

Each EMS system must design an OLMD system that meets its needs for the care of patients. Some have every emergency department within the EMS system prepared for OLMD, while others limit the number and type of physicians who provide OLMD. In communities that have a sufficient number of interested physicians, the solution is easy—share the responsibility. In other communities, EMS-knowledgeable physicians might be scarce, requiring the EMS medical director to develop an on-call list of physicians who are available to the EMS providers. The Pittsburgh EMS system uses a finite number of emergency physicians who are mobile, respond to assist EMS providers in the care of patients, and provide OLMD for all patients regardless of the hospital destination. New York City EMS has a stationary physician in a medical command center who provides OLMD for the entire system. The City of Albany Department of Fire and Emergency Services system functions on a combined standing order and OLMD system, with the OLMD shared among the receiving hospital emergency departments. The city and county of Denver have a single base station with a small group of EM physicians providing OLMD.

8. Do physicians receive training in OLMD?

In some states, such as Pennsylvania, the EMS statutes require that physicians who provide OLMD complete a Base Station Medical Command Course. Other states have also required this training, especially for those physicians who have not been trained in emergency medicine. All emergency medicine residency programs are required to provide EMS education to the physicians in training. While some variability exists between the residency programs with regard to the quality of this training, OLMD is almost uniformly taught with opportunities for supervised experience.

9. What is the advantage of OLMD?

The single most important advantage is the ability to combine or change treatment protocols for patients with complicated medical or surgical problems. The EMS provider, by presenting the salient features of the patient's presenting complaint and the physical assessment, can use the physician's higher medical training to help sort out the best treatment approach. Often, a physician on the radio or the telephone, who is in a more controlled environment, will think of alternative potential causes for the patient's complaints or symptoms and offer suggestions for management. In addition, the OLMD physician may suggest using established out-of-hospital medications in a nontraditional fashion, such as nitroglycerin for hypertensive emergencies rather than only for patients with chest pain. OLMD, therefore, can also become an educational venue for the EMS system. The OLMD physician can speak directly to the patient in those instances when the patient is refusing care and often can convince the patient to accept EMS transport to a hospital. The OLMD physician can also assist the EMT in assessing the competency of a patient who is refusing care. The transmission of timely patient-related information and establishing the responsibility of the physician for the patient are benefits of OLMD as well. Another distinct advantage of OLMD is the opportunity for concurrent quality management of patient care.

10. Are there any disadvantages to OLMD?

There is no obvious disadvantage to OLMD that is measurable or apparent. The criticism most often heard, however, is that there is no clear difference in patient outcome for those who receive OLMD compared with those who do not. Consequently, the opponents of OLMD support the notion that it is time consuming and takes the EMS providers away from patient care. They feel that standing-order EMS systems deliver comparable patient care. From a system standpoint, the only potential disadvantage to OLMD is that sufficient resources are necessary to fulfill the demand for service. The EMS system must have a community of willing and able physicians to assume this important responsibility.

BIBLIOGRAPHY

1. Braun O: Direct medical control. In Kuehl AE (ed): Prehospital Systems & Medical Oversight, 2nd ed. St. Louis, Mosby, 1994, pp 196–216.
2. Paris PM, Roth R, Verdile VP (eds): Prehospital Medical Direction: The Art of On-line Medical Direction. St. Louis, Mosby, 1996.
3. Roush WR: Medical accountability. In Roush WR (ed): Principles of EMS Systems, 2nd ed. Dallas, American College of Emergency Physicians, 1994, pp 227–244.

4. OFF-LINE MEDICAL DIRECTION

Stewart L. Greisman, D.O.

1. How is medical direction relevant to emergency medical services?
Medical direction for emergency medical services (EMS) is based in the belief that all medical care should be directed by physicians.

2. Who would disagree with that?
While most people agree that emergency medical technicians (EMTs) and paramedics practice as physician extenders, there is resistance to the concept of medical control. Generally, disagreement comes from those who (1) were providing response to medical emergencies before active physician involvement and see no need for change and (2) believe that physicians do not understand the realities of medical care delivered in the field and remain skeptical of physicians who assume such authority.

3. What exactly is medical direction?
The supervisory relationship that exists between an EMT or paramedic and the physician who supervises and, in many cases, is responsible for their practice. Other terms that have been used to describe medical direction include *medical control* and *physician direction*. The supervising physician may be called the medical director or the physician advisor.

4. What is off-line medical direction?
The supervision of EMS personnel is, in most cases, remote. Physicians practice in the hospital and provide supervision for many EMS units located outside of the hospital. Physicians may provide direct voice supervision via radio or telephone; this is known as "on-line medical supervision" because the physician is literally "on the line." Off-line medical supervision is medical supervision that is provided *without* on-line contact between the physician and EMS practitioners. This is usually accomplished with written medical protocols.

5. How is off-line medical direction established?
The premise behind off-line medical direction is a combination of good training, clear protocols, and methodical quality reviews after each call. In some systems off-line medical control is augmented by the availability of on-line consultation. Off-line medical direction activities include training, collaboration with field personnel on protocols, and careful retrospective review of calls.

6. Who is responsible for off-line medical direction?
The best medical direction reflects a shared responsibility between the field practitioner and the physician. The EMT is responsible for maintaining proficiency and familiarity with protocols. The physician is responsible for ensuring that protocols reflect contemporary medical knowledge and practice. The physician adviser is involved with EMT training, continuing education, and assuring adequate quality review. The physician is ultimately responsible since the EMT or paramedic is considered to be an extension of his practice.

7. Are national protocols available? Should they be used?
There are no national protocol standards. A number of textbooks have published "model" protocols, and other models may be available from national EMS organizations. Although there is no reason for each locale to "reinvent" protocols for their EMS organizations, model protocols should be adapted to meet the community needs and resources and to reflect the standards of the physicians in the local community.

8. Do protocols need to follow accepted national medical guidelines (such as for advanced cardiac life support, or ACLS)?

There is no requirement that EMS protocols follow any national guidelines such as ACLS. In fact, may locales have developed their own ACLS equivalents. Remember that local medical communities need to be accountable for their level of care as it relates to "reasonable and prudent care" that meets the minimum national standard of care. So it is unusual to find communities whose standards are significantly different from accepted national guidelines.

9. Do protocols need to follow regional training curricula?

Regional training curricula are not mandatory. States have the option of adopting the Department of Transportation EMT curriculum. However, local EMS protocols do need to relate to local training curricula.

10. Why distinguish between off-line and on-line medical direction?

There are major differences in the relationships and logistics between these two varieties of medical direction. Off-line medical direction requires a significant amount of trust in EMS personnel. The medical community believes that EMTs and paramedics can adequately assess patients and will use the appropriate protocol in patient management. On-line direction, on the other hand, limits the decision-making of EMS personnel. Logistically, the use of on-line medical control requires time on scene to contact medical direction, adequate technology to assure communication, and immediate 24-hour access to the on-line physician.

11. Which is better—on-line or off-line medical direction?

There is no right answer to this question because of the varying needs of communities. Medical communities need to be comfortable with EMS protocols and standards. Some are not ready for off-line direction. Some have no choice. Yet off-line medical direction has a number of advantages, including smoother scene management, shorter scene times, and flexibility in geographic areas that preclude the use of radios or cellular phones. There are no data to support the belief that either form of medical direction is better than the other as long as there *is* medical direction.

12. Which do paramedics and EMTs prefer?

We have not seen any studies of field personnel preference, but our experience is that they prefer the trust and latitude that comes with off-line medical direction. But off-line direction does not necessarily imply that medical direction is not available when consultation is necessary. In confusing or complex cases, EMTs and paramedics alike prefer rapid access to medical direction.

13. Is it true that some situations mandate on-line medical direction?

Again, it depends on community standards and the medical protocols that have been created to define the EMS practice. Some states or communities mandate on-line direction for all advanced life support procedures, including intubation, defibrillation, IV insertion, and drug administration. In others, only rarely performed procedures such as cricothyrotomy or chest decompression require on-line direction.

14. What happens if on-line direction cannot be established in these cases?

Two EMS systems with different medical directors may provide different answers. Some states mandate that action without on-line direction is grounds for disciplinary action or revocation of privileges. Other systems allow EMS personnel to perform as they feel appropriate but mandate careful review afterwards of the care that was delivered and the rationale behind the inability to obtain on-line direction.

15. If on-line medical orders contradict off-line medical direction, which takes priority?

This situation is best avoided by making sure that individuals who provide on-line medical direction (usually emergency physicians or nurses on duty in an emergency department) are well-versed in the protocols that define the EMS system. Off-line and on-line directives should follow the same protocols. This sounds simple but may be difficult to achieve in fragmented systems with different EMS services transporting patients to different hospitals with several different base stations. When conflicts occur, priority should be given to on-line direction since it is responding in real-time to the actual patient presentation. The only exception is when the paramedic believes the conflicting order is not in the patient's best interest (see question 21).

16. Does an on-scene physician's order supersede off-line medical direction?

Another situation best avoided. The reality is that on-scene physicians sometimes are helpful and sometimes are not. Many systems have created guidelines for physician-paramedic interactions. Typically, if conflict arises between the off-line protocols and the wishes of the on-scene physician, the on-scene physician is given an opportunity to speak with on-line medical direction or to take complete responsibility for the scene. If the on-scene physician disagrees with the on-line physician or refuses to assume total responsibility for the care of the patient, including the ride to the hospital, the meddling physician may be escorted from the scene.

17. Do any EMS providers operate without medical direction?

Yes. In some agencies basic EMTs operate without any medical direction. Why? Because those regions have decided that the scope of practice for basic EMTs does not involve enough *medicine* to require input from a physician. In some areas there is no physician available or willing to assume the role of medical director.

Is it prudent to operate without medical direction? Probably not. Even routine oxygen therapy or spinal immobilizations have medical implications. EMS systems probably work better when physicians play a role in the education, protocol development, and review of care. After all, EMS stands for emergency *medical* services.

18. Do all EMS practitioners operate with off-line medical direction?

Basically, yes. Even the most restrictive, on-line system empowers EMS personnel to initiate patient assessment and some form of patient stabilization without "calling in." The distinction is in how far they can proceed before getting on-line input or permission.

19. Do patient preference or managed care requirements supersede off-line medical direction?

This is a contemporary issue that will likely be quite vexing for the next several years. The traditional answer has been that the clinician knows what is best for the patient. However, it is getting harder to justify EMS care and destination protocols that leave the patient liable for thousands of dollars of medical care and that is likely to result in nonpayment to the EMS service and the receiving hospital. Like most protocol conflicts, this issue is best avoided through dialogue among all parties involved. EMTs and paramedics should never be asked to perform insurance triage based on ability to pay. Properly prepared EMTs and paramedics may be able to provide valuable assistance to patients concerned with payment issues. Preplanning enables off-line protocols to be modified to reflect the new managed care environment.

20. Does licensure or certification of EMS providers alter the need for medical direction?

No. As long as paramedics practice in a system of medical care under a physician's license there is a need for medical direction.

21. What happens if protocols are in conflict with what the medic thinks is best for the patient?

Health care professionals, which include EMTs and paramedics, are charged with serving as an advocate for the patient and, above all else, doing no harm. This traditional ethic runs deep in our profession and cannot be overridden by the excuse of "I was just following orders." We are all ethically bound to refuse to carry out orders that we believe are not in the patient's best interest.

However, we also need to bear the responsibility for our decisions. If the order really was what was best for the patient, we need to be accountable for the consequences of altering or withholding a care plan or countermanding a base station's verbal order or written protocol.

BIBLIOGRAPHY

1. Corey EC: Medical oversight. Emergency 27:28–33, 1995.
2. Holroyd BR, Knopp RK, Kallsen G: Medical control. Quality assurance in prehospital care. JAMA 256:1027–1031, 1986.
3. Pepe PE, Stewart RD: Role of the physician in the prehospital setting. Ann Emerg Med 15:1480–1483, 1986.
4. Roush WR: Medical accountability. In Roush WR (ed): Principles of EMS Systems. Dallas, American College of Emergency Physicians, 1994, pp 227–244.

5. CONTINUOUS QUALITY IMPROVEMENT

Kevin Chu, M.B., B.S., and Robert Swor, D.O.

1. What is quality?

The American Heritage Dictionary defines quality as a "grade of excellence," but quality has been described in a variety of ways. There is no single uniform definition. Ultimately, quality has been defined functionally. Juran, one of the leaders of the quality movement, describes it as "fitness for use." Others have expressed a more global statement, "We know it when we see it." Virtually all authors agree that quality is what the customers say it is. Ultimately, the definition of quality in health care is subjective, based on both the science of medicine and the accepted art of medical practice.

2. Why do I need quality?

Our patients and communities demand and expect quality health care. As health care providers, we strive to supply services that are consistently high quality and continuously improved. A less philosophic but no less important reason to pursue quality is that the payers for health care are increasingly demanding accounting for the enormous amount of money spent on health care. Payers (insurers, governments) are under intense pressure to reduce health care costs. This translates into demands on the health care and EMS systems for increased efficiency and demonstration that there is significant value for the care rendered relative to the funds allocated for it. The current focus on quality health care has primarily been driven by economic issues.

3. What is quality assurance?

Quality assurance (QA) implies a warranty of quality and a demonstration by the medical community that efforts are in place to review medical care and assure its appropriateness. Its initial emphasis was on individual accountability. This has pervaded medical quality efforts and has perhaps had an adverse impact on efforts to improve quality.

Basically, QA requires a feedback loop involving monitoring (audits, incident reports), assessment, action, reevaluation, and follow-up. QA efforts are outcome oriented, which is an area of intense interest in the era of health care reform. Similarly, QA recognizes that medical practice is an art as well as a science and that review of care by other practitioners in the field (peer review) is a crucial aspect of evaluating care.

4. Why are some people threatened by quality assurance?

Historically, QA was perceived as a method of finding the patterns of individual mistakes, and indeed, there is a focus on individual accountability. Its remedy, focusing on improvement or "reeducation" of the individual, although not intended, was viewed as a form of punishment. Practitioners in EMS and in health care at large were at risk of supplying quality data that could point to themselves as a "problem," or as not participating in QA activities.

Despite well-intended efforts to improve the quality of services, QA programs were often not well supported by the members of organizations. The results of the individual-oriented process were data of suspect quality, poor support for findings of QA activities, and a general decrease in morale despite honest efforts to improve the care within an organization. Not all EMS QA efforts had these results, but significant care and skill were required to prevent QA from becoming a punitive exercise rather than one to improve quality. QA was also crafted as an "add-on" program to many EMS programs, the responsibility of a QA office or individual. The data collection, reviews, and results were all obtained and assessed separately from the rest of an organization. Predictably, there was little support for the findings.

A final reason that QA has been viewed with concern by EMS professionals is that because the focus of QA was on identifying outliers most of time, energy, and effort was focused on the vast majority of providers that were, by definition, providing appropriate care within an acceptable standard range.

5. What is continuous quality improvement?

Continuous Quality Improvement (CQI) focuses not on the individual workers but on the system. A fundamental concept of QI is that a *system* is responsible for most errors (85%) in a given process and that individual errors are far less common than errors in fundamental processes. If processes are improved, efficient, and support individuals, it follows that people's performance and the services delivered (i.e., quality) will improve.

6. What is a process? What are some examples?

A process is the means by which things get done, the steps in getting from point A to point B. A number of different activities in EMS may be thought of as processes: patient flow, information flow, and equipment flow. All require a number of steps to reach the necessary endpoint. For example, a man collapses with chest pain, and his wife calls 911. EMS responds by sending out the necessary first response personnel and higher-level providers with necessary equipment for the emergency. Radio communications with an appropriate physician are in place, and the patient is transported to the facility able to care for that person's condition. Delivering health care to this patient involves screening the call, deploying the appropriate vehicle, getting to the patient, starting medical intervention with direct medical oversight or previously established standing protocols, communication of vital patient care data to the hospital, and the preparation of the appropriate facility and personnel to care for the individual patient. The various steps in this pathway can be thought of as the processes of the system.

7. What is the difference between QA and CQI?

Retrospective reviews, outcome data evaluations, and peer reviews are all a standard part of QA activities. They are limited, however, in their ability to generate genuine system improvements.

Continuous Quality Improvement, in theory, is broader in focus and uses descriptive and analytic methods to improve the processes of EMS organizations. Its implementation requires the participation of a broad cross-section of organizational members. It requires that efforts to improve quality be integrated into the daily functions of an organization and be funded just as other primary processes. In the EMS model, data collection and process evaluation would be viewed as integral components of care delivery, just as dispatch, rapid response, and treatment are integral components.

A fundamental difference of QI is a broad focus on customer service, defining both external customers (patients) and internal customers (hospitals, physicians, and Emergency Departments). This view identifies front-line personnel as key customers as well, so that paramedics would be customers of the dispatcher, and the role of the dispatcher would be to make sure that the customers' needs are met. The QI efforts would focus on improving the service to that customer.

8. What are the costs of quality care?

Not only do we want to deliver quality care to our patients, we need to do it cost effectively. There is a price to be paid for QI in the short run; however, improvements in efficiency can make CQI pay for itself in the long term.

The initial costs of quality improvement are significant. Time, energy, and leadership are required to conceive and develop QI programs. Resources, including technical training and support for staff and investment in data systems, are required. Finally, QI efforts must become a part of the workers' responsibilities, so that part of the time is focused not only on performing work, but also on helping improve the processes of that work.

9. Who should perform CQI?

Deming identifies the front-line workers as key. Those individuals have the most intimate "profound knowledge" of the processes that they perform. Accordingly, they are best able to identify the barriers to quality processes and to suggest data to be collected or solutions to be attempted. The provision of out-of-hospital emergency care is a team effort, so CQI should be a team effort. Provider peer review is invaluable. Physician input is also important, because EMS is patient care. Administrators must also be committed to CQI for it to succeed. They not only must participate in quality activities, such as QI teams, but must also provide resources, such as staff and computer support, data collection expertise, and personnel. Finally, the leadership of the organization must be willing to support the decisions reached by front-line providers if they conform to parameters developed by the leadership.

10. How do I start?

To work to improve quality, there must be a commitment to a new approach to attaining quality. The role of leadership moves from a traditional "top-down" management style to one of devolving control of decisions to front-line personnel within defined parameters. In EMS, the role of front-line workers moves from just providing care to a more active role in QI activities, including assessment and problem solving. The utilization of multi-disciplinary QI teams, which use QI methods and tools, are the heart of QI problem solving.

11. What are the components of CQI?

Juran identified three components of CQI.
1. *Quality planning*—"getting it right the first time."
    • Determine who the customers are. EMS customers are not only patients and their families (external customers) but also individuals working within the system (internal customers).
    • Determine the needs of the customers. This process varies within each portion of the organization but serves to identify and drive which products and processes are of key importance and require attention. The simplest approach to this issue is to identify the customers and ask them to identify their needs.
    • Develop product features that respond to customer needs.
    • Develop processes that are able to produce the features.
    • Transfer the resulting plans to the operating forces to test and improve those processes.
2. *Quality control*—minimize fluctuations so that the system is stable.
    • Evaluate actual product performance. The instruments for its measurement are varied and may range from sophisticated control charts to simple patient surveys.
    • Develop product goals and compare actual performance to product goals.
    • Act on the difference.
3. *Quality Improvement*

To facilitate QI, one needs to identify simple "winning" projects that are necessary improvements but that utilize QI methods to demonstrate their ability to impact change. The selection of such a project is crucial. It must be relevant to caregivers, measurable, relatively frequent, and a process thought to be able to be improved. The data to be collected have to be well defined (or at least measurable), consistently documented, easily retrievable, and able to be analyzed.

12. What outcomes do I measure?

While quality patient care appears to be a readily agreed-upon outcome, there is little consensus in the literature defining what the attributes of that quality are. The most common accepted definition of an improved outcome is an increased rate of survival after a life-threatening event. Generally, outcomes may be defined more broadly to include a variety of changes in the patient's health status. These include the 6D's:

Death: Did the patient survive to hospital discharge?

Disease: Underlying illness and morbidity.

Disability: Was there a better functional patient outcome because of patient care rendered? Examples might include a patient immobilized on a backboard after an accident who had a cervical spine fracture but sustained no spinal cord injury, or a patient who did not require an ICU bed or mechanical ventilation because of field treatment for congestive heart failure.

Discomfort: Relief of patient's symptoms.

Dissatisfaction: Is the patient satisfied with service rendered?

Destitution: Did treatment decrease costs of patient care to the patient, the payer, or society as a whole?

In a survey of paramedics in the Pittsburgh, PA, EMS system, Greenberg asked them to identify what they thought were the attributes of quality and how they should be measured. In addition to patient outcome and symptomatic improvement, a number of other parameters were identified. These included patient satisfaction; provider satisfaction; educational, supervisory, and equipment quality; employee turnover rates; and other measures. These factors could be measured using survey tools, which although not completely objective, can be used in a reproducible fashion.

13. What is a model of CQI in EMS care?

The model most commonly applied to EMS is survival after an out-of-hospital cardiac arrest. This clinical entity is particularly attractive as an outcome measure for a number of reasons:

1. It addresses a clearly definable clinical entity, sudden cardiac death.
2. Treatment is standardized (Advanced Cardiac Life Support).
3. Advanced Life Support (ALS) has been shown definitely to improve outcome.
4. Survival is time dependent.
5. It has a clearly definable outcome (dead or alive).
6. Data definitions are also now more standardized (Utstein).
7. A wealth of literature exists to serve as a benchmark for comparison with other systems.

All of these factors allow a system to use cardiac arrest as a measure of structural components (response), process (is care rendered consistent with existing ACLS protocols?), and outcome (survival to hospital discharge). Limitations of this method of evaluation are also many. Cardiac arrest cases comprise only a small percentage of a system's care. Mortality is high, with survival rates varying from 1–30% depending on case definitions and system studied. Access to hospital outcome data is not consistently available, although death certificates are public documents. An EMS system may not have a large enough number of cardiac arrests from which to derive useful information. All these factors make cardiac arrest survival data useful and identify it as only one parameter of many that may be used to assess system performance.

Other measures of patient survival are more difficult to obtain. Difficulties encountered include standardizing clinical entities for comparison (e.g., multiple trauma patients or myocardial infarction patients) and adjusting for confounders such as age of pre-existing illnesses. Injuries may be identified and classified using the Abbreviated Injury Score (AIS-90) and the Injury Severity Score (ISS), which are standardized scoring systems quantifying the severity of a given patient's injuries. The ISS, in combination with the Revised Trauma Score (RTS), which identifies a patient's initial physiologic status (vital signs), have been used by many authors to calculate a probability of survival (Ps). A comparison of the Ps with patients' actual outcome has been suggested to be a measure in aggregate of a trauma system's care relative to what should be expected. This methodology (TRISS) has come under increasing question in the trauma literature.

The introduction of multiple parameters (which must be adjusted for) produces a degree of complexity and expense that places these evaluations beyond the reach of all but the most sophisticated EMS systems. The time, data volume, and variety of data sources required limit the ability to obtain meaningful results in a relatively short timeline.

14. What tools do I use?

Descriptive Tools

- Process flow charts are a graphic representation of the sequential steps in the process and reveal bottlenecks in flow.

• Fishbone (cause-and-effect or Ishikawa) diagrams categorize and display in groups theories about how and why processes fail. The groups may be internal customers, external customers, supplies, the work environment, or policies and protocols for work.

Data Collection and Display Tools
• Check sheets are used for collection and quantification of data.
• Histograms illustrate the frequency distribution of a process.
• Trends charts display the changes in process over time.
• Pareto charts are histograms graphing the frequency of defects from greatest to least, drawing attention to the former.
• Statistical or control charts show the variability of data around its mean.

Opinion-gathering Tools
• *Nominal Group Processes*—gather opinions from groups to identify theories regarding a given issue or potential solutions to a problem.
• *Brainstorming*—a method by which thoughts may be generated on a given topic to identify potential approaches to problem solving or problem identification.

15. What is the scope of its application?

EMS is patient care, and anything that touches on patient care is within the scope of CQI—personnel, equipment, and all factors influencing the processes of getting the ill and injured patient appropriate care. Personnel issues encompass recruitment, training, certification, continuing education, and recertification. Equipment issues include purchasing and maintenance of items such as vehicles, radios, and defibrillators. Communication issues include access to 911, postdispatch instructions, and communication equipment on ambulances, in hospitals, and at the communications center. Treatments rendered include not only whether performance was up to standard but also include documentation and reporting. Medical oversight, both direct radio control and indirect standing protocols, are within this scope. Looking at the system as a whole, there is an interrelationship between EMS agencies (e.g., who provides the primary and secondary response; who does the transports) and the hospitals (e.g., for the time patient and EMTs spend at the triage area).

16. What happens now that we've started QI?

Is work ever finished? CQI is a continuous process. Although a project may be completed, the system needs to be constantly reviewed.

17. What are some examples of CQI in health care?

CQI is being implemented in a variety of health care environments. Applications may be operational (decreasing the time to admit a patient to a bed), fiscal (decreasing the time to send a bill upon patient discharge), or clinical (decreasing the time to thrombolytic therapy for myocardial infarction patients or decreasing the rate of medication errors).

18. What are some examples of CQI in EMS?

System status management (SSM) is a success story of CQI in EMS. Here, the deployment of ambulances is strategic in time and location. Typically, implementing this sort of process is the result of a leadership initiative to meet the needs of customers (faster response). The process is evaluated, data are gathered, and the process is improved by changes in system structure.

A variety of other QI applications are being tested in EMS. Some agencies are working with teams to facilitate ambulance turnaround in emergency departments. State EMS agencies have applied QI methods to effect more rapid turnaround of licensure applications. Many agencies work with hospitals to facilitate the process of identifying acute MI patients and their treatment with thrombolytic agents. Pinellas County, Florida, reported the use of QI methods to address drownings in their community.

19. Does it improve patient care?

It is often asked whether EMS makes a difference. The answer is evident in cardiac arrest. Whether or not one believes that EMS makes a difference, EMS is demanded by the public and is here to stay. EMS is about patient care, and QI is about improving EMS, thus providing better patient care.

20. Is it research?

CQI and research projects have many elements in common. Research advances medical knowledge and sets the standards for medical care, however, while CQI involves improving the care currently delivered to meet these ever-increasing standards. In addition, research is for publication, while CQI is confidential. Both are disciplined approaches to evaluation and to improving patient care.

21. Would lawyers be interested?

If the purpose of QI activities is to identify areas for improvement, it is clear that the potential exists to identify and document problems that could potentially be used in lawsuits against the organization. To prevent this and to encourage health care entities (including EMS providers), most states have enacted statutes that give protection from discovery of QI activities provided those activities have appropriate safeguards and follow specified processes. There are two fundamental legal issues: confidentiality and liability.

Practical steps to enhance confidentiality

1. EMS organizations need to research and be cognizant of state and federal statutes governing their QI activities.

2. CQI needs to be organized, with the bylaws of the EMS organizations specifying who and what constitute QI activities.

3. The data to be collected should be prospectively identified for the purposes of CQI.

4. Documents generated do not identify patient or provider and are marked confidential and distributed only to people involved in CQI.

Practical steps to reduce risk of liability

1. Follow the CQI bylaws so that review activities are seen as official.

2. The CQI process should not be used for any other purpose than to improve patient care.

3. Preserve the confidentiality of the CQI records.

BIBLIOGRAPHY

1. AMA Council of Medical Services: Guidelines for Quality Assurance. JAMA 259:2572–2573, 1988.
2. Berwick DM, Godfrey AB, Roessner J: Curing Health Care: New Strategies for Quality Improvement. San Francisco, Jossey-Bass, 1990.
3. Crosby P: Quality is Free: The Art of Making Quality Certain. New York, McGraw-Hill, 1979.
4. Donabedian A: Promoting quality through evaluating the process of patient care. Med Care 6:181–202, 1968.
5. Donabedian A: The quality of care: How can it be assessed? JAMA 260:1743–1748, 1988.
6. Gratton M, Campbell J, Lindholm D, Watson WA: Paramedic oral intubation rates in an EMS QI program. Prehospital Disaster Med 9:68, 1993.
7. Greenberg MD, Mosesso VK, Delbridge TR, et al: Quality indicators for emergency medical services: The paramdics' perspective. Prehospital Disaster Med 9:51, 1994.
8. Harrawood D, Gunderson M, Fravels S, et al: Drowning prevention: A case study in EMS epidemiology. J Emerg Med Serv 19:34–41, 1994.
9. Holroyd B, Knopp R, Kallsen G: Medical control, quality assurance in prehospital care. JAMA 256:1027–1031, 1986.
10. Kresky B, Henry MC: Responsibilities for quality assurance in prehospital care. Qual Rev Bull 12:230–235, 1986.
11. Kritchevsky S, Simmons BP: Continuous quality improvement: Concepts and applications for physician care. JAMA 266:1817–1823, 1991.
12. O'Leary DS: Quality assessment: Moving from theory to practice. JAMA 260:1760, 1988.
13. Ryan J: Quality management. In Kuehl AE: Prehospital Systems and Medical Oversight. St. Louis, Mosby, 1994, pp 217–246.
14. Shackford SR, Hollinsworth-Fridlund P, McArdle M, Eastman AB: Assuring quality in a trauma system—the medical audit committee: Composition, cost and results. J Trauma 27:866–875, 1987.

15. Stewart R, et al: A computer assisted quality assurance system for an emergency medical service. Ann Emerg Med 14:25–29, 1985.
16. Swor RA: Quality assurance in EMS systems. Emerg Med Clin North Am 10:597–610, 1992.
17. Swor RA, Hoelzer MH: A computer-assisted quality assurance audit in a multi-provider EMS system. Ann Emerg Med 19:286–290, 1990.
18. Swor RA, Rottman S, Pirrallo RG, Davis EA: Quality Management in Prehospital Care. St. Louis, Mosby, 1993.
19. Townsend PL: Commit to Quality. New York, John Wiley, 1986.

III. System Design

6. EMS SYSTEM DESIGN

William R. Metcalf, EMT

1. What is "modern" EMS?

The modern EMS model has evolved over the last 30 years. Perhaps the most important, fundamental aspect of the modern model is the philosophy of EMS as a *system* of care. It starts with the public and proceeds through a continuum of care, including dispatch, first responders, ambulances, transportation, emergency departments, and definitive care. The term "EMS system" is used to describe how the individual emergency services are organized together to deliver emergency medical care in the community. Many choices need to be made in putting together an EMS system.

2. What do you mean by "system design"? An ambulance is an ambulance, isn't it?

Modern emergency medical services (EMS) systems are much more than just ambulances. Different types of providers, such as first responders, dispatch, and emergency departments, are brought together in a variety of models to provide the complete spectrum of prehospital emergency medical care.

3. What does the public have to do with EMS?

The public is a key component of the EMS system because it is impossible to put trained and equipped medical providers on every street corner. Members of the public will often be bystanders or witnesses when an emergency medical condition occurs. Their ability to recognize quickly the presence of an emergency medical condition, rapidly access the EMS system, and begin initial life-saving treatment are essential to improved patient outcome.

4. Isn't 911 the universal method for accessing EMS assistance?

Not necessarily. 911 is a "universal" emergency access telephone number in most major population centers nationwide. In fact, the vast majority of the population can access emergency services by dialing 911. However, there are still large geographical areas of the country, predominately rural, where 911 service is not available. In these locations, the EMS system is activated by dialing a 7-digit telephone number that may ring in a sophisticated dispatch center or in a volunteer's home.

5. I understand that dispatch plays a part in getting equipment moving, but are dispatch personnel actually involved in medical care?

Absolutely. The current state of the art for dispatch in EMS systems is called "Emergency Medical Dispatch" (EMD). EMD is based on the principle that good information gathering during the dispatch phase of an emergency can better prepare responding EMS providers to deal with the situation at the scene. EMD can deliver basic emergency care instructions to people on the scene. In systems with a variety of potential providers, it can also prioritize requests for emergency medical assistance and ensure that only appropriate agencies or prehospital providers are dispatched.

The dispatch function may be carried out by a variety of agencies, including law enforcement, fire department, EMS agency, or a separate public safety dispatch center.

6. "First responders" were mentioned earlier. Who are they and what role do they play in the EMS system?

First responders are individuals or any non-transport entity, dispatched to respond quickly to medical emergencies to provide initial care until the ambulance arrives. As with EMD, the driving force behind the use of first responders is the motivation to get emergency medical assistance to the patient as soon as possible. First responders have emergency medical training and are able to reach an individual with an emergency medical condition more rapidly than the ambulance.

The first responder concept began almost 20 years ago with the development of a training program for law enforcement called Crash Injury Management (CIM). Police officers were given basic training so that they would be capable of providing initial emergency medical care. This program has evolved into a formal "First Responder" training program that is now provided to a wide variety of potential first responders, including highway workers, school bus drivers, firefighters, and utility workers. The level of care provided by first responders has increased dramatically in recent years with many fire department first responders carrying automatic external defibrillators and other sophisticated equipment. In some systems, the first responders are trained at the full paramedic level.

7. Does the ambulance play a role in the modern EMS system?

Of course it does, but the definition of what an ambulance is and who operates it can be one of the more complex aspects of an EMS system. Ambulances are usually operated within one of four basic organizational models:
- **Private**—May be operated as "for profit" or "not-for-profit" with providers of varying training levels; often financed by fee-for-service.
- **Hospital Based**—Run by one or more hospitals.
- **Municipal Third-Service**—Operated by the local government, not affiliated with fire or police departments.
- **Fire Department**—May use uniformed firefighters (firefighters may serve in dual role, handling fire and EMS calls or EMS calls only) or civilian EMS staff to provide basic to advanced level care; financed by department budget, although many departments bill patients for care and transportation.

8. Where do emergency departments and hospitals fit within an EMS system?

Perhaps the final major component of the EMS system are the facilities that will receive patients with emergency medical conditions. The typical EMS system will include multiple hospitals with varying levels of capability within its geographical boundaries. Some facilities will have special capabilities that are recognized based on national standards, such as trauma centers, burn centers, poison control centers, etc. Others may have special roles assigned by the local, regional, or state EMS system, such as the responsibility to be a "base hospital," a source of on-line medical direction for prehospital personnel.

9. What specialized EMS system components exist?

Many EMS systems also have special response and transportation resources that are not found in every system. These resources may include specialized rescue teams for auto extrication, cave rescue, water rescue, and other unusual situations. Many EMS systems also have air transportation services, either fixed or rotary wing (helicopter), available.

10. What is medical direction?

The final part of the system to be mentioned, which is essential, is medical direction. The practice of providing advanced life support is in reality a form of practicing emergency medicine. In all 50 states, for a paramedic to practice, a physician must extend his or her medical license to the paramedic. A knowledgeable, experienced, interested physician must be actively involved with and responsible for the medical care provided by the EMS system regardless of that system's design or structure.

11. Now that all of the system components have been defined, how are they put together into a "system"?

There are an infinite number of ways that the various potential components can be organized into a successful EMS system. Typically, some state-wide EMS entity will have statutory and regulatory authority over EMS within the state. This office will be headed up by an individual known as the state EMS director. Many states are then subdivided into regional or local EMS areas with governing boards. In the absence of these regional entities, local government usually assumes the responsibility for the delivery of EMS. EMS system design varies. The four basic models include:

- **100% Fire-based System**
- **100% Private System**
- **Public-private Partnership**—Often, the public sector provides first responder services while the private sector offers transportation.
- **Public Utility Model**—Some local municipalities grant a single provider a government-supported monopoly to provide all services.

Decisions about which EMS system components to include and how to link them together usually result from a compromise between medicine, politics, and finances. While it is relatively easy to describe the optimal EMS system from the medical perspective, it is not quite as easy to justify it from an economic or political perspective. Therefore, actual EMS system design is highly variable from one location to another.

12. How can I possibly figure out how the system is designed and how it all fits together in my community?

The simplest approach is to identify the system components one step at a time. Either a top-down or a bottom-up approach should work. Contact the state EMS office which is usually located within the state health agency. The state EMS office will often have information available that describes EMS system structure and function in the state. It can also identify the regional or local EMS entity that is responsible for EMS system design and function in your community. Or, working from the bottom up, contact the local ambulance service. They will be able to describe how the local system works and put you in touch with other system components.

BIBLIOGRAPHY

1. Kuehl AE (ed): National Association of EMS Physicians: Prehospital Systems and Medical Oversight, 2nd ed. Hanover, Mosby Lifeline, 1994.
2. National Highway Traffic Safety Administration: EMS System Development: Results of the Statewide EMS Assessment Program. Washington, DC, US Government Printing Office, 1994.
3. Roush WR (ed): Principles of EMS Systems, 2nd ed. Dallas, American College of Emergency Physicians, 1993.

7. EMS CONFIGURATION AND RESPONSE

Stewart L. Greisman, D.O.

1. What exactly does EMS provide to the community?

EMS configuration and response cannot be understood without a clear understanding of the service the EMS system really provides. In most communities, EMS encompasses a variety of functions, including response to accidents and medical emergencies, critical care transport between health care facilities, nonemergency transport of patients between facilities or their homes, transportation services for wheelchair or other patients requiring special vehicle accommodation, and, in some systems, transport of medical items such as blood, supplies, or equipment. This transportation may be provided by an ambulance or other vehicle. Depending on the nature of the request for service, EMS personnel may need special training in emergency care, critical care, medical instrumentation, communications, and vehicle operation.

2. Aren't all EMS systems alike?

No. A variety of organizations may be involved in the delivery of EMS in a given community:
- Private ambulance companies
- Fire departments
- Municipal ambulance services
- Hospital-based ambulance services
- Air ambulance services (operated by hospital, police, fire, governmental entity, or private vendors)
- Public safety organizations
- Rescue organizations

3. Are all EMS systems created equal?

No. Just as all hospitals do not provide the same quality care, the same applies to EMS systems. Response times, sophistication of EMS care, and quality of care vary from location to location.

4. Why do they differ?

For a variety of reasons, some of which can be controlled and others of which cannot. Some factors that affect EMS systems include:
- Geography. It is more difficult to deliver rapid, efficient care in a large, sparsely populated place than in most cities.
- Population. It may be easier to support a higher level of care in high-volume systems. Typically, greater resources and more funding are available in more populated areas.
- Timing. The development of EMS does not necessarily follow the growth of a community. Communities often expand despite the availability of resources and services and despite the best laid plans. EMS may be an afterthought to the planning process, unless it is actively promoted by a stakeholder in the community.
- Politics. When service and funding and territory and revenue intermingle, those whose interests are not entirely bound by patient care may have conflicting motivations.
- Community commitment. Some communities have spent much time and money assuring that their EMS system is of high quality. Active involvement by physicians, adequate funding, adequate EMT salaries, good equipment, and a commitment to training are all initiatives that promote quality care.

5. Who designs the system?

In many cases, EMS systems are not designed—they just evolve. Like hospitals, EMS systems grow out of local needs and desires and are often unrelated to any master plan. EMS systems are typically developed based on the available resources at the time that the needs are identified. Therefore, if the fire department is willing to provide advanced care at the time that the medical community is ready to train paramedics, the system becomes fire-based. In other communities, private ambulance companies offer their services, local hospitals develop the EMS system, or other ways of providing the service are identified. Economic factors often play a role in shaping systems as well.

6. Why is the EMS system's design important?

The EMS system affects the community in many ways. First, the quality of the system *does* matter to patients and their families, who count on EMS to help them during their worst moments. Hospitals may be affected by the EMS system through transportation and destination policies. EMS programs also impact the local economy by providing jobs for the private or public sectors. Finally, in systems that involve private companies, the design and operation of the EMS system itself may ultimately influence profitability to owners or shareholders. The interaction among stakeholders can influence system design and, ultimately, outcomes.

7. Who runs the system?

In many cases, there really is no one person or entity who is in charge of the EMS system. Systems tend to conform to resolutions that often are published after the system is established. The role of medical authority should be active, credible, and empowered.

8. How can an EMS system operate if nobody is in charge?

The EMS system is made up of many independent parts, including communications, police departments, fire departments, rescue groups, ambulances, medical directors, base stations, and destination hospitals with varying capabilities and staff. It would be extremely unusual for all these components to be part of the same organization and hence to be under the control of the same individual. So, in most EMS systems, there really is not anyone "in charge" because EMS is provided collaboratively by many different groups. In a few systems, a county or regional agency coordinates the efforts of all the EMS providers; however, in most cases their role is coordination rather than control.

9. Does every EMS system have a medical director?

No.

10. Should all systems have a medical director?

There is a fair amount of controversy regarding this issue, for two reasons. First, philosophically and operationally, many EMS organizations are based in public safety groups, not health care systems. Their traditional focus has been on fire or police functions, and their paperwork, training, and quality efforts reflect this public safety orientation. Public safety organizations may not have a medical director. Also, the role of a medical director who is not an officer or even an employee of a department can create legal issues beyond the scope of this question. So, they do not see the need for a medical director.

The second reason has to do with the delivery of care. Organizations that operate at a basic EMT level may argue that their functions are merely first aid and do not require the intervention of a physician. Because there is no delegation of advanced practice, physicians may not argue for involvement. However, EMS organizations without medical directors miss out on the educational opportunities, quality reviews, and protocol revisions that can best be led by someone with a strong foundation in medicine.

11. What is a tiered system?

A tiered EMS system delivers care at a variety of levels. For example, the first rescuer to approach a person who is in cardiac arrest might be a nearby police officer who could start CPR. Then, several minutes later, the local fire department might arrive and might be able to continue

CPR, administer oxygen, and defibrillate. Then a transporting ambulance might arrive, perhaps from a private company or from a different fire station, with paramedics who could intubate the patient and initiate advanced life support care as well as transport the victim to the hospital. Each level of care (police, fire, ambulance) is a tier.

12. How many tiers can there be?

There is no definitive answer to this question. In some rural areas patients might be cared for by many tiers as they move toward the hospital. For instance, a county sheriff might be the first tier, followed by a volunteer rescue group. A basic life support ambulance from a nearby town might be the next tier and could start transport. The ambulance might be met on the highway by an advanced life support ambulance or aeromedical unit, which would continue care to the hospital. Or a single agency can provide response, advanced care, and transport as a single tier.

13. Is there shared responsibility or obligation between tiers?

Whether the providers belong to one agency or come from different organizations, the ultimate shared responsibility is a cooperative effort to care for the patient. Medical direction should focus all providers on the patient regardless of their position in the hierarchy of response.

14. Is there a risk in tiered systems related to transferring a patient's care?

Absolutely. Patient "hand-offs" increase the risk of the loss of information about the patient's complaint, mechanism of injury, or past medical history. Hand-offs also increase the potential for a treatment to be administered twice or to be skipped because one tier thought the other had done it.

15. Given this risk, why would an EMS system have tiers? Would it not be better to have a single responding agency to eliminate the risk of hand-offs?

Yes and no. A single responding agency *would* decrease the hand-off risk. But a single-tiered system might dramatically increase response time, cost, or consumption of valuable resources. Tiered systems work because they use resources that are close to the patient to initiate care and actively manage the transfer of care in a prudent fashion.

16. What does "first response" mean?

First response is a function, and it represents the first tier to reach the patient. Implied in the term *first response* is that another, more sophisticated level of care is on the way. To some, bystander CPR or instructions provided by a trained emergency medical dispatcher may be considered first response.

17. What is a first responder?

A level of training that may be required in some states or systems for individuals who are performing the first response function. Some protocols require that these providers be trained in advanced first aid, some as EMTs. In some states or systems there is a dedicated level of training and even certification for the first responder, which is more specific to the first responder function but not as intensive as EMT training.

18. What is the difference between fixed and dynamic deployment?

Fixed deployment refers to having a constant number of EMS units, such as ambulances or rescue units, respond from fixed locations such as fire stations. Dynamic deployment involves having varying numbers of EMS units respond from mobile locations, strategically selected to be close to where the need is anticipated. Police cruisers are good examples of dynamic deployment.

19. How does the approach to EMS differ between fixed and dynamic deployment?

Fixed deployment and dynamic deployment represent radically different approaches to EMS delivery. The philosophy, tenets, and logistics of each require a commitment to purpose that is controversial across the country. This controversy has helped to highlight the differences: between change vs. the status quo, profit vs. nonprofit, public vs. private, union vs. nonunion, and in some cases has pitted provider against provider. A common concern is the rationale behind deployment. Is it to enhance the management and effectiveness of the resources (which it can)? Or is it to enhance the profitability (which it can)? Is profitability bad especially if the profits contribute to a better system of care? To a large extent it depends on which uniform you wear.

20. What is system status management?

A concept developed by EMS system expert Jack Stout, system status management is a dynamic deployment model that attempts to match the anticipated demand for services with the supply and placement of vehicles and staff. Simply stated, system status management means having the right number of EMS units in the right place at the right time. Therefore, during peak periods, more EMS units are in the appropriate locations than in slow periods.

21. What is the point of system status management?

The assumption behind dynamic deployment is that vehicles will be strategically placed at the location where and when they are most needed. This is achieved through system status management, which involves a detailed analysis of EMS demand based upon hour of day, day of week, month of year, and factors such as historical call patterns and traffic-related issues.

22. Why do not all EMS systems use system status management?

For two simple reasons. The first is tradition. Some EMS and fire organizations have built organizations around well-placed real estate. They provide constant, station-based staffing. Crews work fixed shifts. During peak times they work like crazy, often traveling far from their stations; during slow times they wait in the station for the next call. This tradition continues. The emotional and capital cost of changing this model would require a huge investment. Many believe that the fixed based model is still the best model for their community, if not universally.

The second impediment is knowledge and technology. Effective system status management requires the EMS system to have a firm understanding of the timing, location, and nature of its workload. These types of data, typically computerized, are not available in many EMS organizations and may be cost-prohibitive to install.

23. What is "unit hour utilization"?

As applied to EMS, a *unit hour* refers to an EMS unit (e.g., an ambulance) that is stocked, trained, and ready to provide high-quality EMS care for 1 hour. Utilization is measured by the number of calls run. Unit hour utilization (quantified against the number of calls run an hour, i.e., 0.36) is a tool that is used to evaluate the effectiveness of system status management. The efficient system has achieved a balance between the available unit hours and their utilization.

24. What is a CAD system?

CAD stands for computer-aided-dispatch. It is a high-technology tool that can aid in achieving the highest unit hour utilization from an EMS system through dynamic deployment. In other words, CAD can help keep track of and effectively manage the EMS resources in a dynamic deployment system. For example, CAD systems can automate the process of moving EMS units to the region of greatest need and can quickly identify the unit that is closest to an incoming call.

25. Do CAD systems work?

It depends. If the measure of success for CAD is the absolute best unit hour utilization, yes, it can work. Systems that use CAD can maintain good response times while minimizing the consumption of EMS resources that are not being used. However, whether system status management, dynamic deployment, and CAD have a positive, neutral, or any effect on the quality of patient care delivery is unclear and controversial.

26. Is it true that EMTs and paramedics are now connected to satellites?

Not exactly. Global positioning system (GPS) technology was originally developed by the military. It is a satellite-based technology that identifies any point on the earth by intersecting co-ordinates. Using GPS technologies, CAD systems can keep track of the locations of their EMS resources. GPS systems positively identify and track units automatically and display their locations on a screen to assist in the CAD process.

BIBLIOGRAPHY

1. Narad RA: Emergency medical services system design. Emerg Med Clin North Am 8:1–16, 1990.
2. Roush WR, McDowell RM, Pons PT: Emergency medical services systems. In Roush WR (ed): Principles of EMS Systems. Dallas, American College of Emergency Physicians, 1994, pp 11–24.
3. Smith JE: Administration, management, and operations. In Roush WR (ed): Principles of EMS Systems. Dallas, American College of Emergency Physicians, 1994, pp 103–122.
4. Valenzuela TD, Goldberg J, Keeley KT, et al; Computer modeling of emergency medical system performance. Ann Emerg Med 19:898–901, 1990.
5. Weigand JV: Prehospital ground transport: System structure and function. In Roush WR (ed): Principles of EMS Systems. Dallas, American College of Emergency Physicians, 1994, pp 165–182.

8. THE PREHOSPITAL ENVIRONMENT

Mike Smith, MICP

1. Do I really need to read this chapter?
Not if all your patients are going to walk into your firehouse or ambulance quarters. If you are planning to actually get in the rig and respond to emergency scenes, however, you should definitely read on.

2. What makes the prehospital environment so unique and so challenging?
The fact that it is a huge collection of variables. Take your garden-variety call for assistance involving a single car off the road on the exit ramp of the interstate at high noon on a sunny summer day. Change day to night. Go from sun to rain. Add some wind for good measure. Instead of a paved interstate, let's try a gravel road. Roll the car over on its roof. You see what I mean . . . and the list goes on. There is an almost limitless array of possibilities that you may encounter in the prehospital setting. That's what makes the field so interesting, and it is certainly part of the lure of EMS. In the same light, the corresponding challenge is formidable as well.

3. Why do seasoned emergency medical services (EMS) providers often say that the prehospital setting is a wealth of information?
Because it's true. If a provider is observant, is attentive to detail, and puts forth the necessary effort, he can ferret out a virtual gold mine of information at the scene of an emergency. The list of possibilities includes:
- The mechanism of injury
- Eyewitness accounts
- How the patient initially presents
- Crime scene clues (i.e., homicides, child abuse)
- Current prescription and over-the-counter medications

4. Of all the variables that I may encounter in the field, about which should I be most concerned?
People. The biggest factor that can destabilize a scene is people. Any number of factors can push a person's buttons. The stress of the emergency. Alcohol or illicit substances. Peer pressure. Anxiety, anger. And that's only a partial list of what makes people lose control.

You should always keep in mind that when emotions run high, judgment usually runs low. The person may have been in a fit of rage when he pulled the gun and is later truly sorry that he fired it. You could still be shot, however, and "sorry" does not bring you back, so stay on your toes.

5. When can an urban area take on one of the main properties of the rural setting?
Either during rush hour, when you respond at single-digit speeds, or when you take a mass of people and stack them vertically in a high-rise office or apartment building. In either case, your response time can increase exponentially; often, that is a key determinant of a rural response (e.g., dispatch to on-scene time > twenty minutes).

6. When I'm searching for medications in a house or apartment, where should I look?
Try the bathroom window first, then the medicine chest. Next, try the bathroom vanity drawers before you move to the drawers in the nightstand in the bedroom. Try the purse if the patient is a woman. Take a quick look in the refrigerator.

7. What percentage of dogs bite?

All of them, given the right stimulus. Quite a few of the procedures performed in the field can make a patient pull back or cry out. That may be all it takes to turn a passive pooch into a protective predator. Save yourself future problems. Have the patient or a family member secure Fido somewhere so that he won't be tempted to turn you into a buffet item.

8. When should I enter an unsecured, dangerous scene?

Never. We've all heard the old adage *fools rush in where angels fear to tread*. That's neither a trite phrase nor silly philosophy. The nature of prehospital medicine involves incurring a degree of risk, however, sometimes minimal, sometimes more. Therefore, the only way to avoid all risk in EMS is simply not to respond. That not being a practical alternative, you may choose to risk your life now and then, but keep in mind that no one can order you to throw your life away. It is prudent to have police "clean" all potentially dangerous scenes prior to entry. It comes down to an analysis of risk versus benefit.

9. How troublesome are motor vehicles at emergency scenes?

Very. Remember, motor vehicles *always outweigh you* and more often than not *have more velocity*. That's a double whammy, and you can bet that you'll come up on the short end of the stick.

In urban areas where bumper-to-bumper traffic is a daily affair and cars move at a snail's pace, passing on the right or on the shoulder of the highway or driving up on a sidewalk is illegal, but it still occurs.

In a suburban housing development, daytime traffic may be infrequent. Because of that, drivers may drive too fast and be inattentive because they expect the kids to be at school, the adults to be at work, and the roads to be empty.

Rural America has its own subculture of backroads race drivers. Excessive speeds; thin two-lane highways or, in many cases, gravel roads; plants and trees of every size and shape that obscure curves; and poor or no streetlights can make a rural emergency scene lethal.

Try to use your emergency vehicle as a defensive barrier whenever possible, and work behind it. Always leave yourself an out as well.

10. How important is it for me to learn to read a map?

Until all EMS response units are equipped with Global Positioning System technology, it's very important. If and when that occurs, map books will not be obsolete; they will just be slightly less useful. You can't help anyone until you can get to where they are located, can you? More importantly, you should become very familiar with your response geography so that you rarely have to refer to a map.

11. Of the urban, suburban, rural, and wilderness settings, which is the most dangerous for the prehospital provider?

The answer to that question depends on your understanding and appreciation of each of those four settings. Each of them presents with unique dangers and pitfalls just waiting for the inattentive, ill-informed, or unprepared EMS provider. A man with a gun in an inner city alley who wants your drug box is an obvious threat to you. By the same light, a 2000-lb bull with his mind on a cow in heat can take you out if you cross his path. It is your responsibility as an EMS professional to take the time to know the potential dangers of your response areas.

BIBLIOGRAPHY

1. Dernocoeur K: Streetsense, 3rd ed. Lang Communications, 1996.

IV. Personal Safety and Wellness

9. INFECTIOUS DISEASE EXPOSURE

Kevin L. Crumpton, M.D.

1. What are pathogens and communicable diseases?

Pathogens are microorganisms that cause disease; these include bacteria, viruses, fungi, and parasites. Communicable diseases are diseases that can be transmitted from one person to another by transfer of a pathogen. Transfer can occur by such routes as blood-to-blood contact (bloodborne), inhalation of infected airborne particles, ingestion of infected food (foodborne), or sexual contact.

2. Which communicable diseases can be transmitted to prehospital personnel?

As with all health care workers (HCWs) who provide direct patient care, the prehospital provider is at risk for a number of diseases, including bloodborne infections (such as hepatitis B, hepatitis C, AIDS/HIV infection, and syphilis), and airborne infections (such as tuberculosis, pertussis, chickenpox, and bacterial and viral meningitis). Diseases transmitted solely by foodborne routes (Salmonella, *E. coli* infection) or sexual activity (gonorrhea, chlamydia) would obviously not pose much risk to the prehospital provider.

3. But can't modern medicine treat and cure these illnesses?

Only some; that's why this chapter is so important. Curable diseases include pertussis, tuberculosis (most strains), and syphilis, but many (such as hepatitis B, hepatitis C, and human immunodeficiency virus) can only be curtailed with treatment and eventually may cause significant morbidity and even death.

4. Who is OSHA, and what does it have to do with prehospital care?

The Occupational Safety and Health Administration (OSHA) is a federal government agency responsible for enacting and enforcing safety guidelines in the workplace. The OSHA Bloodborne Pathogen Standard requires that states and employers develop plans to protect HCWs, including prehospital personnel, from the risk of transmittable diseases. These plans must include training, provision of personal protective equipment (PPE) for universal precautions, vaccination against hepatitis B (free of charge), and postexposure medical care.

5. What are universal precautions?

With "universal precautions," the HCW assumes that every patient potentially has a communicable disease, and he or she wears appropriate PPE for the situation. This is important because it is not possible to know from the history, appearance, or examination whether a patient has a transmittable disease. *Latex or plastic gloves* are recommended for all potential exposures to bodily fluids, including blood and open wounds. *Protective eyeware* and *gowns* are recommended for all potential splashes, including spurting blood, childbirth, intubation, and airway suctioning. *Masks* can protect the oral mucous membranes as well as filter potential airborne pathogens and thus are recommended for the splash settings and for patients with coughing who are suspected of having a communicable respiratory disease.

6. With bloodborne pathogens, what other specific precautions should be taken to minimize risk of transmission?

- Wash hands thoroughly after patient contact.
- Cover open skin lesions and sores (of the prehospital staff) with an adhesive bandage.
- Never recap or directly handle open needles.
- Clean ambulance after patient transport with a disinfectant known to kill infective organisms (when in doubt, a 1:100 mixture of bleach to water will work).

7. With airborne pathogens, what other specific precautions should be taken to minimize risk of transmission?

- Use particulate respirator masks (prehospital staff) when available.
- Place a surgical mask over the mouth and nose of the patient.
- Open the vehicle windows if possible.
- Set air-conditioning or heating of transport vehicle to nonrecirculating mode.

8. How is tuberculosis transmitted? Why is the stage of the disease important?

Tuberculosis (TB) is an airborne illness caused by a bacterium, *Mycobacterium tuberculosis*. It is generally a pulmonary disease but may also affect other organs such as the kidneys, lymph nodes, vertebrae, or adrenal glands. It is spread by "droplet nuclei" from a coughing or sneezing patient with *active* disease. Proper drug treatment may contain a primary infection with scar tissue and make the disease inactive. Reactivation of the disease can occur in immunosuppressed patients, such as those with AIDS, cancer, or advancing age. The drug arsenal against TB is limited to five or six primary drugs. Recent development of multi-drug resistant (MDR) TB has been seen. Development of MDR TB can be lethal, so the utmost attention must be paid to protective mask wear, especially particulate respirators, when transporting high-risk patients.

If the patient being transferred has known active TB or is highly suspected of such, the transferring facility is under legal obligation to notify prehospital staff on transport. This knowledge should be communicated to the receiving facility, preferably before arrival, so that respiratory isolation rooms can be arranged.

9. How are hepatitis B and hepatitis C transmitted?

Hepatitis B virus (HBV) and hepatitis C virus (HCV) are organisms transmitted by the bloodborne route or by sexual contact. Both viruses cause inflammation of the liver in the acute phase of infection and sometimes cause long-term effects. Hepatitis can also be caused by the foodborne route (hepatitis A) or by chemical toxicity (alcohol).

10. What is the course of hepatitis?

Up to 50–75% of transmitted cases of HBV or HCV will be minimally symptomatic (or asymptomatic). Of those with acute HBV, 5–10% will develop chronic hepatitis, cirrhosis (scarring of the liver), or liver cancer, 25% of minimally symptomatic "carriers" will develop some of these long-term effects. HCV infection will produce such long-term effects in 20–60% of cases. Currently, HBV infection can be prevented with the hepatitis B vaccine, which is provided free of charge by employers. No such vaccine for HCV currently exists.

11. How is AIDS transmitted, and what is the course of disease?

The acquired immunodeficiency syndrome (AIDS) is caused by human immunodeficiency virus 1 or 2 (HIV-1, HIV-2) and is transmitted by the bloodborne route or by sexual contact. Both viruses cause a disease spectrum ranging from asymptomatic infection to AIDS. AIDS generally develops 3 to 8 years after HIV infection as the virus decreases the ability of the body's immune system to fight infection. The specific illnesses seen with AIDS (thrush, *pneumocystis* pneumonia, Kaposi's sarcoma) are fought off quite well by people with competent immune systems. Recent breakthroughs in drug therapy have markedly decreased the progression of HIV and AIDS, but a cure for the disease remains elusive.

12. What clues may indicate that a patient has a communicable disease?

Tuberculosis (TB)—persistent cough, cough productive of bloody sputum, fever, night sweats, weight loss, and family or personal history of previous episodes of TB. Groups at high risk include alcoholics, immigrants from countries with a high prevalence of TB, and nursing home patients.

Pertussis—persistent hacking nonproductive cough; most often pediatric patients.

Meningitis—fever, stiff neck or neck pain, muscle aches, rash on extremities, "flulike" syndrome.

Syphilis—primary genital lesions, rash on palms or soles, lymphadenopathy.

Hepatitis B/hepatitis C—fever, nausea, jaundice (yellowing of the skin), fatigue.

AIDS—depends on stage of illness. Acute illness may manifest with symptoms of fatigue, fever, rash, lymphadenopathy, and weight loss. Like hepatitis B and C, HIV occurs more frequently *but not always* in high-risk groups such as intravenous drug abusers, homosexuals, bisexuals, those who received blood transfusions before 1985, and those with heterosexual exposure or maternal-neonatal exposure.

13. With a needle stick, what are the actual risks of transmission of hepatitis B virus, hepatitis C virus, and human immunodeficiency virus?

Exact data are unavailable, but current estimates are as follows.

HBV—6–43% for needlestick exposure, depending on the state and activity of the virus in the transmitting patient.

HCV—2.6% for needlestick exposure.

HIV—0.3–0.5% for needlestick exposure.

The risk of transmission from a splash exposure (eye or mucous membrane exposure) is probably 5 to 10 times less in each instance mentioned.

14. What should be done after a needle stick or suspected TB or meningitis exposure?

Needle stick—Recent management has changed based on studies that have shown that the risk of acquiring HIV after needlestick exposure to an HIV-positive individual can be decreased tenfold if prophylactic medicines are begun. A counselor should be available to you for discussion of your needle stick within hours of exposure. Because there is a "window period" between infection with HIV, HBV, and HCV and the ability of blood tests to detect infection, testing is usually recommended at the time of infection and at 6 weeks, 3 months, and 6 months after exposure.

Tuberculosis—TB skin test at 3, 6, and 12 months. Conversion with a large reddened lesion at the site of injection will require prophylactic medicines usually for at least two months, and sometimes longer.

Meningitis—Follow-up with the infectious disease counselor to see if prophylactic medications are warranted (as for meningitis caused by *Meningococcus*).

15. What are the current recommendations by the Centers for Disease Control (CDC) for a needle stick involving a high-risk patient or one known to have HIV?

A high-risk exposure must first be determined. If the patient is known to be HIV positive or is at high risk for the disease and a needle stick, splash, or other potential transmission occurs, the HCW should be seen immediately by a counselor or available physician (often an emergency physician) with regard to prophylactic medicines. If prophylaxis is chosen, the medicines should be given as soon as possible, preferably within 2 hours of exposure. Current recommendations include a combination of two antiretroviral medicines (AZT and 3TC) and a protease inhibitor (indinavir). These medicines often cause side effects including headache, fatigue, and gastrointestinal symptoms.

BIBLIOGRAPHY

1. Aledort LM: Consequences of chronic hepatitis C: A review article for the hematologist. Am J Hematol 44:29–37, 1993.

2. Barillo DJ: Infection control. In Pons PT, Cason D (eds): Paramedic Field Care: A Complaint-Based Approach. St. Louis, Mosby, 1997, pp 131–144.
3. Carco D, Srivastava P, Ciesielski C: Case-control study of HIV seroconversion in health care workers (HCW's) after percutaneous exposure to HIV-infected blood [abstract]. Infect Control Hosp Epidemiol 16(suppl):20, 1995.
4. Deinstag JL, Isselbacher KJ: Acute hepatitis. In Wilson JD, et al (eds): Harrison's Principles of Internal Medicine, 13th ed. New York, McGraw-Hill, 1994, pp 1458–1477.
5. Deinstag JL, Isselbacher KJ: Chronic hepatitis. In Wilson JD, et al (eds): Harrison's Principles of Internal Medicine, 13th ed. New York, McGraw-Hill, 1994, pp 1478–1490.
6. Dooley SW, Castro KG, Hutton MD, et al: Guidelines for preventing the transmission of tuberculosis in health-care settings, with special focus on HIV-related issues. MMWR CDC Surveill Summ 39(RR-17):1–27, 1990.
7. Guidelines for preventing the transmission of Mycobacterium tuberculosis in health-care facilities. MMWR 43(RR-13):1–55, 1994.
8. Mullan RJ, Baker EL, Bell DM, et al: Guidelines for prevention of transmission of human immunodeficiency virus and hepatitis B virus to health care and public safety workers. MMWR 38(S6):1–37, 1989.
9. Perlmutter BL, Harris BR: New recommendations for prophylaxis after HIV exposure. Amer Fam Phys 55:507–512, 1997.

10. CRITICAL INCIDENT STRESS

Patricia L. Tritt, R.N., M.A.

1. I've been in this business a long time, and I've seen a lot. I've always been able to handle it, so why can't everyone else do the same?

This is a two part question. First, we all have different tolerance levels for stress. Several types of stress may affect emergency responders, which we shall address shortly. Some individuals may go their entire careers without experiencing a particularly stressful or distressing call or event. However, studies have shown that approximately eighty-five percent of emergency personnel have experienced acute stress reactions after working in one or more situations that meet the criteria of a critical incident. Approximately two to four percent may experience longer term, more profound effects on their lives.[4]

Recently, there has been a growing realization that some of the things that emergency responders thought did not bother them were merely buried deep in a mental file drawer. Sometimes those files pop out later with worse effects than originally felt. What we experience is rarely truly forgotten. The important point is to deal with the event or situation effectively at the time, rather than postpone the inevitable. It is like overdrawing your checking account. You may be able to write checks for awhile, but eventually the bank will discover the fact and the repercussions are inescapable.

2. Why is critical incident stress suddenly such a big deal?

This is largely a matter of perspective. The critical incident stress "movement" officially began in 1983 with the publication of an article on the subject by Dr. Jeffrey T. Mitchell.[3] Emergency responders began to realize and acknowledge that some events are critical incidents, and personnel deserve methods to effectively cope with the aftermath. The proof of the perceived need lies in the development of over three-hundred critical incident stress management teams throughout the United States and teams in numerous other countries. Seventeen nations were represented at the 1995 Third World Congress on Stress, Trauma, and Coping in the Emergency Services Professions. Emergency responders from all specialities have adopted the critical incident stress management philosophy.

3. What is a critical incident?

Critical incidents are powerful events with significant impact which overwhelm the usual coping mechanisms of the individual or group. Critical incidents tend to occur suddenly and are outside the range of normal human experience. Emergency responders are typically in the "right place at the right time" to encounter these profound traumatic events.

4. I have heard it said that emergency responders may be victims of things they experience in their profession. How can that be? Are not the victims the people to whom we respond?

There are three categories of victims.

- **Primary victims**—those most directly affected by a traumatic event, usually considered the direct or immediate victims of accidents, disasters, and non-accidental trauma.
- **Secondary victims**—observers of the immediate traumatic effects on the primary victims—e.g., emergency responders, witnesses.
- **Tertiary victims**—those indirectly affected by the traumatic event, either by later exposure to the traumatic scene or to the primary or secondary victims—e.g., family members of both the initial victims, emergency responders.

Critical incident stress management services, as discussed in this chapter, are focused on the emergency responder and the emergency responder's family. The critical incident stress process over the past decade has clearly demonstrated that these individuals and groups do become victims and deserve rapid and timely psychological "first aid."

5. What is so different about the everyday stress we experience in our lives and critical incident stress?

Good question. We are inundated daily with talk of stress in the workplace, schools, families, and society. Many of us have probably tuned out the talk of stress and stress management. When everyone else is stressed, who wants to hear about it? Our everyday stress level is affected by many factors, events, and people in our lives. Our stress level may go up and down frequently or rapidly, like springtime temperatures. Or, our stress level may remain fairly high (or fairly low) for long periods, depending on what is going on in our lives. Various factors have been shown to directly affect the stress level, including:[2]

- Stressful emotions, thoughts, and beliefs
- Psychosocial causes such as adaptation, frustration, overload and deprivation
- Bioecological stressors, including biorhythms, eating and drinking habits, drugs, noise pollution, and climate and altitude
- Personality causes, such as self-perception, patterns of behavior, anxious personality type, and the need for control
- Occupational stress and stressors

Critical incident stress (CIS), on the other hand, is usually incident specific. Alternately, multiple incidents of lesser psychological impact may occur in rapid succession or in close time proximity to cause an acute stress reaction.

6. Is stress like caffeine? Most of us need it to get us going in the morning.

Yes, most of us do need a little stress in our lives to get us going and keep us mentally sharp. Not all stress is bad. The positive, productive aspect of stress is called eustress. Eustress enhances health, performance, and productivity. It provides motivation, overcomes lethargy, and facilitates coping. For any individual, at any particular moment, there is an optimal level of stress, however. When stress becomes negative and debilitating, harmful distress ensues. Distress interferes with normal performance and coping. The key to staying on the right side of stress is learning to recognize the signs of distress when they occur in ourselves and others.

7. Are critical incidents just the "really big ones" like plane crashes, building collapses, and large scale natural disasters?

Early discussion of critical incident stress highlighted experiences of emergency responders following disasters such as plane crashes; natural disasters, including hurricanes and tornados; building collapses; mass murder scenes; and other large scale responses. The nature and enormity of these events helped bring to light both the short and long term effects on rescue personnel. Many emergency responders still equate critical incidents with the "Big One." However, the vast majority of critical incidents occur when the incident is of a much smaller scale, but is extraordinary for one or more reasons. Examples of critical incidents include:

- Death of a coworker in the line of duty
- Serious injury to an emergency worker in the line of duty
- Suicide of a coworker
- Death of a civilian as a result of emergency service operations
- Mass casualty incidents resulting in serious injury or death
- Death or serious injury to a child
- Responding on calls when the victim is known to the emergency service worker
- Threat to the safety of the responders, i.e., hostage or sniper situation, hazardous materials, or other threat to personal safety
- Situations with excessive media interest or criticism
- Loss of a patient following prolonged rescue or resuscitation efforts
- Personal identification with the victim or circumstances

• Incidents in which the sights and sounds are particularly distressing

This list of critical incidents is not exhaustive. A variety of circumstances may combine to produce acute stress reactions in responders.

8. Is this stress stuff all in your head? Can't you just think or talk yourself out of it if you really want to?

Stress is all in your head. Or at least the stress response *starts* in your head. The cortex of the brain receives input from the senses and interprets the data at both the conscious and subconscious levels. The midbrain and limbic system are stimulated which adds emotional interpretation, such as fear or anger. When a stressor is identified, the hypothalamus is activated, initiating a chain reaction resulting in stimulation of both the sympathetic and parasympathetic nervous systems. Stress hormones, including epinephrine, norepinephrine, cortisol, and aldosterone, are released. Once the stress response is initiated, arousal continues until the stress products are absorbed. Since the process operates at both the conscious and subconscious levels, your conscious mind may say "Don't sweat it" but your subconscious may not agree. Guess who wins.

9. I hear a lot about burnout in our profession. What is burnout and how does it happen?

Burnout is an overused, and frequently misused term, that refers to cumulative stress reaction. This phenomenon is usually the result of multiple stressors occurring over time. Factors typically include job-related stress, family and relationship issues, and interpersonal stresses. A high chronic level of stress often exists. The individual's coping mechanisms and ability to adapt to a changing environment may be slow to respond or inadequate. The onset of cumulative stress reaction may be insidious, developing over months or years. The syndrome is characterized by physical and emotional exhaustion and negative, cynical attitudes. The quality of the individual's life and the ability to enjoy family, friends, and social life is decreased. Job performance eventually declines, physical illness and work absences increase, and emotional distress becomes more apparent. Other symptoms may include substance and alcohol abuse, disillusionment, apathy, withdrawal, chronic irritability and anger, disrespectful attitudes towards others, and an increase in interpersonal conflict. Resolution of cumulative stress reaction may be complex and require psychological and career counseling.

10. Do emergency responders have certain personality characteristics that make us immune to critical incident stress?

Does the job create the personality profile, or does the job attract individuals with certain personality traits or characteristics? Probably some of both. Either way, there are characteristics that are common among emergency responders. Each factor can produce a positive effect, or can actually increase one's stress level. Characteristics of emergency responders include:

• Strong need to be in control
• Risk taking, action orientation (easily bored)
• Detail oriented
• Idealistic
• Dedicated and loyal
• Suppression of emotions

None of these characteristics makes us immune to stress. Knowledge of how our personal characteristics work for, or against, us helps us to recognize those times we may need additional support.

11. Why can't I just forget about what happened? Why do I need to drag it all up again by talking about it? It seems to me that the less said, the better.

"Reveal and heal" is the watchword here. Remember the subconscious mind mentioned earlier? The subconscious stores what happens to us in greater detail than the conscious mind does. You may think it is past, or "filed," but all the details are waiting in your stored memory. Sometimes, out of nowhere, with a single unintentional key stroke, the entire event from years earlier is back.

Mitchell and Everly identify several possible mechanisms of action of critical incident stress debriefings (CISD), including early intervention; opportunity for catharsis or venting; opportunity to verbalize the traumatic event; behavioral and psychological structure of the critical incident stress debriefings; group support; peer support; stress education; and opportunity for follow-up.[5] The chance to ventilate emotions and verbalize specific traumatic elements is a key concept. Mitchell and Everly explore numerous studies documenting the importance and efficacy of early effective intervention with individuals and groups who have experienced traumatic events. Reduction of stress arousal and improved immune system functioning result from release of emotions. Suppression of emotions leads to increased anxiety and depression over time.

12. By admitting that I am occasionally affected by critical incidents, doesn't that mean I am crazy or have post traumatic stress disorder (PTSD)?

The answer to both is no. You are having normal reactions to abnormal situations. Emergency responders may routinely be called to some pretty awful scenes and situations, *but this does not mean they are normal life events!* Emergency responders are in a unique situation to be routinely exposed to great human misery, tragedy, and suffering. A protective shell and coping mechanisms develop, but they may not always be adequate to protect you from what you encounter on your job.

Post traumatic stress disorder is a formally recognized psychological disorder which may result from exposure to a traumatic event, an event outside the range of normal human experience. This diagnostic label includes specific criteria in four areas: the traumatic event, re-experiencing the event, avoidance and numbing reactions, and symptoms of increased arousal. The term PTSD is often used casually, and erroneously, to refer to any exposure to a psychologically traumatic event. PTSD is a complicated diagnosis that can only be made by a competent mental health professional. The thrust of the critical incident stress management process is to prevent the development of PTSD through early, and effective, intervention.

13. What is the difference between critical incident stress debriefing (CISD) and critical incident stress management (CISM)?

Critical incident stress debriefing (CISD) refers to only one of the interventions involved in the critical incident stress management (CISM) process. A CISD is a structured group meeting between personnel directly involved in a critical incident and a CISM team. A debriefing is a confidential, non-evaluative discussion of the involvement, thoughts, reactions, and feelings resulting from the incident. The formal debriefing allows for ventilation of feelings by the responders and an assessment by a CISM team mental health professional and other CISM team members of the intensity of the stress response. A debriefing provides support, reassurance, and education. It stimulates mobilization of individual and group resources and allows the design of a plan of action, if needed. Formal debriefings have both psychological and educational components. Debriefings accelerate recovery in normal people who are having normal reactions to abnormal events. Other CISM interventions include:

- Pre-incident education
- On-scene support services
- Demobilizations
- Defusings
- Family and significant other support programs
- One-on-one crisis intervention
- Stress management and trauma management education programs
- Follow-up programs

14. How do I know when I or my coworkers are experiencing the effects of critical incident stress?

Evaluation of the need for CISM services may be obvious, as in the case of a line of duty death. However, more often indications for CISM services may be less clear. Here are some questions you may consider in making an evaluation.

• How many individuals are affected, one or many?
• What reactions or symptoms are being reported by participants in the event? Continuation of symptoms of acute or delayed stress reactions or intensification of symptoms are key indicators for interventions. Acute stress reactions may include physical, cognitive, emotional, and behavioral signs and signals. Common physical reactions include: fatigue and exhaustion; gastrointestinal upset, elevated blood pressure and heart rate; and headaches and muscle aches or twitches. Cognitive reactions involve: poor concentration and attention span; memory problems; poor problem solving; nightmares; and intrusive images. Emotional reactions may appear as: anxiety; guilt; grief; denial; loss of emotional control; depression; inappropriate emotional response; apprehension; feeling overwhelmed; intense anger; and irritability. Behavioral reactions include: change in activity; withdrawal; emotional outbursts; change in usual communications; loss or increase in appetite; alcohol consumption; inability to rest; antisocial acts; hyperalert to environment; startle reflex intensified; pacing; and erratic movements.
• Has there been a change in the behavior or affect of the participants in the event?

Only debrief events that require debriefing. Do not dilute the process by debriefing events that do not have significant emotional impact.

15. How important is prior education in making CISM interventions more effective?

Prior education is beneficial, but not essential. Pre-incident education about the nature of the stress response, possible reactions, and appropriate management techniques raises the level of awareness of emergency responders. Education helps to dispel the "it's all in your head" myth. Education encourages open expression of thoughts, reactions, and feelings among coworkers and significant others. And, education makes us more aware of our resources, and when to activate or use those resources, including a CISM team. Emergency responders are action oriented individuals; providing management techniques for acute stress reactions can be extremely beneficial, in both the short and long term.

16. What can and/or should be done when the effects of critical incident stress are recognized?

The menu of CISM interventions was listed earlier. The appropriate intervention will depend on the incident and the amount of time elapsed. For example, in a large mass casualty situation the CISM team should be called on scene to assist in psychological support of personnel. If the event is prolonged, a series of demobilizations should be organized. Debriefings should be scheduled following on-scene response and involvement. Follow-up services should be available to all personnel. Debriefings for significant others would be appropriate.

For other, smaller scale events, a defusing the same day of the incident is beneficial. If scheduling a defusing is not possible, consider a debriefing within 24–72 hours. A one-on-one may be needed if only one individual is affected. Consult with your local CISM team for the most appropriate interventions.

17. What is the difference between a debriefing and a defusing?

The format of a debriefing was described in the answer to question 13. The formal debriefing is ideally scheduled within 24–72 hours following the critical incident. This provides a normalizing period and an opportunity to internally process the experience. It also affords an opportunity to invite all emergency and healthcare personnel involved in the call to the debriefing. One of the unique advantages of this inclusive approach is the opportunity to share information and generate support within the group.

The defusing is a small group intervention following a traumatic event. Defusings differ from debriefings in timing and number of individuals involved in the group. The defusing is held the day of the incident before the personnel leave their duty shift. The immediacy of the defusing allows for early ventilation and education on anticipated effects of the stress response. Due to the close proximity to the traumatic event, personnel may not have yet had an opportunity to assess the depth or degree of potential reactions. However, evidence suggests that immediate intervention may be more beneficial than waiting for a later debriefing.[5] The rapid scheduling of a defusing may make it impossible for all personnel involved to attend the defusing. A defusing may eliminate the need for a debriefing or a debriefing may be an important CIS management component. These decisions should be made between the requesting personnel and the CISM team.

18. Just what happens in a CISD? Is it the same as a critique of the call?

Critiques and psychological debriefings are opposites. The critique focuses on the cognitive: what went right, what went wrong, what we will do next time. The critique is meant to be a logical, thoughtful evaluation of events. The psychological debriefing consists of seven phases and is structured to transition from the cognitive to the emotional level, returning to the cognitive plane. The phases of a formal debriefing include: introduction; fact phase; thought phase, reaction phase; symptom phase; teaching phase; and reentry. The appropriately run debriefing should steer participants away from critique and evaluation to a safe expression of thoughts, reactions, and feelings. All group members must respect the expressions and feelings of others. Material divulged in a debriefing may not be used outside the session by other members of the group (command personnel, peers, or CISM team members).

19. I know that occasionally a call gets to me. But I do not take my work home and I keep my family insulated from the distressing things I encounter on the job. There really is not any need to bother them with that side of the job, is there?

Most of us would like to think that we can compartmentalize our lives and leave work at work and home at home. The reality is that the subconscious (remember that function?) is always with us. We are all a sum of our parts and experiences, which we carry around with us. Consider who knows you best. Is it not the family and other loved ones who are the first to spot when something is amiss with you? When you show signs of distress, be assured that those closest to you will notice. And, unless they have information to the contrary, what or who will they consider is causing the problem? Right on the first try. Your loved ones will assume the problem is with them or with your relationship. The best approach is open communication. Discuss how to handle these situations *before* traumatic events occur. Find out how much information your spouse or significant other wants to hear or can handle. Discuss your needs and usual style; for example, do you typically withdraw, seek comfort, talk, or keep silent. You have a stressful job. Understand that the job stress translates to your family and preplan for how you can handle the stress as a family.

20. There isn't any hurry to have a CISM intervention, is there? There are so many things to do following most calls, can't the CISM part just wait? Shouldn't we do our critique first?

Critical incident stress management is a preventative strategy aimed at preventing or mitigating traumatic stress syndromes. Early intervention is crucial. Same day interventions, such as defusings, have proven to be extremely effective in decreasing the level of acute distress in emergency responders. The analogy is early attention to a physical wound. Proper early wound management leads to primary healing with minimal discomfort and disability. Delayed treatment often results in infection and other complications which may end in scarring, continued discomfort, and even disability.

Emergency responders are trained to continually evaluate their performance and response. Critique and continuous quality improvement activities are important processes. Following critical incidents, however, psychological debriefing should occur **before** a critique. The debriefing process allows the emergency responders to deal with the emotional impact and aftermath of the event. The critique or evaluation that is scheduled at a later date following a debriefing will be more constructive, objective, and beneficial to the individuals and the organization.

21. Will the same approach to providing CIS services work for all situations? What is different about interventions for a disaster versus a fatality of a child, for example?

Experience has taught us that all types of critical incidents are not the same and different approaches to interventions are needed. Each situation requires careful assessment of the most appropriate response. The usual approach of defusings and debriefings may be inappropriate, or even counterproductive, in the disaster situation requiring long term disaster recovery efforts. This is especially true if the emergency responders were also primary victims, as in the case of a natural disaster such as a hurricane or flood. Event stressors for disaster workers may include: the type of disaster; continued threat of recurrence; personal loss or injury; continued exposure to traumatic stimuli; and mission failure or human error.[1] Consultation with an experienced CISM team is essential in structuring appropriate CISM disaster intervention strategies.

22. Is CISM just another name for therapy? I do not feel like I am crazy. Well, at least not most of the time.

By now it should be clear that CISM interventions are preventive strategies and not therapy. A key concept in the CISM model is to avoid doing therapy. The CISM process focuses on a specific work related incident, or accumulation of incidents, that created an acute stress response in the emergency providers. CISM focuses on returning the individuals and group to their previous level of functioning, protecting them from further psychological harm, and preventing further harmful reactions. The CISM process was developed for the psychologically healthy to assist them in maintaining and enjoying that state.

23. I have heard that we have a regional CISM team. What is it and what does it do?

The CISM team is normally a multidisciplinary, multijurisdictional, regional team of volunteers trained in all aspects of the CISM process. The core team members include mental health professionals, EMS personnel, law enforcement officers, firefighters, and healthcare personnel (nursing and other healthcare providers). Other disciplines may include chaplains, dispatchers, search and rescue personnel, ski patrol, corrections officers, victims' advocates, and other specialty personnel in the region. The CISM team is trained to provide all interventions discussed in this chapter. The team may be part of a larger state or regional organization, and may also be registered with the International Critical Incident Stress Foundation (ICISF). For more information, contact the ICISF at 410-750-9600.

24. Do we really need to use a CISM team? Can't we just take care of things "in-house"?

One form of CISM intervention is called the initial discussion. Emergency responders are encouraged to use their work group to explore their initial thoughts, reactions, and feelings regarding troublesome calls. This is often all that is needed in a supportive environment that encourages open sharing of feelings. The initial discussion can be accomplished "in-house" without outside facilitation. It is occasionally beneficial, however, to bring in a team from outside the organization to provide defusings or formal debriefings. Experience has demonstrated that the most effective debriefings and defusings are inclusive of all personnel involved in the incident and facilitated by an experienced, outside CISM team. Participants generally experience a higher level of trust and confidence in a regional team. There is less concern about how information in the debriefing or defusing will be used or if it will become part of an internal investigation or critique. Using CISM team members who are not familiar with incident personnel is psychologically protective for both the team and the impacted personnel.

25. You know, this call did not seem to bother me, but it sure seems to have hit some of my coworkers hard. What can I do to help them?

Peer support is an extremely important component of the critical incident stress management process. The most important part of peer support is listening. Frequently emergency responders are reluctant to offer assistance or support to distressed coworkers because "I don't know what to say." The key is to say little, listen a lot, and allow the individual his or her feelings. It is okay to feel angry, sad, frightened, overwhelmed, or depressed. Validate feelings as normal. Do not try to talk the individual out of feeling the way they feel. Do not give pat advice such as "It will be okay, try not to think about it, you'll get over this, or I know just how you feel." As a supporter, ask yourself this question: "What would help me the most if I were in his or her position?" If only one individual seems to be affected by the call, spend time one-on-one. If you are uncomfortable in that role or feel unprepared, find another co-worker to provide peer support. If several of your team members have been impacted, contact your local CISM team.

26. I believe in the CISM process, but administration sure does not seem to. What can I do to help convince them it is needed?

Pre-incident education provides an excellent opportunity to educate administrative personnel on the effects and costs of critical incident stress. A well prepared presentation on the topic can illustrate the potential costs to an emergency responder team and organization. Even administrative personnel who have "been there, done that, and it never bothered me" can be made to realize that critical incident stress can result in increased sick time, decreased productivity, increased mistakes and errors, increased on-the-job injuries, and ultimately increased turnover in personnel. Each of these effects is costly for an organization. Turnover is very expensive in any industry with extensive training and experience requirements, such as emergency services. Aside from financial motivation, attention to psychological well being should be the concern of every employer.

27. Okay, so if I attend debriefings and defusings that will take care of all the stress in my life, right?

There is no simple solution. The issue of stress in all spheres of our lives is complex. Critical incident stress debriefings and defusings are only part of the answer. A regular stress management program and attention to diet and exercise are musts. Developing and maintaining a strong and supportive social network provides on-going support. Tending to important relationships in our lives with spouses, significant others, children, parents, and others close to us is essential. Tending to relationships includes striving to improve our communications and becoming more open and sharing. Recognition of both acute and chronic stressors in our lives allows us to develop appropriate ways of dealing with stress on a long term basis. Evaluate your current methods of coping with stress. Are they healthy and helpful, or are they self damaging and destructive? Stress management and mitigation is an ongoing process. Most of all, find ways to enjoy your life, your job, and your family.

BIBLIOGRAPHY

1. Everly GS Jr (ed): Innovations in Disaster and Trauma Psychology. Vol 1: Applications in Emergency Services and Disaster Response. Ellicott City, MD, Chevron Publishing Corporation, 1995.
2. Girdano D, Everly G Jr, Dusek D: Controlling Stress and Tension: A Holistic Approach, 4th ed. Englewood Cliffs, NJ, Prentice Hall, 1993.
3. Mitchell JT: When disaster strikes . . . The critical incident stress debriefing process. JEMS pp 36–39, 1983.
4. Mitchell JT, Bray G: Emergency Services Stress: Guidelines for Preserving the Health and Careers of Emergency Services Personnel. Ellicott City, MD, Chevron Publishing Corporation, 1990.
5. Mitchell JT, Everly GS Jr: Critical Incident Stress Debriefing: An Operations Manual for the Prevention of Traumatic Stress Among Emergency Services and Disaster Workers. Ellicott City, MD, Chevron Publishing Corporation, 1994.

11. SCENE SAFETY

Tom Tkach, NREMT-P

1. Isn't too much emphasis placed on scene safety? Don't most people want my help? Why would they want to hurt me?

Providing emergency medical care is frequently fraught with peril for EMS providers. While most calls for assistance place us at little personal risk, we do respond to shootings, stabbings, domestic violence events, and countless other violent scenes that place personal safety in jeopardy. Gang- and drug-related activity is increasing, and weapons are proliferating in society. Not only is the criminal element of society arming itself, but many law-abiding citizens are arming themselves in response. Other environmental variables can cause virtually any situation to deteriorate and become unsafe. Because of the changing nature of society, EMS providers should have great concern for these issues and must always be accountable for their own safety.

2. Isn't it the responsibility of the police to make sure I am safe?

Although police take the role of protecting EMS providers seriously, there is no mathematical formula to determine how much police cover is enough. On occasion, the police do not feel safe themselves and call for additional officers to assist or simply tell the EMS team that it is time to leave. Clearly, EMS providers must never assume a scene is safe just because the police are present; they should always make their own independent judgment on the safety and stability of a scene.

3. What are the most perilous calls?

One of the common misconceptions is that the most dangerous calls are shootings and stabbing scenes. In fact, these calls may present little risk simply because most perpetrators leave the scene after committing their crime. Calls that probably hold the greatest risk involve alcohol, drugs, and psychiatric patients, because the behavior of the patients and bystanders is unpredictable. Domestic violence calls are also very unpredictable; more police officers are killed or injured on domestic violence calls than on any other type of call.

4. Who are the problem patients?

Reviewing emergency department diagnosis of violent patients clearly shows that the most common cause of violent behavior is alcohol and drug intoxication, with the most common drugs being cocaine, amphetamines, and phencyclidine. Patients with psychiatric problems are the next most common type of patients prone to violence. Even patients with medical problems such as hypoglycemia or head trauma can become violent. EMS providers must anticipate violent behavior when faced with these situations.

5. What is situation awareness?

The ability to see the big picture. The term is derived from military pilots who fly combat missions. To ensure survival, a pilot in combat must be aware of everything going on around the aircraft at all times. We can draw a direct analogy between the pilots in combat and an EMS call. EMS providers must be aware of the big picture on every scene. Unfortunately, most EMS providers fall into an awareness category called patient-oriented, leading to increased personal risk on hazardous scenes.

6. What does *patient-oriented* mean?

All through our EMS education, we learn to be patient-oriented: to observe a patient's clinical presentation, take a history, perform a physical assessment, and provide technical procedures.

Little of our education is focused on reading the big picture. Ultimately, EMS providers unconsciously tune out the scene and focus on the patient. For most calls this is not a problem, but this patient-oriented mindset can lead to tunnel vision. Tunnel vision increases personal risk because it can prevent or delay a response to danger. All EMS providers should strive to become scene-oriented, allowing them to read not only the patient but the entire scene for potential problems.

7. How do I learn to become scene-oriented?

As with any other skill, you must pay conscious attention to this ability. Practice scanning the entire situation as you approach. Eventually, this skill will become a conditioned response. Total situation awareness requires continual scanning since scenes are constantly changing. A scene that was initially safe may not remain safe. One must keep that "mental searchlight" moving and assess all the environmental variables: the patient, the patient's family, the bystanders, the physical setting. This will maximize your safety by allowing you to recognize a scene that is dangerous or deteriorating.

8. How do I approach a high-risk scene?

When you arrive at a scene, you are guaranteed of becoming the focus of the neighborhood's attention; everything you do will be under a microscope. No one in EMS likes to perform for crowds. When approaching a high-risk scene, shut down the emergency lights and sirens several blocks away to allow for a discreet arrival and to enable you to survey the scene before announcing your presence. Choose a strategic parking location that will provide a safe approach to the scene and a quick exit should the need arise. Approach houses and doors from the side instead of directly. During the approach, scan for any signs of danger and listen for sounds of violence taking place.

9. Shouldn't I just wait for the police before entering a high-risk scene?

Many EMS systems have policies that direct their personnel to wait for police to secure a violent scene before entering. This type of policy ignores the fact that the most hazardous calls can start out innocently and deteriorate rapidly. EMS providers usually make the decision to wait for police based on the initial dispatch information and usually never hesitate to enter a "routine" scene. This can lead to major risk, because even routine calls can turn bad.

10. Are there any red flags that can help me identify potential danger?

A dark house at night, an open door, and signs of violence such as blood and broken glass and furniture are major indicators of an unsafe scene. Great caution must be used in the face of such findings. Once on the scene, you should read the bystanders for signs of hostility. Identify the "bad actors" immediately and ascertain the presence of any type of weapon. Learn to "feel" the scene and trust your instincts. If something doesn't feel right, it probably isn't. If the scene is unsafe or potentially unsafe, applying the lion tamer theory is an effective way of minimizing risk.

11. What is the lion tamer theory?

One of the most effective techniques for controlling a high-risk patient or a high-risk scene. The lion tamer at a circus enters his large cage and then watches as the lions and tigers are brought into this cage one by one. By bringing these dangerous cats into his cage, the lion tamer establishes a psychological advantage over the animals. The lion tamer will *never* go into the lion's cage, because it's the lion's home, a place where the lion has an instinctive psychological advantage. Problem patients maintain a similar advantage when we enter their "cage." By moving such a patient quickly into our cage, the ambulance, or by simply moving them out of their environment, we can reverse this psychological edge.

12. How do I recognize when I'm losing control of the scene?

The first sign is that the scene starts to get noisy. Bystanders stop following directions to stay out of the way. If you're the medic in charge, you'll notice that things start happening that you didn't direct, because another EMS crew member perceived a control vacuum and began to take action. You will hear comments from the crowd such as, "Why don't you do something!" Any scene with hysterical family or bystanders has high potential for escalation. Remember that perception is reality. If the crowd perceives that you are not in charge, you're not. Once this happens, it's time to get the patient out of there. Once you lose control of a scene, rarely can you get it back.

13. What are the red flags signaling that a patient may become violent?

You must learn to read not only the scene but also your patients by observing their body language and verbal comments. Common forms of aggressive body language include the boxer's stance, where the patient "squares off" to fight. Another form is a stance taken when one is feeling threatened, called blading; the patient will turn at an angle toward you, "blading his body." The "1000 yard stare," where the patient is "looking right through you," is seen when a patient is mentally preparing to fight—the calm before the storm. Any patient showing obvious anxiety and lots of agitated motor activity is also at high risk for becoming violent. You may observe "target glancing," with the patient stealing furtive glances at the trauma scissors on your belt or the door. This patient is telegraphing his intention to grab your scissors or try to escape. Verbal cues, with the patient screaming or using pressured speech, also can help to predict violent behavior.

14. What should I do if I observe these warning signs in my patient?

Even sober people dislike anyone violating their personal space. Intoxicated or psychiatric patients are especially prone to violence if you approach them too quickly and violate their personal space. Take extra time to evaluate the patient's potential for violence before approaching. If the patient seems safe to contact, approach slowly from an angle instead of from directly in front and be ready to move back if the patient reacts negatively. Have the police ready to assist if necessary. Most of these patients can be controlled verbally without resorting to physical control.

15. How do I verbally control problem patients?

Most potentially violent patients can be controlled verbally. Set the proper tone for the call by being a "good guy." Being verbally aggressive with these patients is counterproductive. Escalating your tone should be a last resort. If you start out with a hard guy approach, you have no place to back down to. The patient may call your bluff and you will end up in a fight.

16. Which patients need to be restrained?

Anyone who is violent needs to be restrained, and anyone who you feel is going to become violent probably needs restraints, but this is clearly a judgment call. There are no hard and fast rules, but a good guideline is to restrain anyone who you feel is going to be a problem. It usually takes six or more people to restrain a patient in full combat. Have a team approach, with each member of the team assigned to restraining a certain portion of the patient. Four-point restraints, at a minimum, are recommended. Chemical restraint is also a good option.

17. What is chemical restraint?

Intravenous administration of various sedatives will take the steam out of any fighting patient. The easiest times to get injured by a violent patient are when you are initially restraining him and when untying him from the ambulance stretcher to transfer him to the hospital bed. Many EMS systems carry drugs such as droperidol for this purpose. Other drugs that can be effective are diazepam, morphine, and diphenhydramine. Consult medical control regarding the protocols for use in combative patients.

18. Do I need to search my patients?

Any patient that you consider high risk needs to be searched. A search for weapons can always be incorporated into the physical assessment of the patient. If you are not comfortable performing a search, ask a police officer to do it. Remember to search the patient's belongings if you feel it is necessary.

19. What is combat medicine?

The most hazardous scenes, such as shootings, stabbings, and gang fights, require a different approach to prehospital care than usual. Obtaining a history and performing a physical exam are obviously out of the question. A combat style approach to these scenes is advisable. Rapid extrication of the victim to the ambulance before beginning assessment and management will minimize risk. Don't hesitate to cut some corners when you are on a scene that is perilous.

20. Do I need to wear concealed body armor?

The decision to invest in concealed bullet-resistant body armor is a personal one. Most employers do not fund the purchase, which can cost $300–500. Many EMS providers, like most police officers, would never work without their vest. Soft body armor is hot and uncomfortable but gives great protection. It also keeps you warmer in the winter.

21. What's the greatest danger the prehospital provider will face in the field?

Exposure to infectious diseases. Always take appropriate precautions to avoid any potential exposure, and always wear gloves and protective eyewear. Mask and gowns should be donned situationally.

22. Besides the personal risk from violence, are there other safety concerns?

There are always risks beyond the obvious threat of violence. Be careful when attending to motor vehicle accident victims in active traffic lanes. Strategic parking of the ambulance is important on such scenes. For instance, block traffic to protect you while you are attending to the injured. Remember to park upwind of fire scenes. Approach hazardous material scenes cautiously, parking upwind and surveying the scene from a distance to identify the material. Specialized protective gear will be required, along with special training. Refer these incidents to your local HazMat experts or call CHEMTREC for specific protocols.

BIBLIOGRAPHY

1. Dernocoeur K: Streetsense: Communications, Safety, and Control. Bowie, MD, Brady, 1985.
2. Mizell LR Jr: Streetsense for Women: How to Stay Safe in a Violent World. New York, NY, Berkley Books, 1993.
3. Remsberg C: The Tactical Edge: Surviving High Risk Patrol. Northbrook, IL, Calibre Press, 1986.
4. Thompson GS, Jenkins JB: Verbal Judo: The Gentle Art of Persuasion. New York, NY, Quill Publishing, 1993.
5. Whitfield RG: Dealing with violence. Int J Offender Ther Compar Criminol 26:255–262, 1982.
6. Winfree L, Williams L: Call security: The effects of fear and public image on staff-security contacts in a public hospital. J Police Sci Admin 13:310–329, 1985.

V. Communications

12. PREHOSPITAL COMMUNICATIONS

Thomas R. Cribley, MSHA, EMT-P, and Pam Copeland, EMT-B

1. This chapter title is quite broad. What is covered under prehospital communications?

Information about various aspects of communications, including 911 systems, radio systems, emergency medical dispatch, medical dispatch protocols, and field/hospital communications.

2. Do I need to be a radio geek to understand prehospital communications?

No, unless you want to understand the really technical stuff. The information presented in this section is intended to help the emergency medical services (EMS) provider understand some of the concepts used in prehospital communications. Thus, the information should give you some background for understanding how some of this stuff works. The technical details have been summarized to allow readers to apply the concepts to their own situations.

3. Why is dispatch referred to as the heart of the EMS system?

The dispatch center is the focal point for all EMS system activity. With the exception of direct field medical control (between field personnel and the base station physician) and some hospital notifications, the balance of emergency medical services is coordinated through the dispatch center—system access for the emergency caller, resource management (unit availability and positioning), response unit assignment, response monitoring and support, hospital availability, and hospital notification. The communications center is essential to and involved in virtually every part of the emergency response.

4. What is 911?

The nationwide emergency telephone number. It was developed by the telephone utilities to allow people quick, easy access to emergency services, regardless of where they may be. It is a number that is well publicized and easily remembered. By virtue of its nationwide implementation, people needing help don't have to search for a telephone book to find a seven-digit telephone number to call for help.

5. Will 911 work everywhere?

Unfortunately, no. While most of the country has the 911 system in place, there are still some areas, mostly rural, where 911 does not work. Most of these areas are moving toward 911 service, trying to satisfy the funding and legal and political conditions that are necessary to implement an efficient service. Until a 911 system is implemented, people who need help still have to dial a seven-digit telephone number.

6. Why is 911 better than dialing "0"?

Dialing "0" (for "Operator") is a good second choice if 911 doesn't work. The operator can connect the caller with an emergency communications center; however, it is not as efficient as 911, for a couple of reasons. First, there is an additional call and routing process, which takes time. Second, the caller may not be connected with the correct jurisdiction or service that he needs. Operators (or calltakers) on the 911 system, on the other hand, are trained to manage the emergency caller, quickly eliciting the information necessary to send an appropriate response.

7. What is E911?

The "E" in E911 stands for "Enhanced." The first implementations of 911 simply routed the caller to an emergency communications center. The communications center was generally determined by the location of the telephone company's central office that managed the caller's telephone prefix. (The telephone prefix is the first three digits of the telephone number.) Telephone service areas do not follow political boundaries. Therefore, while the call was routed to an emergency communications center, it may not have been the correct one, perhaps in the "wrong" city, county, or other response jurisdiction.

"Enhanced" 911 routes the caller to the correct emergency communications center. When the call is received in the telephone company's central office, several things happen. First, the telephone company identifies the telephone number from which the call is being placed. This is referred to as ANI, or Automatic Number Identification. Many people have a similar service on their own telephones known as Caller ID.

Once identified, the phone number is matched to a database that includes the basic information—name of the responsible party, billing address, apartment or suite number, and response jurisdiction for police, fire, and EMS. This information is referred to as ALI, or Automatic Location Information. In most cases, the ALI information is the same as the telephone location. The call is then routed to the communications center responsible for that location. Thus, in the vast majority of cases, the E911 call is routed to the correct emergency communications center.

8. What if it's not the correct center?

E911 systems have the capability of transferring all the information, both ANI and ALI, to another E911 center. For example, let's assume you live in Gotham City. Your aging mother, who has a "heart condition," lives in neighboring Pleasant Valley. Unfortunately, she calls *you* instead of 911 and tells you she's having a heart attack. "I'll call 911" you say, and you do. Your call is appropriately routed (for your Gotham City phone) to Gotham City—the wrong jurisdiction. Fortunately, your astute 911 calltaker recognizes the situation and transfers your call to Pleasant Valley, allowing you to talk directly to the "correct" communications center and allowing them to get the necessary information directly from you.

9. I often hear the term "peesap" around the communications center. What is it?

PSAP stands for *P*ublic *S*afety *A*nswering *P*oint. This is the initial site where 911 calls are answered. A PSAP may be for a single jurisdiction or may answer calls for multiple jurisdictions and agencies. In either case, the initial answering point is called the "primary" PSAP. If the calls are subsequently routed to other jurisdictions or agencies, those secondary answering points are referred to as "secondary" PSAPs.

10. What if I'm calling for help that is needed somewhere else?

E911 can identify the location of only the calling party. It cannot identify where help is needed. It is the calltaker's responsibility to verify the location where help is needed. The calltaker cannot simply rely on the E911 information displayed automatically on the E911 terminal but must question the caller to be sure that the appropriate assistance is being sent to the right place.

11. I just got a new phone. Will E911 work for me?

Maintenance of the E911 databases across the country is an enormous task. While the telephone companies strive to keep the databases up-to-date, there is occasionally a lag of a few days, although they make every effort to enter new numbers (and remove old ones) as rapidly as possible.

12. What is EMD?

EMD stands for Emergency Medical Dispatch. This is a formal program that in its most generic form is intended to help the emergency calltaker to gather as much important information as quickly as possible, determine the appropriate response level, and give instructions to the caller to provide appropriate medical assistance to the patient.

13. What information is most important to calltakers/dispatchers?

The person answering the emergency wants to gather three pieces of information as quickly as possible. It is usually gathered in this order, for the noted reasons.

1. Event location. The dispatcher must know where to send the unit. Even if no other information is obtained, at least someone can go to the scene to make an assessment of what's going on there.

2. Callback number. This is really helpful in the event that the original address is incomplete or incorrect. If the responders can't get there, they can't provide help.

3. Problem or nature. Once the calltaker can assure a response to the scene, information about what is happening there will allow him to make a good decision regarding who to send and how to send them. The calltaker should also gather information about scene safety and any information particular to the event that will affect the responding units.

14. What safety functions do dispatchers provide?

Dispatchers/calltakers provide several safety "nets" for emergency responders. First, the calltaker will try to make some assessment of scene safety. This includes, among other things, electrical wires down at auto accidents, the presence of an assailant at scenes of violence, or wind and weather conditions in the case of hazardous materials incidents. The dispatch center will endeavor to warn the responders of impending danger. Second, the dispatcher will try to make responding units aware of other units responding to the same or nearby incidents. This is a warning to anticipate and watch for other emergency traffic to avoid accidents. Finally, dispatchers monitor on-scene times of responding units. They do this to assure the responders' safety or assistance while on scene. Most centers use a certain time period, possibly related to the type of event, as a cue. If a responder has been on the scene in excess of the allotted time, the dispatcher will attempt to contact the responders and verify their safety. If they cannot be contacted, additional personnel (usually law enforcement personnel) will be dispatched to assure their well-being.

15. Who decides which services are sent to a call?

This is essentially the calltaker's responsibility. Most EMS communications centers provide their personnel with basic guidelines or protocols to help determine an appropriate response. Certain situations, such as stabbings and assaults, require a law enforcement response in addition to the medical responders. Other situations, such as cardiac arrests, may require more personnel than those sent on the transport unit; thus, a fire unit or other support personnel may be sent. Some calls require that the "cavalry" (a whole bunch of advanced life support folks) be sent. Others may require only a nonemergency basic life support response. The key is the training and experience of the calltaker, whose goal is to assure an appropriate response for the patient and the safety of responding personnel.

16. How are dispatch protocols different from field protocols?

They are similar, yet different. They are similar in that they give the provider a consistent set of guidelines to apply to a given set of circumstances. They are different in that the circumstances and the information available to the provider vary dramatically. The field provider is afforded the luxury of multiple types of sensory input in evaluating a patient. The EMS calltaker has only one—hearing. The calltaker must make a decision based solely on the information presented to him over the phone. He can't see it, can't feel it, can't smell it, and can't taste it. (Yes, even taste is used by the field provider.) Thus, dispatch protocols tend to be more conservative, opting for safety, expecting the worst, sending more resources rather than less in an uncertain situation. The difficult part is balancing the safe approach with the risks associated with sending too many resources.

17. What risks?

The risks of sending too many resources fall into two categories. First, there is the actual risk of injury or property damage. Emergency responses are dangerous and put people at risk. This includes responders, civilians, and patients who may suffer from actual, or even near-miss, vehicle accidents. The second category is more subtle. It is the risk of not having the right resource available for the real emergency. If we send too many resources to a call in which they are not needed, they may not be available for the call in which they actually are needed. Other units must be dispatched from further away. What is the cost? Who "pays" for increased response times and possible increases in morbidity and mortality when it takes longer to get to a scene?

18. What is a "zero response time"?

"Zero Response Time" is a phrase used in conjunction with emergency medical dispatch (EMD) and PreArrival Instructions. A calltaker who is well trained in EMD can actually deliver care immediately to a patient by giving instructions to the caller on how to initiate care for the patient, even before response units are dispatched. This has been well documented and can even include such complicated medical procedures as cardiopulmonary resuscitation. Thus, in many situations, by instructing the caller to initiate treatment, medical care is provided to the patient with a "zero response time."

19. Does EMD work all the time?

No. There are many factors that affect EMD outcomes. Even if everything goes just as it is supposed to, there are no guarantees. We've probably all heard the comment, "The procedure was a success, but the patient died." We can do every part of the EMD process correctly and still not save the patient. It is, however, the success that we are after, which won't happen unless we are willing to accept the failures, too.

20. Are EMT-D and EMD the same thing?

No, they are not. EMT-D stands for Emergency Medical Technician—Defibrillator. This is an EMT who has received special training in the use of a cardiac defibrillator. This is a qualification for all field personnel. EMD, on the other hand, includes training and certification in the use of emergency medical dispatch protocols and procedures. This function is unique to dispatch.

21. What is "megahertz"?

A technical term used in identifying radio frequencies.

22. What does it mean when a radio system is "trunked"?

This is a high-tech system that allows agencies to optimize the use of radio frequencies. With older technology, agencies were assigned to particular radio frequencies, and all their communications took place on those particular frequencies. Some agencies even shared the frequency with another. This generally meant one of two things: (1) Since the frequency was dedicated to a particular agency, any time that agency was not talking was "dead air." This was, in some respects, a waste of available air time on the particular frequency in a world that is using more and more forms of wireless communications. (2) One agency had to wait while another agency completed their business. This competition for air time occasionally delayed emergency communications.

"Trunked" radio is a solution to help rectify both these problems (dead air and delays). It is a fairly complicated process. Basically, the various radios in the system have the capability to function on a variety of frequencies. The radios are programmed to talk to a particular set of radios, and a computer manages frequency assignments. When one radio wants to "talk" to other radios, the computer determines which frequency is available. It then directs all the radios in the set to go to that frequency. The frequency assignment lasts only as long as the radio transmission, and the frequency is then made available for other radio sets. The reply to the original transmission may occur on the same, or more likely, a different frequency.

This is a very simple and superficial attempt at explaining trunked radio. You can probably see, however, that a computer system has the wherewithal to coordinate the communications of several groups of radios, minimizing "dead air" by allocating the time to live communications, and thus reducing the number of frequencies needed.

23. What is CAD?

CAD stands for Computer Aided Dispatch. There are many different systems in use around the country, but they all provide some common functions. They are a tool for dispatchers to use to keep track of EMS units and their status (whether available, out of service, or involved in a response). The systems keep track of call information, as defined by the agency. Most record location, callback number, type of problem, responding unit(s), relevant times, and a disposition for each call for service. Some are much more sophisticated, collecting much more information regarding individual calls. Some deal with unit positioning, response recommendations, and call loads per unit. Some systems have an integrated EMD system. Some systems have mapping capabilities, and some of those are integrated with Automatic Vehicle Location systems. Some are integrated with Mobile Data Terminals (MDTs) or Mobile Computer Terminals (MCTs) in the response units. There are far too many system designs to describe here. Every one is unique. If you have a CAD system and you really want to know more, go to your communications center and ask for a demonstration.

24. What does the dispatcher have to do with transport destinations?

The transport destination for a field unit is generally determined by the field unit in conjunction with standing destination protocols and medical control personnel. There are some happenings that draw the communications center into the decision. First and perhaps most common is a change in hospital divert status. Hospitals may, for a variety of reasons, become unable to accept certain types of patients. If this happens before a transport unit can be notified and the unit goes to that hospital, it is the responsibility of the communications center to advise the transport unit of a divert status. This will allow the unit to change its destination in a timely manner and assure that the patient can receive proper care when it arrives.

The second situation is also quite common. By virtue of its view of "the bigger picture," the communications center is generally aware of significant events within the jurisdiction. If an event or other situation such as construction or traffic signal problems makes the preferred destination difficult or even impossible to access, the transport unit must be notified.

Finally, the communications center acts as a resource, especially in those situations in which a transport unit is unfamiliar with local destinations. This is perhaps most likely in mutual aid situations. The communications center can identify the nearest appropriate receiving facility and provide routing assistance.

25. Do all dispatchers do the same thing?

No. Some personnel in the dispatch center work only as calltakers. Some work only as dispatchers. Some do both. Some work only for a particular agency. Some provide services for multiple agencies. Some provide administrative support as well. The only way to know what the dispatchers in your center do is to ask.

26. Why doesn't the dispatcher have better information to give me about the type of call?

Telephone triage is a one-sense function. The only way a calltaker gets information about what is happening at a particular scene is by listening (hearing). He does not have the advantage of additional types of sensory input that field personnel have—sight, smell, touch, and even taste in some cases. Try to imagine what your patient "sounds" like, in most cases through the eyes and ears of a third party, an untrained, frightened caller. Complicate that situation with telephone static, slang or cultural words, and foreign language, and perhaps you can understand why what you responded to was not quite what you thought you were dispatched to.

27. Why don't they answer the radio right away?

While it may seem like dispatchers have nothing to do but answer the radio, that is usually not the case. While some centers have the resources to assign an individual to do nothing but handle radio traffic, most do not. Dispatchers have other responsibilities. Some monitor multiple radio channels, some are responsible for hospital notifications, some have administrative responsibilities, and some have to answer emergency telephone calls. If it's not an emergency, be patient. They're listening (probably) and will get to you as soon as they can.

28. What do doctors have to do with dispatch?

Medical dispatch should have medical control, just like a field medical unit. It is important that emergency medical responses meet the standard of care for the community. This applies to both the types of resources that are sent and the way in which they are sent. It also applies to any directions that a calltaker may give to a caller or patient. The Medical Director for the medical dispatch center is responsible for assuring that the medical aspect of the dispatch services that are provided is appropriate.

29. Is a biophone like a batphone?

Kind of. In both cases, you use the phone to contact a particular resource to get help. In the case of the batphone, you get Batman. In the case of the biophone, you get a prehospital medical control person, usually based at a hospital. Even though the term includes the word "phone," it has become more broad in its definition to include both phone and radio media.

30. What is a "biocom"?

A "biocom" is essentially the radio version of a biophone. It was the term used when most field/hospital communications were accomplished via radio. That was before cellular phones. Even with cellular communications, a great deal, perhaps even the majority, of field/hospital communications still happen on the radio.

31. What is telemetry?

Telemetry in EMS is generally the transmission of electrocardiograms (EKGs) via radio from field units to a hospital for assistance in EKG interpretation and treatment. Some systems around the country require the use of telemetry for all cardiac patients; some use it selectively for physician support in difficult situations; and some systems do not use it at all, relying on the training and judgment of field personnel. The recent development of field cardiac monitors capable of high-quality 12-lead EKGs is resurrecting the use of telemetry. Quality EKGs from the field may allow for the field use of thrombolytic therapy in the setting of the acute myocardial infarction.

CONTROVERSY

32. Is CAD a good thing?

CAD has mixed reviews. Some say that it actually lengthens the dispatch process because the calltaker has to type in all the information in the right place and in the right way, which takes too much time. They feel that the old way was better and faster. Others say that CAD allows them to ensure that the dispatch information is accurate and complete, that there is virtually no potential for misunderstanding, and that the information can be transmitted to multiple dispatch centers simultaneously, actually improving the overall dispatch process.

BIBLIOGRAPHY

1. The Associated Public Safety Communications Officers: The Public Safety Communications Standard Operating Procedure Manual, 22nd ed. New Smyrna Beach, FL, Associated Public Communications Officers, 1990.

2. Clawson JJ: Quality assurance: A priority for medical dispatch. Emerg Med Serv 18:53–63, 1989.
3. Culley LL, Clark JJ, Eisenberg MS, et al: Dispatcher-assisted telephone CPR: Common delays and time standards for delivery. Ann Emerg Med 20:362–366, 1991.
4. Curka PA, Pepe PE, Ginger VF, et al: Emergency medical services priority dispatch. Ann Emerg Med 22:1688–1695, 1993.
5. McMillian J, Rhett JR: The Primer of Public Safety Telecommunications Systems. New Smyrna Beach, FL, The APCO Institute, 1990.
6. Steele S: Emergency Dispatching: A Medical Communicator's Guide. Englewood Cliffs, NJ, Prentice-Hall, 1993.

VI. Destination Issues

13. DESTINATION GUIDELINES AND HOSPITAL DESIGNATION

Catherine B. Custalow, M.D., Ph.D.

1. Besides my assessment and treatment of a patient, is there anything else that is an important determinant of patient outcome?

One of the most important decisions to be made at the time of transport, in addition to determining the interventions to be performed, is the choice of destination. In those communities with only one hospital, the selection is easy. In those EMS systems that have more than one facility to choose from, however, the patient should be taken to the hospital that can best provide for that patient's medical need.

2. How do I know which hospital to go to?

Although we would like to believe that all hospitals are created equal, in fact some provide specialized services that others do not. The EMS system should have a mechanism in place for identifying which hospitals have specialized services available and which patients would qualify for transport to those facilities directly, even if it means bypassing other, closer hospitals.

3. Are there any national guidelines to help identify these hospitals?

A number of organizations (such as the American Burn Association and the American College of Surgeons) have developed guidelines and recommendations that describe the equipment, facilities, and personnel that are needed to provide optimal care for victims of burn or traumatic injury. These organizations also provide a rigorous on-site review process to verify the preparedness of the hospital that desires to be identified as a specialty care center.

4. What factors determine whether a trauma patient should be transported emergently to a trauma center?

There are various organizations (such as the American College of Emergency Physicians and the American College of Surgeons) that have published prehospital triage criteria for evaluating trauma patients. While there are minor differences among them, all agree on the key determinants of high risk for serious injury. All patients determined to be emergent trauma patients should be transported to the highest-ranking available trauma center. Following are injuries and trauma mechanisms commonly recognized as indicators of serious injury.

Injuries
Significant blunt trauma with unstable vital signs
Penetrating trauma to head, thorax, abdomen, neck, or proximal extremities
Altered mentation after trauma
Flail chest
Pelvic fractures
Open or suspected depressed skull fracture
Spinal cord injury with neurologic deficit
Multiple long-bone fractures

Amputation
Burns > 15% or involving face, airway
Mechanism
Auto-pedestrian hit at > 20 mph or victim thrown 15 feet
Falls > 20 feet
Death of occupant in the same vehicle
Ejection from vehicle
Automobile accident with significant vehicular body damage
Motorcycle accident > 20 mph or with separation of rider from bike
Significant bicycle or all-terrain vehicle impact

5. What is a level I trauma center, and how is it different from level II, III, and IV centers?

Trauma facilities are designated as level I to IV after a thorough application and review process. Level I trauma facilities must have in-house general surgery, neurosurgery, emergency services, and anesthesia 24 hours a day, as well as many other surgical and medical subspecialties on call and promptly available. Level I facilities must also have a trauma research program and active teaching programs. Level II facilities do not have the same research or teaching requirements and are not required to have as many subspecialties on call. Level III trauma centers must have 24-hour emergency services but are not required to have in-house surgical services at all times. Level IV facilities are primarily rural hospitals that would help stabilize a patient in anticipation of transfer to a higher-level trauma center.

6. What is the difference between a pediatric trauma center and a trauma center with pediatric commitment?

A pediatric trauma center is a children's hospital that meets level I trauma designation criteria, with a pediatric emergency department, ICU, and trauma service having appropriate personnel, equipment, and facilities to meet the needs of an injured child. A trauma center with pediatric commitment is a general hospital that meets level I or II criteria for adults and has the capabilities and commitment to care for pediatric as well as adult trauma patients.

7. Does trauma care in rural areas differ from that in urban areas?

Yes. Trauma care in the rural setting is a challenge based on the differences in the distance to trauma facilities, the surrounding terrain, and the occurrence of accidents in isolated and wilderness areas. Motor vehicle accidents may go unrecognized for long periods of time in sparsely populated areas. Each EMS agency should have predetermined protocols for how and where to transport patients from all locations within their jurisdiction.

8. When should helicopters be dispatched directly to the scene of an accident?

There are various guidelines for the timing of dispatching an air medical team. Trauma patients with critical injuries need to be transported to a regional trauma center as quickly as possible. When transportation time by ground to the trauma center is more than 15 minutes; when ground transport time would be longer than helicopter transport time; in wilderness areas with difficult access; or when ground ambulance access is impeded by road conditions, weather, or traffic, an air medical team should be dispatched, if available.

9. What are the destination guidelines for patients with extremity amputations?

Patients with proximal finger or extremity amputations should be taken to the nearest facility with reimplantation capabilities. Treat every amputated part as if it will be reimplanted, with urgent transport and appropriate handling of the amputated part. As always, address life-threatening injuries first, and if the patient has multiple injuries, transport him or her to the highest-level trauma center available. Exceptions to this are toe amputations or distal finger amputations that occur at or beyond the distal-phalangeal joint.

10. How are destinations assigned during a mass casualty?

Category I (critical) victims should be transported to and distributed among the available trauma centers. Patients with less serious injuries may be taken to nontrauma centers. Whenever possible, the goal is to distribute victims to all available hospitals and avoid overloading any one hospital.

11. When should burn victims be taken to a hospital with a burn center?

Burn victims benefit greatly from transport or early transfer to hospitals with burn centers. The following criteria may be used as guidelines to determine which patients benefit most.

Second- or third-degree burns > 10% body surface area (BSA) in patients < 10 or > 50 years old

Burns > 20% BSA in all age groups

Third-degree burns > 5% BSA

Inhalation injury

Circumferential burns

High-voltage electrical burns

Severe chemical burns

12. What are the guidelines for the destination of patients with medical emergencies?

All emergent medical patients generally should go to the nearest hospital. This includes those with such problems as acute myocardial infarction, cardiac arrest, and massive gastrointestinal hemorrhage. Nonemergent medical patients may go to the hospital requested by the patient, family, or private physician, so long as the EMS service is capable of honoring that request.

13. Should patients with significant carbon monoxide exposure be taken to the nearest hospital?

Patients with significant smoke inhalation or carbon monoxide exposure require treatment in a hyperbaric oxygen chamber. Signs of significant exposure include loss of consciousness, altered mental status, seizures, and arrhythmias. Therefore, when possible, these patients should preferentially be taken to a hospital with a chamber. The only exception is that patients with burns and smoke inhalation associated with multisystem trauma should go the highest-level trauma facility available in order to deal with the major injuries first.

14. Do destinations differ for victims of scuba-diving accidents?

Victims of diving accidents with symptoms suggesting air embolism or decompression sickness also require treatment in a hyperbaric oxygen chamber and therefore also should be taken to a facility with a chamber.

15. What should I do when a hospital is on divert or ambulance bypass, particularly if I have a patient in cardiac arrest?

As a general rule, a hospital's divert status should be honored and the patient transported to another facility. Ideally, cardiac arrests should go to the nearest hospital, regardless of divert status. In reality, if the patient has not been resuscitated in the field, there is very little likelihood of being resuscitated at the hospital. Thus, there should be little impact on the limited resources.

16. Can a physician at the scene alter destination guidelines?

A physician at the scene should not be allowed to change the destination as determined by the paramedics, in accordance with EMS agency protocol, unless approved by the base-station physician. In addition, if an on-scene physician wishes to intervene, the physician should be advised that he or she will need to accompany the patient in the ambulance to the hospital.

BIBLIOGRAPHY

1. Benson NH, Prasad NH: Rural EMS. In Tintinalli JE, Ruiz E, Krome RL (eds): Emergency Medicine: A Comprehensive Study Guide, 4th ed. New York, McGraw-Hill, 1996, pp 7–11.

2. Hankins DG: Alternatives to ground transport. In Tintinalli JE, Ruiz E, Krome RL (eds): Emergency Medicine: A Comprehensive Study Guide, 4th ed. New York, McGraw-Hill, 1996, pp 11–15.
3. March JA, Benson NH: Prehospital care of the trauma patient. In Harwood-Nuss AL, Linden CH, Luten RC, Shepherd SM, Wolfson AB (eds): The Clinical Practice of Emergency Medicine, 2nd ed. Philadelphia, Lippincott-Raven, 1996, pp 375–378.
4. Prehospital Triage Criteria: Advanced Trauma Life Support Student Manual. American College of Surgeons, 1993, pp 317–318.

VII. Legal Issues

14. MEDICOLEGAL ISSUES

S. Scott Henderson, J.D., EMT-P

1. Can you practice your entire career and never be sued?

Yes, but it will take thoughtful consideration on your part. Bad outcomes are a part of practice. Try as we may to deliver the best of care, patients sometimes still "crash" and successful intervention often can be fleeting and transient. The fastest way to assure that a patient or family will call a lawyer is to stop talking to them when a bad outcome occurs. Health care providers often are too busy to spend enough time to explain the unavoidability of adverse outcomes to patients and relatives. Worse, we tend not to spend the time when disaster strikes to demonstrate genuine concern and the acknowledgment that illustrates that not all morbidity or mortality is preventable. The "treatment" that is required when adversity or, worse, catastrophe, results is as important to the EMT or paramedic as it is to the patient and family. It is "legal prophylaxis" that, if withheld, may result in a purulent propensity for "infectious litigation" that can be just as persistent and unmanageable as the most aggressive strains of streptococcus. Indeed, no one who has been through the legal process ever hopes to do it again. A lawsuit can sap your self-esteem, reputation, self-confidence, marriage, money, and worst of all, your life.

2. What can I do to try to prevent a lawsuit?

The simple truth is that health care providers who have the best bedside manner or people skills and keep talking to their patients even when adversity strikes have fewer lawsuits filed against them. Good bedside manner is akin to the good manners that fuel interpersonal interactions, resulting in less friction and confrontation than abrasive words or conduct. Abrasiveness communicates that the health care provider is too busy to listen and respond to the needs of the person for whom he provides his professional services.

3. Should the notice of my deposition make my "blood run cold"?

There are three good reasons why depositions are taken during the discovery phase of a lawsuit: (1) to discover the facts and who has them, (2) to pin down the witness so you can hold them to the story, and (3) to assess the credibility of the witness and estimate how a jury is likely to respond to the testimony. This final analysis is particularly important when the plaintiff's lawyer deposes the defendant health care provider. The demeanor of the defendant is one part of the equation that enters into the valuation of the case and whether the case should be tried or settled. As in all aspects of life, "nice people" are generally treated better than others. An EMT or paramedic who is arrogant, self-righteous, and egotistical is an inviting target for the plaintiff's lawyer; the lawyer will try to cast him as uncaring, cavalier, and disrespectful to his patients and try to get the defendant to show the traits in front of the jury. By contrast, the plaintiff's attorney will lose credibility by trying to paint a courteous, compassionate, and soft-spoken provider as a callous person.

4. What else can I do to minimize my risk of being sued?

The single most important step you can take to avoid being sued is to document thoroughly. Medical malpractice cases are often referred to as "records cases." This means that, from the plaintiff's lawyer's viewpoint, there must be documentary evidence of the breach of the standard of care, either in the form of a documented wrongful act or evidence of an omission. The documented wrongful act is clear and obvious, albeit hotly contested. The omission is identified by a document that fails to show that, for example, a neurologic exam was performed before a patient at risk of head injury was released.

5. How extensive should the documentation be?

Although not all care is documented, the essential information must be recorded. Sometimes the pace of emergency medical services (EMS) moves so quickly that important care that was rendered doesn't always make it onto the chart. However, you may count on spending considerable time in deposition and in the courtroom while the plaintiff's lawyer highlights the void in the record and grills the hapless medical witness. The lawyer will resonate the phrase, "If it's not documented, it wasn't done," in the courtroom. Although a failure to document can sometimes be defended through testimony that the provider's custom, pattern, habit, and practice is to *always* perform a particular examination or test for a patient with the particular complaint at issue, a jury may view such statements as self-serving.

By contrast, the medical record that is painstakingly complete and well-documented will signal a plaintiff's lawyer to decline the case. Three factors could send up a red flag for declining the case:

1. If the history is complete, even if it is factually wrong but shows that time and effort were taken to acquire it.

2. If the physical examination is thorough and not filled with routine, stock phrases, and is instead tailored to the patient.

3. If the assessment and plan are reasonable given what was known or, in the exercise of the reasonable practice of medicine, what should have been known.

6. What is the statute of limitations in most jurisdictions?

The time within which a medical negligence suit must be filed or else barred forever is often 2 years from the date on which the patient discovered the harm and its cause. Therefore, these cases are often filed about 2 years, or a little less, following the event to avoid fights over when the harm was discovered. Since your memory for the patients that you treated two or so years ago is probably not good, it is the medical record that limits your likelihood of being sued and reduces your chance of losing if you are sued. Disciplined, thorough record-keeping means that the odds of ever having to get to the issues of causation and damages are substantially less.

7. What does it take for the plaintiff to win?

The plaintiff must establish that the defendant owed the plaintiff a legal duty, breached the duty, that the breach of duty is what legally caused the harm that came to the plaintiff, and that, in fact, harm or damage to the patient actually resulted. Successful proof of all four elements is both intellectually and factually difficult to demonstrate.

8. What constitutes "legal duty"?

The issue of whether the health care provider owed the plaintiff/patient a legal duty is a question of law for the courts to decide. Generally, when a patient, by words or conduct, accepts the offer of health care delivery from a health care provider, a legal duty to provide reasonable care arises. The duty of reasonable care requires the health care provider to give that degree of care based upon the health care provider's knowledge, skill, training, education, and experience that any reasonable health care provider, similarly trained and situated, would provide under similar circumstances. This "reasonable person" measure of appropriate conduct has been tagged the "Ward Cleaver" standard from the "Leave it to Beaver" television series because Ward, the father, always seemed to have a reasonable, logical, and thoughtful response for every complicated, jagged, and truly heart-wrenching situation that his sons could bring home.

9. Describe breach of duty and causation.

Although negligence is shown when the jury is persuaded that the defendant health care provider had a duty and unreasonably acted or unreasonably failed to act on the duty owed to the patient, it is not enough for the lawyer simply to show negligent conduct. Causation must be satisfied. It is necessary to demonstrate that the breach of duty (collectively known as "violation of standard of care") is what caused the patient's damages.

10. Does "standard of care" apply to prehospital providers?

Absolutely. In a medical negligence lawsuit, the jury is asked to determine what the reasonable health care provider with the same level of expertise would have done under the same or similar circumstances. An important point is what is meant by the phrase, "the same or similar circumstances." The answer to the question is dramatically affected by the "yardstick" that is used to measure the conduct. If the site of the alleged wrong is a small community, the defense will want the defendant to be held accountable to the level of care customarily provided in that community; thus, the "community standard" or the "locality rule." On the other hand, since a national standard of care may be more clearly defined and be more stringent, the plaintiff will most likely argue that a national standard is appropriate.

The plaintiff probably will argue that the national standard is appropriate if the health care provider is certified by a national standard such as the National Association of Emergency Medical Technicians. Consideration of this issue is important because a rural health care provider who is certified to a national standard will be held to the same standard as an urban provider who may have had the opportunity to amass much more experience.

11. How hard is it to show causation?

Causation is complicated and tricky. Although there may be "cause-in-fact," it does not necessarily follow that the law will recognize legal cause, meaning legal liability. "Legal cause" takes one of two forms: (1) "but for" causation and (2) "substantial factor."

"But for" causation means that the defendant's conduct caused the harm to the patient in a natural and probable sequence of events, the cascade of which directly flowed from the defendant's wrongful conduct and would not have occurred "but for" the defendant's culpable behavior.

"Substantial factor" causation arises when two or more concurrent causes exist, any one of which is sufficient to bring about the damaging result. In such instances, causation is satisfied if any defendant's action or failure to act was a substantial factor in producing the harm.

12. Describe an example of substantial factor causation.

Imagine that two distinct fires have destroyed the plaintiff's house and either one would have resulted in the damage absent the other. If Defendant 1 negligently set one fire and Defendant 2 negligently set the other, who is responsible and for how much of the harm? If the first fire was negligently set by Defendant 1 and the second fire set by Defendant 2 was not started by negligence, who is responsible? Finally, where the first fire is negligently set and the second fire is caused by a lightning strike, is Defendant 1 responsible for damages? Does the analysis change if the first fire is caused by lightning and the second is the result of the defendant's negligence? Does it matter when each of the fires began and when the actual damage occurred?

13. How does the plaintiff reach the damages stage?

It is not sufficient to simply claim that damages occurred. Actual injuries or losses must be shown, and it is these that are compensable. In other words, the level of proof required in a civil lawsuit for negligence means that actual harm must exist that likely resulted from the wrongful conduct.

14. Is the concept of being innocent until proven guilty applicable, or must the defendant prove that he wasn't negligent?

The burden of proof is on the plaintiff to prove each of the four elements of the negligence action "by a preponderance of the evidence." Words and phrases that connote that the preponderance of the evidence is satisfied include "likely," "probable," "to a reasonable degree of medical probability," "more likely than not," and, in some jurisdictions, "to a reasonable degree of medical certainty." These terms mean that each of the four elements of a negligence claim must be proved to the 51% standard of probability: the jury must be persuaded that the plaintiff has prevailed on each element in even a slightly more convincing way than not.

15. Describe DNRs, living wills, and durable powers of attorney.

So-called DNRs (do not resuscitate orders) living wills, and durable powers of attorney are laws enacted by state legislatures; thus they vary from state to state. As a result, the appropriate statutes in a particular jurisdiction must be carefully examined. These statutes go by various names. For instance, in Colorado, the relevant statutes are (1) the Colorado Medical Treatment Decision Act, which is the living will statute and includes an approved form entitled the Declaration As To Medical Or Surgical Treatment; (2) the Proxy Decision-Makers for Medical Treatment article, which delineates the circumstances under which a person may substitute for the patient in decision-making; (3) the Directive Relating to Cardiopulmonary Resuscitation, which specifies appropriate circumstances for DNRs, and (4) the Medical Durable Power Of Attorney section.

16. These laws sound the same. Is there a difference?

Although they are similar in some ways, there are important differences. For example, the living will becomes active after a patient has become incapacitated, but in many states there is a delay in that the patient must be incapacitated for a certain time before the provisions of the living will can be implemented. On the other hand, the proxy decision-makers for medical treatment and the medical durable power of attorney become active immediately upon the incapacitation of the patient. Finally, the directive relating to cardiopulmonary resuscitation is active immediately upon signature of the patient.

17. What happens if state law is not followed?

Policies, procedures, and protocols guiding EMS operations must be consistent with the statutory requirements of the laws in a particular state. Failure to abide by the legislated requirements may result in negligence per se if deviation results in foreseeable harm to the patient. Negligence per se means that there is a presumption of negligence as a matter of law (disregarding other factual disputes) if a law is violated that is intended to protect the group of persons that includes the harmed patient and the violation is the cause of the harm.

For example, imagine the following scenario. A patient is found unconscious and in need of advanced life support. A person on the scene tells the EMS crew that the patient doesn't want heroic efforts and also thinks that the patient has signed a living will to that effect. The EMS crew doesn't insist on inspecting the living will before electing to not resuscitate. Most statutes state that health care providers may not be held liable if the document "appears on its face" to be validly executed. If, as in this hypothetical case, there was no inspection of the document and none, in fact, exists, the EMS crew may be found presumptively negligent and liable for the resulting harm if advanced life support was withheld.

18. Explain informed consent.

Patient autonomy means that in law and ethics the patient has the right to make decisions concerning the extent of medical care that the patient will accept. The law has long recognized that patient autonomy includes the right to make "bad" medical decisions.

In 1914, Justice Cardozo, writing for the highest court in New York, stated that "every human being of adult years and sound mind has a right to determine what shall be done with his own body, and a surgeon who performs an operation without his patient's consent commits an assault for which he is liable in damages." Actually, the wrongful conduct that was just described is a battery, but assault and battery have been muddled for years. The point is that wrongful, actionable conduct occurs by any contact with a patient's body without the patient's consent, and the health care provider becomes responsible for *any* damages. This is of great concern because a medical procedure can be done without negligence and with all reasonable care, but the health care provider remains liable for even unforeseen, untoward reactions and even known risks of the procedure.

19. What is actually required to obtain informed consent?

Four items must be shown. The health care provider must convey to the patient (1) the ailment, (2) the treatment or procedure that is being suggested, (3) alternatives to treatment, and (4) the risks associated with treatment and nontreatment. The patient must be informed of this information to the extent a reasonable health care provider would under the same or similar circumstances.

20. How do these legal issues apply to prehospital providers in the field?

Any patient you are going to treat must give permission for that treatment. The problem in EMS is that many patients are unable to give consent, either because of their emergency or other confounding factors such as intoxication. In an emergency situation, it is important to determine whether delay would endanger the patient, whether a careful health care provider would do the same as the defendant, and whether the patient was unable to consent. If so, the health care provider may proceed under the concept of "implied consent," meaning that most people would want to receive appropriate medical care; therefore, consent is implied and the provider can treat the patient. In the second case, the intoxicated patient may not be competent to give consent. Legal capacity to consent or refuse is not the same as medical capacity to consent or refuse. The patient need not be legally adjudicated as incompetent for patient rights to be disregarded in the emergency medical setting. An example is alcohol impairment. In 1993, the Rhode Island Supreme Court examined this issue and held that a patient's intoxication may render him incapable of giving informed consent and, in an emergency, a health care provider may dispense with obtaining the patient's informed consent.

21. How do issues of consent apply to patients who refuse care?

Just as the medical caregiver must obtain informed consent to treat a patient, informed refusal must also be obtained if the patient decides to refuse care. Thus, any competent adult may refuse medical services, but the provider must explain the potential ramifications of the decision and be sure the patient understands the risks. By the same token, the patient must be competent in order to refuse care. An intoxicated patient would be considered incompetent and unable to refuse medical care until the intoxicant wore off.

22. How do issues of consent apply to minors?

A minor's medical capacity to accept or refuse treatment is a thorny area for EMS providers and varies among the states. In general, a minor has recognized legal impediments; a minor can't enter into a contract and generally can't vote, but can a minor consent or refuse medical treatment? Kansas held in 1970 that there is a difference between a legal and a medical capacity. The Kansas Supreme Court held that a minor can verbally consent to medical treatment. Tennessee followed the same reasoning in 1987. The cases are fact-specific and the EMS provider needs to know the law concerning a minor's capacity to accept or refuse medical treatment for the state in which he or she practices.

23. What is the key to avoiding lawsuits?

Provide good care, provide good documentation, and be nice to the patients. These maxims won't prevent you from getting sued, but they will make it more difficult for a plaintiff to win.

BIBLIOGRAPHY

1. Ayres RJ Jr: Legal considerations in prehospital care. Emerg Med Clin North Am 11:853–868, 1993.
2. Frew SA: Emergency medical services legal issues for the emergency physician. Emerg Med Clin North Am 8:41–56, 1990.

3. Goldberg RJ, Zautcke JL, Koenigsberg MD, et al: A review of prehospital care litigation in a large metropolitan EMS system. Ann Emerg Med 19:557–561, 1990.
4. Selden BS, Schnitzer PG, Nolan FX: Medicolegal documentation of prehospital triage. Ann Emerg Med 19:547–551, 1990.
5. Shanaberger CJ: Case law involving base-station contact. Prehosp Disaster Med 10:75–81, 1995.
6. Siegel DM: Consent and refusal of treatment. Emerg Med Clin North Am 11:833–840, 1993.
7. Sullivan DJ: Minors and emergency medicine. Emerg Med Clin North Am 11:841–852, 1993.
8. Wood CL: Historical perspectives on law, medical malpractice, and the concept of negligence. Emerg Med Clin North Am 11:819–832, 1993.

VIII. Disasters and Multiple Casualty Incidents

15. DISASTERS AND MULTIPLE CASUALTY INCIDENTS

Jon R. Krohmer, M.D.

1. What is a disaster?

Any situation that disrupts normal community function; it overwhelms the community's ability to respond to the situation and threatens the safety, property, or lives of the citizens. It may stress the area's ability to provide public health resources, utilities, communications, food, shelter, and clothing. A disaster also may involve more injuries than the local emergency medical services (EMS) system or local hospitals can care for. However, not all disasters result in injuries or illnesses.

2. How is a multiple casualty incident different from a disaster?

A multiple casualty incident (MCI) is any situation in which multiple injuries occur from a single event. Several events occurring simultaneously or a large MCI may qualify as a medical disaster. Although an MCI technically is any situation involving more than one patient, most systems do not consider it a MCI until there are more than 5–10 injuries. When these situations require more resources than are immediately available to provide the necessary care, a disaster plan may need to be activated. MCIs are sometimes called medical disasters.

An individual incident may be both a disaster and an MCI, but it does not always have to be both. For example, a flood may affect a large geographic area and displace many people from their homes while destroying farms, homes, stores, and utilities. Such a situation could easily qualify as a disaster. However, without a large number of injuries or illnesses, it would not qualify as an MCI. Likewise, a motor vehicle collision involving a school bus and a small van that injures 18 people with varying degrees of severity would be an EMS MCI requiring many prehospital resources and possibly requiring the activation of the EMS disaster plan. However, a disaster response is unnecessary if the hospitals are able to adequately care for all of the patients. Many of the components of a disaster plan will be used in smaller MCIs; the principles are the same, but the magnitude of the response will vary depending on the size of the event and the availability of local medical resources.

3. What are examples of disaster situations?

Natural disasters include hurricanes, tornadoes, floods, earthquakes, severe winter storms, and volcanic eruptions. Man-made disasters are airplane, train, or motor vehicle crashes, industrial explosions, fires, terrorists attacks, and hazardous materials incidents such as chemical spills and radiation leaks. It is possible that natural and man-made events may occur at the same time, as when a tornado causes a hazardous materials incident.

4. Why is it important to understand the principles of MCIs and disasters?

Most emergency care personnel, including emergency medical technicians, paramedics, emergency physicians, and nurses, will find themselves in situations in which they will need to handle MCI situations. Many will never have to handle situations such as a plane or train crash, but the principles of the response to both the MCI and the larger disaster are the same.

5. How is the focus of medical care during an MCI different from the routine daily focus of medical care?

During daily medical care, there are a limited number of persons for whom care must be provided and providers tend to commit a large level of very intensive resources to each of those patients. During an MCI, many persons require care, and it must be provided with relatively limited resources. The goal of care during an MCI is to provide the greatest amount of good for the greatest number of potentially survivable victims. This change in philosophy (e.g., not trying to resuscitate someone in cardiac arrest or intubating someone with a fatal head injury) is often difficult for emergency medical personnel to adopt in disaster situations.

6. Who should participate on the disaster management team?

Representatives from all groups who will be providing services during the disaster: the local, state, or national government, police, fire services, EMS, hospitals, utilities and public works departments, emergency management, Red Cross, social services, and mental health services. All of these representatives will be responsible for coordinating the activities of the respective disciplines to ensure that the needed services are provided to the community. They should work together to develop a response plan to use in the event of a disaster.

7. Why is the development of a disaster response plan important?

To ensure successful response to a disaster, which depends on the coordination of the activities of many agencies, including the government and public and private organizations. Plans must be developed prior to the incident to ensure that (1) lines of authority are established, (2) appropriate communications will occur, and (3) all agencies and personnel will understand their areas of responsibility. The plan should include a risk analysis of potential disaster-producing factors, such as chemical plants, nuclear power plants, busy airports, and train routes. A survey of available resources also should be made. The disaster plan should structure response activities as closely as possible to the daily operations.

Once the plan has been developed, it is important to regularly conduct disaster exercises to test the plan so that everyone involved understands what is expected of them during a disaster response.

8. What are the four phases of a disaster response?

Activation, implementation, mitigation, and recovery.

9. Describe the activation phase of a disaster response.

The activation phase includes the initial notification of the incident, the response, and the establishment of the command structure. The first responders should quickly assess the scene to ensure that their safety and the safety of other responders is maintained. They must then determine the nature and magnitude of the event, an estimated number of victims, and an idea of the resources that will be needed to handle the situation. This information must be communicated to the dispatch center or medical command facility to initiate the remainder of the response. Additionally, a command structure must be established to assure proper communication and use of resources.

10. What are the components of the implementation phase?

The implementation phase initially involves a search for victims and rescue, which is usually provided by the fire department or specially trained search and rescue teams. This is followed by triage and beginning the stabilization and transport of victims to hospitals.

11. What does the mitigation phase involve?

The hazards are controlled, and treatment is provided to patients. The treatment provided at the scene is generally limited to airway, breathing, and circulation issues and immobilizing patients for transport to hospitals. The purpose is to provide care to preserve life and function.

Occasionally, if there is a delay in transporting patients from the site, additional treatment may begin in the field. Sometimes, trained medical teams from the hospital may assist with medical care.

12. What happens during the recovery phase?
The responders leave the scene and return to normal operations. They restock equipment and supplies. A debriefing session should be held to review the response to the event, to determine if the disaster plan must be modified, and to address any psychological issues that rescuers or victims may be experiencing. Also, displaced persons are sheltered until they can find other places to live or return to their homes.

13. Explain the command structure of a disaster response.
The command structure most commonly used in the United States is called the incident command system (ICS) or incident management system (IMS). This concept was developed in the fire service to outline a structure for coordinating all activities that occur during a major incident. It is routinely used in the fire service and has been found useful and easily adaptable to a disaster response.

Under the ICS, one person assumes overall responsibility for coordinating the activities of the response. The role of incident commander usually is filled by the fire chief. All of the functions that must occur during the response are then assigned to others to coordinate, but they report to and are responsible to the incident commander. The various functions are referred to as sectors. EMS personnel generally are responsible only for the medical aspects of the response and fall under the operations sector.

14. What is the triage process?
Triage is a process of prioritizing patient care based on severity of injury or illness, the patient's prognosis, and the availability of resources. The goal of triage is to select the patients in greatest need of immediate medical attention and arrange for that treatment with the currently available resources. The concept of triage is best represented by Charles Dickens' phrase: "The needs of the many outweigh the needs of the few."

Triage should be started as soon as possible by the most trained medical person available. It is a rapid survey to determine the number of victims, any hazards to victims and rescuers, and what additional resources are needed.

15. Why is triage so important?
When faced with many persons who are injured or ill but with limited resources to care for them, the rescuers must decide which patients have the best chance of survival and should be taken care of quickly with the available resources. This often means that some patients will not get the care they need and will likely die. Triage decisions are the most critical decisions that medical personnel make during an MCI.

16. How does triage affect treatment and transport of patients?
The triage category determines how quickly a patient receives treatment in the field and how rapidly he or she is transported to the hospital. Triage is a continuous process that is repeated when patients are prepared for transport and when they arrive at the hospital. Triage is repeated because the patient's condition may improve with treatment or may deteriorate.

17. What does "triage category" mean?
A patient who is assessed during triage is assigned to an urgency category based on the severity of the injury or illness. The most common scheme uses four categories: immediate, delayed, minimal, and expectant. Patients in the *immediate* category have injuries or illnesses that require immediate care for life-threatening situations but have a high likelihood of surviving if the situations are corrected. *Delayed* category situations can be treated within hours to days without

an expectation of significant deterioration or morbidity. *Minimal* conditions generally can be treated by the patient or require minimal medical care. Patients who are declared *expectant* have such severe injuries that they will die; if resources allow, they receive comfort measures only.

18. What are triage tags?

Triage tags are sometimes used to identify the patient's triage category to other rescuers. The most commonly used tags are color-coded to identify the patient's category: immediate (red), delayed (yellow), minimal (green), and expectant (black). Once the patient is triaged, the tag is attached to the patient. Many people do not believe that triage tags work well during a disaster. Some people simply place a piece of colored tape on the patient's forehead to identify the triage category. Whether tags or tape are used, some method of identifying the category should be used.

19. Is it important to have doctors and nurses on the scene?

There is no concrete answer. Generally, care can be provided quite well by EMS personnel. Occasionally, it may be necessary or helpful for physicians and nurses to assist with patient care in the field. This is particularly important if significantly advanced care, such as limb amputation, is needed. Additionally, if there will be a long delay before transport, physicians and nurses can further stabilize patients until they can be transported. In situations in which hospital personnel do respond to the scene, they must be very knowledgeable about providing medical care out of hospital.

20. How do the responders communicate with each other?

Although communication is very important during a disaster response, it is the factor that often causes the most problems.

Many people must be able to communicate with each other, whether by radio, telephone, or in person. The incident commander must be able to talk with those coordinating the various sectors, including EMS personnel. The EMS coordinator must communicate with those coordinating triage, treatment, and transportation as well as with the medical control facility or hospital coordinating center. The transportation coordinator also must communicate with hospitals or the coordinating center.

However, with so many people needing to talk with each other, radio frequencies can become overcrowded. Aggravating that situation is the fact that many different agencies are responding to the situation; the agencies often have individual frequencies, which makes it impossible to communicate between agencies. Land-line telephones and cellular circuits are often tied up with disaster-related activities—from disaster responders as well as citizens using the phones to get information.

21. How can such problems be overcome?

Responders should try to talk face-to-face with each other. When dedicated radio frequencies are available, they can be used effectively. The use of messengers and amateur radio operators also can be effective. Information can be shared using bullhorns in relatively controlled areas. Disaster responders are starting to use computers for communications.

22. When the radios are busy, how can EMS personnel call the hospital to discuss patients and receive medical care orders?

Usually, in disaster situations, there is little communication between the EMS personnel and the hospitals. Much more emphasis is placed on the personnel taking care of patients by standing orders in the protocols.

23. Once the transport of patients begins, how are victims assigned to receiving hospitals?

This component of MCI management is often overlooked. The common tendency is for the transporting personnel to want to bring the patient to the closest hospital so they can quickly turn around to get the next patient. Before too long, the MCI has been transferred from the disaster site to the closest hospital. Part of any disaster plan is appropriate distribution of patients and hospital destination assignments. Victims in the *immediate* category should be transported to trauma centers. Patients with less severe injuries can be taken to nontrauma centers. Although dispersing patients to multiple hospitals will entail longer transport times, care will generally be improved by not overwhelming one facility.

24. How can the media be kept out of the way at the disaster site?

The media can be very important and helpful during a disaster. Initially, the media can provide public information about the situation, announcing potential hazards and educating the public about evacuation routes if necessary. The media, if given proper information, can inform the community about health care issues and threats. They can announce to medical personnel the need to return to hospitals or other care facilities. A public information officer should be identified whose responsibility is to regularly provide the media with reliable and accurate information. The media will not go away; they should be used constructively.

BIBLIOGRAPHY

1. Doyle CJ: Mass casualty incident. Integration with prehospital care. Emerg Med Clin North Am 8:163–175, 1990.
2. Gans L: Disaster planning and management. In Harwood-Nuss AL (ed): The Clinical Practice of Emergency Medicine, 2nd ed. Philadelphia, Lippincott-Raven, 1996, pp 1511–1514.
3. Mahoney BD: Disaster medical services. In Tintinalli J (ed): Emergency Medicine. A Comprehensive Study Guide, 4th ed. New York, McGraw-Hill, 1996, pp 20–25.
4. Noji EK: Natural disaster management. In Auerbach PS (ed): Wilderness Medicine, 3rd ed. St. Louis, Mosby, 1994, pp 644–663.
5. Schultz CH, Koenig KL, Noji EK: A medical disaster response to reduce immediate mortality after an earthquake. N Engl J Med 334:438–444, 1996.
6. Waeckerle JF: Disaster planning and response. N Engl J Med 324:815–821, 1991.

16. SMALL-SCALE MULTI-CASUALTY INCIDENTS

Tom Tkach, NREMT-P

1. What is a multi-casualty incident (MCI)?

Any situation in which the number of patients overwhelms the ability to the initial EMS responders to care for them is defined as an MCI. This could be a motor vehicle accident (MVA) with as few as three patients or an airliner crash with hundreds of patients. Whenever multiple ambulances respond to the same incident, the normal dynamics of scene control change.

2. Are there different levels of MCIs?

Since patient volume varies from MCI to MCI, and EMS systems have variable resources, the dynamics of managing MCIs also varies. For this reason, MCIs are often broken down into three categories: Level 1, Level 2, and Level 3. It is helpful to think in these terms, since the EMS action plans must vary based on the magnitude of the event.

3. What is a Level 1 MCI?

A Level 1 MCI is any event in which the volume of patients overwhelms the initial responding ambulance but the EMS system has enough resources to respond and transport the patients. Extra ambulances are readily available and arrive in a short time, allowing for rapid evacuation of the patients. These types of MCIs are quite common, usually as a result of motor vehicle accidents. Level 1 MCIs are usually quick "in and out" calls in which time at the scene is minimal and patients receive quick and efficient care. In a Level 1 MCI, the most efficient use of time by the initial responding ambulance is to focus on treating primary life threats only, then "packaging" patients for incoming ambulances.

4. What is a Level 2 MCI?

With a Level 2 incident, the initial responding EMS crew is again overwhelmed by the patient volume. In direct contrast to Level 1, however, there aren't enough resources to respond to the scene, thereby creating a delay in transporting patients. The initial crew is faced with the potential for extended scene times, requiring the need to establish treatment zones at the scene. Most Level 2 incidents occur as a result of fire and smoke inhalation in large buildings or hazardous material exposures, creating large volumes of patients. Another common cause of Level 2 MCI is bus accidents, which generate a larger volume of patients than the responding EMS agency can transport.

5. What is a Level 3 MCI?

A Level 3 event is also known as a Multi-Casualty Overload (MCO). This describes a true disaster, such as a large airline crash or a tornado touchdown in a trailer park. All the resources in a jurisdiction become overwhelmed, from the EMS agencies to the receiving hospitals. In an MCO, the local disaster plan is usually activated, enabling regional resource response. Please refer to the chapter on "Disaster Management," for more information regarding management of MCOs.

6. Why can't I apply my usual EMS disaster plan to the small-scale MCI?

All EMS agencies have some form of disaster plan, usually found collecting dust somewhere on a shelf. These plans tend to be complex documents that are difficult to digest, much less put into practice during a disaster. Another disadvantage is that a disaster plan is somewhat like a nuclear missile: once you launch it, it's pretty hard to call it back. You must be sure that you want to activate a full-scale disaster response. Small-scale MCIs do not require such massive mobilization of resources, so one must use discretion before requesting a disaster response. Fortunately, true disasters are rare enough that most EMS providers will never respond to one in their entire career. Those who do, however, are expected to utilize a disaster plan they probably have never seen. Many EMS systems use the incident command system (ICS), which is an effective tool that allows for a unified command structure and enables additional resources to be layered on the event as needed. The ICS format is geared more toward command personnel, however, than initial responders.

7. Will the time of day an MCI occurs affect the level of MCI that I declare?

In many EMS systems, available resources vary based on the time of day, especially in agencies that use system status management. It may take longer to get additional ambulances in the middle of the night, since there may be fewer staffed and they may be on other calls or more distant locations. An MCI that would be a Level 1 MCI during the day could be a Level 2 at night, requiring the initial ambulance crew to focus more on treatment at the scene rather than just packaging patients for transport.

8. What are the common types of calls that create multiple casualties?

Motor vehicle accidents, by a large margin. Building fires, especially large apartment buildings, can create multiple patients, along with other unique scene management problems. Hazardous material exposures can produce large numbers of patients as well. Also, the specter of domestic terrorism with the potential for mass casualties from weapons of mass destruction must be acknowledged. A thorough understanding of the unique problems encountered with the various scenarios will enable you to anticipate and respond to each MCI.

9. What are the most common errors made in managing a small-scale MCI?

A typical problem that occurs is failure to identify and contain rapidly the total number of patients in an incident. A classic example is a multiple-vehicle auto accident with injured passengers wandering around the scene, making it easy to miss patients during the initial scene survey. Patients must therefore be rapidly identified and sequestered on any MCI scene.

Another problem is failure of the initial responding EMS crew to establish strong scene control. The initial minutes of an MCI response are crucial to success. If control isn't established immediately, before additional crews begin arriving, a "control vacuum" will occur, creating chaos at the scene. Another problem that occurs is when the additional incoming EMS crews don't follow the directions of the scene commander, essentially "free-lancing" their own scene management. This causes a breakdown in scene control.

10. What is a "mission conflict"?

This term describes the inevitable conflict that occurs whenever numerous response agencies interact at an MCI scene, each with their own "mission" as a goal rather than the ultimate goal of providing patient care. This phenomenon seems to occur at all MCIs to some degree. Perhaps the police had to finish the accident report before letting the ambulance transport the patient or a tow truck driver tried to climb into the ambulance to get a tow slip signed by the patient, hampering the ability to care for patients. Responders must be aware of the potential for mission conflicts and work to avoid them. One proactive solution is to have your agency develop policies dictating scene control responsibilities and outlining task-specific functions. Since small-scale MCIs are common, these policies should simply be an extension of your normal operating policies, separate from your disaster policy.

11. What is meant by "first-in—last out"?

This is a concept regarding the first ambulance to arrive at the scene of an MCI. The initial responding ambulance essentially becomes the triage team and assumes medical command of the scene. The crew performs the survey of the scene, triages the patients, determines resource needs, and develops the action plan for managing the event. If the first ambulance simply grabs a couple of patients and immediately transports them, not only does this cause a control vacuum at the scene, but also some other EMS crew will have to come in and start from scratch. The first crew to arrive therefore should be the last one to leave, transporting the least injured patients at the end of the event. Since the first ambulance crew set up the plan, they should see it through all the way to the final "cleanup sweep."

12. Why can't my supervisor respond and take control of the scene?

Many EMS agencies have established policies regarding this issue. This really only applies to the Level 3 incident, when scene times will be prolonged. On a Level 1 MCI and on many Level 2 MCIs, the call should be over before a supervisor can arrive to take control.

13. Since the first-arriving crew is so important, can you provide some more detail about their responsibilities?

The crew of the first-arriving ambulance has enormous responsibilities including scene assessment, communication, triage, and choreography of the scene. They are the ones who set the tone and structure that will guide the entire EMS response. First, they need to just step back and get an overall impression of the magnitude of the event, the potential number of victims, and the medical needs, then relay that information back to dispatch. The first-arriving EMS crew becomes the triage crew. An effective technique for the initial triage of the scene is having crew members split up, triage patients separately, then meet to determine resource needs. The technique is especially effective when dealing with a scene that is spread out. It is essential that both crew members have communication capabilities if they split up, for obvious reasons. Once the volume of patients and their acuity have been determined, the crew must make a decision regarding the number of additional transport ambulances needed. Resources are then requested. Based on the information from the dispatcher regarding available resources, the triage crew can then declare the call a Level 1 or 2 incident. This decision will drive the focus of scene management toward either packaging patients for immediate transport or formal treatment at the scene. Another primary responsibility is scene "set-up."

14. What is meant by "scene set-up"?

This concept involves identifying any hazards at the scene that the incoming resources must be made aware of. It also involves notifying them of appropriate ingress and egress routes as well as any other specific information about the scene they might need. Level 1 MCIs usually don't require formal staging and triage areas, but Level 2 incidents may require their use. Incoming resources must be notified if these components are in use at the scene and directed to the appropriate areas.

15. What do I need to know about triage?

As we all know, triage is the process of sorting patients according to the acuity of their medical needs. This is essential for prioritizing patients for transport. Ideally, the patients with the highest acuity needs will be transported first and the lowest acuity patients sent out last. Triage is an intimidating task for those who have never done it. Textbooks and classes on multi-casualty responses can sometimes leave EMS providers with the impression that one is "playing God" by having to decide who lives and who dies. One can minimize the mystique of triage if one realizes that we essentially perform triage on every call. Even on routine calls, we learn to determine patient acuity quickly by performing a primary survey. This is an instinctive skill for an EMS provider. On an MCI, the same principle is used, except that there are more patients needing this assessment.

16. How long should it take me to triage a patient?

Whether dealing with a single patient or with multiple patients, triage is performed by assessing for primary threats to life. A rapid ABC assessment can be performed in less than 10 seconds, easily identifying primary threats to life that require immediate intervention. Medical care should be limited to treating these immediate life threats only, such as opening an airway and controlling obvious external hemorrhage. On a scene involving multiple patients, the provider doing the triage must fight the tendency to get involved with delivering complex medical care to one patient. It is more important to continue the triage of the entire scene.

17. What are the triage categories?

Patients must be triaged according to their acuity to determine priority of transport. There are many variations in EMS systems regarding triage categories and their labels. Some systems use four categories, and some use five. Some systems use colors to identify a category. Regardless of these system variations, there is fundamental agreement regarding priority of transport. High-priority patients, those with immediate threats to life, are transported first. These patients should have minimal scene times. Next priority of transport are patients without immediate life threats but who may have significant injuries. These patients should be able to withstand a short delay in transport. Last priority is the walking wounded, those patients without systemic injuries. These patients could conceivably be transported by means other than an ambulance, such as a bus. Finally, dead and mortally wounded are the last priority.

18. What is meant by "retriage"?

During a Level 2 MCI, transport is delayed owing to a lack of resources, allowing more comprehensive treatment at the scene. Depending on the length of the delay, patients must be triaged again to determine if their status has deteriorated, necessitating upgrade of their transport priority. Retriage should not be necessary on a Level 1 MCI, since there is no delay in transport.

19. If I am the triage officer, at what point should I begin treating patients?

Once triage and primary intervention are complete, you can begin performing more time-consuming tasks. If the call is a Level 1 MCI, you should focus on packaging patients for transport by securing them on backboards. Your focus on a Level 2 MCI should be on providing standard prehospital care for your patients while awaiting transport vehicles.

20. What unique problems will I encounter with an MCI involving a motor vehicle accident?

As alluded to previously, patient containment is difficult because of the natural tendency for patients to wander around the scene. The initial EMS crew must rapidly determine how many occupants were in each vehicle so that they can determine resource needs. Rescue vehicle gridlock is a concern, since there will usually be multiple fire trucks, police cars, ambulances, and tow trucks at the scene. Strategic parking is important, therefore, with concern given to ingress and egress for other ambulances. Another problem occurs when patients are trapped in vehicles and require extrication. Usually, the goal is to transport the worst injuries first. Unfortunately, critically injured patients from an MVA may be the last ones transported, owing to the delay in extrication. This must be taken into account when setting up receiving emergency departments so that they know to reserve their critical care rooms for the more seriously injured patients still to come.

21. What kinds of problems should I anticipate at a fire in a large building?

The most important thing to keep in mind about fire scenes is the potential for multiple evacuation points from the building. If you station yourself on one side of the building without anticipating patients fleeing the building from other exits, you are bound to miss people. Another problem that occurs is that people with smoke inhalation don't always exhibit symptoms immediately; in fact, symptoms may take hours to evolve. Therefore, anyone who has inhaled smoke must receive a thorough assessment and must be educated about the possibility of worsening symptoms if he is allowed to refuse care initially. People trapped in a burning building will do anything to escape from the fire, even jumping from the roof of a 20-story building. You must anticipate injuries such as major trauma from such falls along with burns and smoke inhalation.

22. What about MCIs involving violent trauma, such as shootings and stabbings?

It is not uncommon in our society to have to respond to scenes with multiple victims of violent trauma. Clearly, your safety as a rescuer is the primary concern. These scenes tend to be the most chaotic scenes we manage and can easily slip away from you. One unique problem is that violent trauma victims seem to refuse to limit the size of the scene and tend to ambulate all over the neighborhood, making patient containment difficult. This can create a setup for missing victims on your initial assessment of the scene.

23. When should I contact Medical Control during an MCI?

As soon as you determine that your are dealing with an MCI, notification of Medical Control should occur. The sooner the receiving hospital(s) receive word of multiple incoming patients, the better prepared they will be. The initial call can be a simple set-up advising about the potential for multiple casualties and does not necessarily require great detail about the types of injuries. Once the scene has been completely triaged, Medical Control can be updated as needed.

24. What are the responsibilities of the incoming ambulances?

First, it is crucial that the incoming crews receive as much information about the scene as possible. The initial crew should advise the communications center exactly how to approach the scene, where to park, and especially where the patients are located. The communications center is responsible for advising all the incoming crews, minimizing the need for the busy triage crew to be on the radio. Once the incoming crews have been advised, they need to follow these directions. Once on the scene, the incoming crews should be directed immediately to their patients so they won't be tempted to wander around the scene. Once their patients are loaded, on-scene treatment should be avoided. The loading area at an MCI tends to become hopelessly gridlocked if the incoming crews sit on the scene, taking up valuable space in the action zone.

25. Do I need to have a separate radio frequency activated during an MCI?

Most EMS agencies have tactical frequencies available for use during MCIs or other major incidents. Some MCIs require little radio traffic, while others can be quite radio intensive. The decision to move the MCI to its own channel can be made by the person in charge at the scene if the need arises. This can also be done at the request of the dispatcher if normal operations cannot be performed on the same channel.

26. Should I be concerned about destination assignment of multiple casualties?

Most Level 1 MCIs don't generate enough patients to make this a problem, but a Level 2 MCI can. Many EMS systems have established destination policies to assist in assigning destinations. In the absence of policies regarding hospital destination, concern must be given to the special needs of the patients so that the right patient is transported to the right place. Finally, one must be cautious about overloading a single emergency department with casualties. In a system that has but one emergency department, this issue should be addressed in advance, with procedures in place to address resource mobilization at the hospital.

BIBLIOGRAPHY

1. Beinin L: Medical Consequences of Natural Disasters. New York, Springer-Verlag, 1985.
2. Caroline NL: Emergency Care in the Streets, 5th ed. Philadelphia, Lippincott-Raven, 1995.
3. Caroline NL: Emergency Medical Treatment: A Text for EMT-As and EMT-Intermediates, 3rd ed. Philadelphia, Lippincott-Raven, 1991.
4. Haynes BE, et al: A prehospital approach to multiple victim incidents. Ann Emerg Med 15:458, 1986.
5. Rund DA, Rausch TS: Triage. St. Louis, Mosby, 1981.
6. Schwartz TJ: Model for prehospital disaster response. J World Assoc Emerg Disaster Med 1:78, 1986.

IX. Mass Gatherings

17. MASS GATHERINGS
Jedd Roe, M.D.

1. What is a mass gathering?

One dictionary defines a mass as a "large body of persons in a compact group" and a gathering as an "assembly or meeting." Those involved in the planning of prehospital care generally consider any event that involves at least 1000 persons to be a mass gathering.

2. Why should medical care be provided at mass gatherings?

Most mass gatherings will involve substantially more than 1000 participants. For example, sports stadiums generally hold at least 70,000 occupants. Thus, for several hours, the population of many small to medium-sized cities is confined to a relatively small area. With a population base of this magnitude, a significant number of medical events are likely to occur. Most medical complaints involve only first aid, but it is important to be prepared to deal with the truly emergent problems that might occur, from cardiac arrests and childbirth to true mass casualty situations. In addition, if medical care is not provided onsite, the local emergency medical services (EMS) system will be called for every medical complaint. This could easily overburden the EMS system and seriously impair its ability to meet its routine responsibilities.

3. What is the framework for providing care at a mass gathering?

Essentially, one must create a microcosm of an EMS system. Each component of the system, including communications, personnel, medical equipment and supplies, onsite response, and transport capability, will be required in order to provide care at a mass gathering.

4. Do physicians need to be involved?

A strong case can be made for physician involvement at mass gatherings. First, most of the published research on the medical care provided at mass gatherings has been done by the physicians who have designed and implemented plans for such events. While most of the medical care can and will be provided by paramedics or nurses, the emergency physician's greater medical expertise is occasionally required. Perhaps more importantly, the physician can accept the responsibility for treating and releasing patients who might otherwise require transport when common prehospital protocols are followed. Reducing the number of transported patients results in reduced costs of care and greater satisfaction for patients and event organizers.

5. Where should planning begin?

Usually, the event organizer is contacted first to ascertain his or her expectations for the medical care that may be required. Those planning for the medical care should share the results of their prior experiences and those published in the literature for similar events to be sure that the expectations of the event organizers are reasonable. Financial issues regarding the cost of the medical care need to be addressed. Many for-profit events have funds budgeted for emergency care, and even if volunteer personnel are to be used, supplies may need to be purchased or donations solicited. Perhaps the most important issue to clarify is who will be in overall charge of all medical care. This is particularly important for events that will use personnel from different agencies or volunteer groups. Many bands, sports teams, or speakers may have their own medical personnel with them. Determine the level of responsibility for their care that you will assume and how to meet other requirements they may have, such as transport.

6. What other agencies or organizations are likely to be involved?

For any large gathering, local police and possibly fire departments generally will be involved. Events may have their own security details or customer service representatives. Education of, and liaison with, each of these groups will enhance the ability of event participants to access medical care. Interagency communication may be facilitated by the use of a command post, usually containing a representative of each agency, for event coordination. In the case of events involving a head of state or other security concerns, agencies such as the U.S. Secret Service may be involved. Joint planning is especially important in such instances so that medical personnel receive appropriate clearances and care can be provided under the auspices of these special security concerns.

7. How does the physical site of the mass gathering influence the planning for medical care?

Planners must become familiar with the site in detail. Where will the concentrations of people be, and what are the points of access? This will aid in determining the required number and location of first aid stations. Plan for the ingress and egress of ambulances to the first aid room(s). What are the barriers to EMS response to event participants or access to first aid rooms? Determine where your responsibility for medical care ends and where those of the local EMS system begins. For instance, whose responsibility is the event participant who has collapsed in a distant parking lot? Arrange for public service announcements or signs that clearly identify the location of first aid rooms and how the public can access medical care.

8. Is a first aid room necessary?

Yes, at least one. First aid rooms serve as a central source of supplies and operations. They should be clearly identified and easily visible and accessible to the public. Cots or beds should be present so patients may lie down and, ideally, should allow for privacy from walk-in traffic. An EMS provider should always be in attendance at the first aid room—to be present for walk-in patients and prevent unauthorized use of supplies and equipment. If several first aid rooms are being used, it may be helpful to designate the largest room with best access to ambulance transport as the main first aid room where most of the supplies may be stored and seriously ill patients may be attended to while awaiting transport.

9. Are outdoor events handled differently than indoor events?

Yes. Outdoor events allow for exposure to the elements and may have additional special requirements. Sites near large bodies of water may require water rescue capabilities. The largest environmental factor is usually temperature. While hypothermia can be a concern for events held in cold temperatures, mass gatherings held in warm climates generally produce larger numbers of patients who experience dehydration and heat exhaustion. Most indoor events are climate-controlled and involve seated participants, thus decreasing the potential for medical problems.

10. Can the estimated attendance at a mass gathering be used to help determine staffing levels?

Generally, yes. While there have been a number of published recommendations, there is some consensus to provide one physician for 40,000–50,000 people and one emergency medical technician-paramedic or one nurse for 10,000 people. Ideally, if a similar event has been held at a similar venue, one should have good data on which to base future planning. If this information is not available, other event characteristics become important in determining staffing levels.

11. What other characteristics of a mass gathering are important?

The type of event has been shown to influence the volume and categories of medical problems. For instance, one is likely to see more patients with sequelae of alcohol and drug use at rock concerts than at classical music concerts. The risk of violence or trauma varies greatly among events and rises dramatically at auto racing events or pubic demonstrations. Reported rates of medical encounters have varied from 16 per 10,000 people at the 1994 Los Angeles Summer Olympics to 185 per 10,000 people at the 1991 Super Bowl in Tampa, Florida.

The age of attendees may be an important factor. More significant medical problems could be anticipated from an older population. The environment and duration of an event can also be a potent factor. For instance, at one stadium, on a hot August day with a 12-hour rock concert, 10 times the number of patients were contacted than during an average 5-hour National Football League game at the same stadium. Severity of illness also increased, as evidenced by a similar rise in the number of patients requiring transport to a hospital.

12. How much medical capability is needed at a site?

While medical problems will be minor, such as requests for first aid or acetaminophen, most authorities agree that preparations should be made for personnel and equipment to deal with life-threatening problems such as cardiac arrest, respiratory complaints, and traumatic injuries. At a minimum, if advanced life support is not available, automated external defibrillators and emergency medical technicians trained in their use should be present.

13. Functionally, how would a medical response take place at a mass gathering?

First, pre-established lines of communication are paramount. An EMS representative in the command post might be notified of an incident by a security representative. While it is helpful for the EMS representative to have radio contact with the local EMS system, medical operations should be conducted on a separate frequency or talk group (800 MHz). A paramedic is notified by radio and could respond by electric cart or on foot. Many systems have recently implemented responding by bicycle. In Denver, paramedics on mountain bicycles have achieved a 50% reduction in response time at many mass gatherings. Depending on severity of illness, a patient may be transported to the first aid room by wheelchair, stretcher, or electric cart for observation and therapy. Hospitals can be notified by radio of impending patient arrival, but telephone communication eases the quality of communication.

14. Does every patient contact need to be documented?

Yes. For minor first aid and analgesic requests, one may elect to merely record demographic data (time, name, age), chief complaint, treatment, and disposition. Any complaint of greater severity requires the usual complete documentation required of an EMS response or emergency department visit. Compulsiveness in this area allows for greater medicolegal protection and data gathering for future planning and quality improvement.

15. Besides the typical events, do any other special situations warrant this sort of planning?

Most major airports should be considered in the same context as a mass gathering. They tend to be isolated from major metropolitan areas, up to 23 million passengers may pass through annually, and as many as 15,000 employees may be onsite. Yearly call volumes have ranged from 800 to 6,000. Some airports staff onsite medical clinics with physicians and nurses, and others provide paramedic first response and first aid rooms. An independent system of providing onsite medical care should be established that conforms to Federal Aviation Administration regulations. Depending on distance to a hospital, helicopter transport may be necessary for severely ill or injured patients.

16. What's the worst case scenario?

Each mass gathering is a mass casualty event waiting to happen. The local EMS disaster plan can be initiated in such circumstances, but each mass gathering has a specific set of logistics that can be anticipated and analyzed beforehand. Fixed sites, such as stadiums, can have site-specific disaster plans, which can be tested by the use of tabletop and full-scale exercises.

BIBLIOGRAPHY

1. Cwinn AA, Dinerman N, Pons PT, et al: Prehospital care at a major international airport. Ann Emerg Med 17:1042–1048, 1988.
2. Leonard RB: Medical support for mass gatherings. Emerg Med Clin North Am 14:383–397, 1996.
3. Parrillo SJ: Medical care at mass gatherings: Considerations for physician involvement. Prehosp Disaster Med 10:273–275, 1995.
4. Paul HM: Mass casualty: Pope's Denver visit causes MegaMCI. J Emerg Med Serv 18(11):64–75, 1993.
5. Sanders AB, Criss E, Steckl P, et al: An analysis of medical care at mass gatherings. Ann Emerg Med 15:515–519, 1986.

X. Special Situations

18. WATER EMERGENCIES

Catherine B. Custalow, M.D., Ph.D.

1. What groups of people are at risk for drowning?
Children younger than 4 years old are the victims in nearly half of all drownings and near-drownings, with the highest rate in children 1 to 2 years old. Teenage boys are the second most likely group to be at risk for drowning, related to risk-taking behavior and alcohol use. It is estimated that 40–50% of drownings are associated with alcohol use. Epilepsy is also a risk for drowning, with a four- to fivefold increased risk among seizure patients.

2. What is the sequence of events in drowning?
There is considerable variability in the sequence of events leading to drowning. As the patient sinks below the water, he or she gasps and coughs, and a small amount of water is aspirated. This leads to laryngospasm, which prevents more water from entering. Asphyxia results, and in most patients, the glottis then relaxes and water again enters the lungs. In 10–15% of cases, patients suffocate and do not aspirate. The final consequence with or without aspiration is hypoxemia, leading to death.

3. Does it make a difference whether the person drowned in fresh water or salt water?
Theoretically, hypotonic fluid aspirated during fresh water drownings passes through the lungs into the intravascular space, causing fluid overload and electrolyte abnormalities. Aspiration of hypertonic salt water would be expected to cause fluid to be drawn into the lungs, creating pulmonary edema and hypertonic serum. Whether the drowning or near-drowning occurred in fresh water or salt water, however, the initial prehospital resuscitation is the same, with attention to respiratory and circulatory support.

4. Are there any special techniques for extricating drowning or near-drowning victims from the water?
If the patient is conscious, first attempt to throw a flotation device to the victim, or extend a pole or rope to tow the victim to shore. If unsuccessful, then attempt to rescue the victim with a boat. Only after all these measures have failed should a swimming rescue be attempted. Swimming rescues are the most dangerous of all to the rescuer and should only be done by individuals who can swim and are trained in water rescue and lifesaving techniques. Always wear a personal flotation device.

5. Are cervical spine precautions necessary?
Yes. Suspect spinal cord injuries, especially if drowning potentially resulted from a diving accident. The neck should be supported in a neutral position and the patient placed on a backboard in the water with the head, neck, and body moved as a single unit into the supine horizontal position.

6. Should rescue breathing and CPR be initiated in the water?
Rescue breathing may be initiated as soon as the safety of the rescuer can be insured. There are special appliances (snorkels, buoyant devices) that allow for deep-water rescue breathing for

those with special training. If the patient is pulseless, CPR should be initiated in the water only if the rescuer has special training in the techniques of in-water CPR, which include using special equipment to support the back. It is difficult to perform adequate CPR in the water. The priority should be rapid transport to the shore so that CPR may be promptly initiated on land.

7. What are the treatment priorities during transport?

Remove the patient promptly from the water. Clear the airway by suctioning. Administer oxygen. Assist ventilation and intubate when necessary to protect the airway in an unconscious victim. Establish intravenous access. Cardiac monitoring is essential. Treat arrhythmias and institute early CPR when indicated. Remove wet clothing and wrap the victim in blankets. Obtain details of the accident at the scene, such as submersion time and symptoms.

8. Should the Heimlich maneuver be performed to expel water?

The Heimlich maneuver is not recommended under current ACLS guidelines. Attempts to remove water from the lungs with methods other than suction may prove dangerous because gastric contents may be ejected and cause aspiration. The Heimlich maneuver may be used only if it is suspected that foreign matter is obstructing the airway.

9. Do all near-drowning victims need to be transported to the hospital, even if they seem to have recovered at the scene?

Yes. Patients need to be monitored closely because they can deteriorate. Pulmonary edema may develop secondary to aspiration and may not be clinically evident for several hours.

10. When should resuscitation efforts be discontinued in the field?

Patients who have experienced submersion in cold water should be transported even if they are pulseless and apneic after 30 minutes of CPR. Patients have been successfully resuscitated with full neurologic recovery after prolonged submersion (more than 60 minutes) in cold water. Continue CPR until you reach the emergency department, where a physician can make the determination to discontinue CPR. The only exception is when there are obvious signs of death (dependent lividity or putrefaction).

11. Are there any special considerations for ice rescue?

Yes. Keeping the victim in sight is very important. At least two observers should be assigned to posts a moderate distance apart to keep visual contact with the victim at all times. Throw a flotation device to the victim so that he or she does not have to expend energy treading water or swimming. When rescuing a victim over thin ice, rescuers should be prepared for ice water immersion themselves: They should be wearing wet suits, have flotation devices, and be attached by a lifeline to the shore.

12. What is an air embolism?

Air embolism occurs when a diver ascends rapidly while holding his or her breath. Air inside the lungs expands, causing alveoli in the lungs to rupture. Ruptured air can cause pneumothorax by entering the pleural space or pneumomediastinum by entering the mediastinum. Air can also leak into blood vessels.

13. What are the signs and symptoms of air embolism?

Dyspnea, hemoptysis, chest pain, and cardiac arrest (from coronary occlusion). Neurologic manifestations can range from subtle mood changes to dizziness, vertigo, aphasia, syncope, visual disturbances, complete blindness, paralysis, and numbness.

14. What is decompression sickness?

Decompression sickness results when nitrogen bubbles form in blood vessels and body tissues during rapid ascent while diving. Symptoms are similar to those of air embolism; most notably, patients experience extreme joint or abdominal pain. The brain and spinal cord are especially susceptible, with more than 80% of individuals having neurologic symptoms. Decompression sickness can occur after diving if patients fly in an unpressurized airplane or drive up a mountain.

15. How should patients with air embolism be managed during transport?

The patient should be removed from the water, and 100% oxygen should be administered by nonrebreather mask. If the patient is intubated, hyperventilation is recommended to decrease intracranial pressure. Establish intravenous access and administer intravenous fluids. Seizures may be treated with diazepam.

16. What is the definitive treatment for decompression sickness and air embolism?

The treatment is the same for both conditions: Basic life support measures followed by recompression in a hyperbaric oxygen chamber.

17. Does the hospital destination differ for diving victims?

Yes. Victims of decompression sickness and air embolism should be transported to the nearest hospital with a hyperbaric oxygen chamber for definitive treatment. Learn the locations of recompression chambers in your area.

CONTROVERSY

18. What is the best position for transporting a patient with air embolism?

This has been a subject of controversy over the years. When patients are positioned with the head up, air distributes primarily to the cerebral circulation, while in the head-down position, air distributes primarily to the coronary circulation. When supine or in the left lateral decubitus position, air distributes equally. Placing the patient supine with the head neutral is probably the best transport position so that arterial and venous blood can flow unrestricted.

BIBLIOGRAPHY

1. Advanced Cardiac Life Support. Dallas, TX, American Heart Association, 1994.
2. Heckman JD (ed): Water hazards, extrication and rescue. In Emergency Care and Transportation of the Sick and Injured, 5th ed. Park Ridge, IL, American Academy of Orthopedic Surgeons, 1991.
3. Jerrard DA: Diving medicine. Emerg Med Clin North Am 10:329, 1992.
4. Olshaker JS: Near drowning. Emerg Med Clin North Am 10:339, 1992.
5. Ornato JP: The resuscitation of near-drowning victims. JAMA 256:75, 1986.
6. Smith DJ: Diagnosis and management of diving accidents. Med Sci Sports Exerc 28:587, 1996.
7. Weinstein MD, Krieger BP: Near-drowning: Epidemiology, pathophysiology, and initial treatment. J Emerg Med 14:461, 1996.

19. DECOMPRESSION ILLNESSES

Jonathan D. Apfelbaum, M.D.

1. What is decompression sickness?

Decompression sickness (DCS) is a disorder caused by the expansion of nitrogen bubbles in the tissues and circulation. There are two types of DCS. Type I is called "pain only" or musculoskeletal DCS, causing pain in joints, bones, and soft tissues. Type II is central or neurologic DCS, affecting the brain, spinal cord, and cardiopulmonary system. Other names for DCS are the "bends" or the "staggers."

2. How does it happen?

It is seen primarily in underwater divers. The compressed air mixture breathed by most self-contained underwater breathing apparatus (SCUBA) divers is 21% oxygen, 78% nitrogen, and 0.03% carbon dioxide. As a diver descends, the pressure increases one atmosphere for each 33 feet descended. This means the volume of air in the SCUBA tank at sea level is half that at 33 feet, but each breath the diver takes continues to be the same volume because the tank is pressurized and the regulator is set to compensate for ambient pressure. Therefore, the amount of nitrogen absorbed is greater at depth than at sea level. Excess oxygen can be metabolized, but excess nitrogen cannot and may be released from solution upon decompression. Divers plan dive "profiles" based on tables or dive computers that calculate how much nitrogen they can absorb safely. The excess nitrogen is released during a controlled ascent or during safety stops at various depths to "off gas." If the rate of ascent exceeds the body's ability to release the nitrogen, it can "boil out" in the tissues and produce bubbles in tissues anywhere in the body. This can occur in persons ascending too rapidly in an aircraft or altitude chamber as well.

3. Is DCS the only decompression illness?

No. Barotrauma and nitrogen narcosis also may occur. Barotrauma occurs when the pressure is not equalized across any volume of free gas in the body. Known as a "squeeze," any area of free gas may produce pain or injury upon compression or decompression. Classically, the middle ear is a primary example. Remember that the same volume of gas occupies half the volume at 33 feet that it does at sea level. If a diver is unable to clear the ears, the ear drum will retract painfully or even rupture as he descends, or it may bulge and pop on ascent. Other affected areas include dental work with air pockets, sinuses, or lungs. Divers are cautioned never to hold their breath on ascent for this reason.

Nitrogen narcosis, otherwise known as "rapture of the deep," occurs when the amount of nitrogen absorbed by the body causes a euphoric intoxicating effect with altered mental status and judgment. It can occur at any depth but is classically seen on deeper dives.

4. I live in a landlocked state. Why should I care?

With the increased popularity of SCUBA diving and the ease of air travel, DCS can be seen in any state. Also, diving is not limited to the ocean, and free water diving occurs in every state (including Alaska!). Nor is barotrauma limited to deep diving; it can occur in a swimming pool.

5. What is the worst form of DCS?

Arterial gas embolism (AGE) is the most extreme form of DCS. In this case, the nitrogen forms bubbles in the arterial system. It is second to drowning as a cause of diving-related deaths. The bubbles move through the circulatory system until they lodge in a vessel, blocking further blood flow. Almost all cases present within 5 to 10 minutes of ascent. Symptoms include neurologic deficits (essentially a dive-related stroke), pneumothorax or pneumomediastinum, hemoptysis, seizures, and total vasomotor collapse.

6. You are on a diving boat when a diver is observed to have a seizure in the water imme-diately after surfacing. You get him on board and find him obtunded but without other focal findings. After assuring his ABCs and while awaiting assistance, what should you do?

Of course in any circumstance like this, the ABCs are the first thing to be addressed. After that, high-flow oxygen, which is felt to reduce the size of air emboli, should be administered. In addition, the patient should be placed in the left lateral (Durant) or feet up (Trendelenburg's) po-sition. This is to try to trap any systemic or venous air bubbles in the right ventricle and prevent their further migration. The use of positioning is controversial and may not be possible on a pitching boat, but it should be considered.

7. You are called to the home of a 36-year-old male who complains of a blotchy rash on his arms and an "itchy" feeling on his arms and thorax. He states that he returned home yesterday after a diving trip. His last dive was two days ago. He observed his dive tables strictly and had no diving complications that he can recall. His symptoms have been pro-gressing over the last day. Is thee any particular facility to which he should be transported?

Absolutely. He needs a recompression, or hyperbaric oxygen (HBO), chamber. Most cases of Type I DCS present 36 hours after symptoms develop. Whether this is due to lack of recogni-tion, denial of symptoms, or other factors is not known. Unless there are other contraindicating circumstances, any diver who presents with complaints that could be considered DCS should be transported to an HBO facility.

8. So how deep is deep? How deep does a diver have to go to place himself at risk for DCS or AGE?

Unfortunately, not very deep. Cases of AGE have been reported in 12 feet of water. Although the dive tables used by most SCUBA divers have been around for many years and were worked out by the Navy, they are not absolutes. Divers can still get the bends, despite staying within dive profiles. Also, the increased use of dive computers, which provide an ongoing calculation of ni-trogen absorbed and have variable integrated profiles, may increase the risk of DCS.

9. I'm in a remote location and am getting a diver with the bends ready to transport to a recompression facility. Anything special I need to do?

Assuming the patient is going by aircraft, further depressurization should be avoided at all cost. The aircraft should be capable of full pressurization (1 atmosphere) or should fly no higher than 1000 feet above sea level. Endotracheal tube and Foley catheter cuffs should be inflated with saline so that they do not compress with HBO. Consultation with the Divers Alert Network (DAN), (919) 684-8111, is recommended.

10. I've heard that free divers can't get the bends. Is this true?

Yes. Free divers, or breath-holding divers, are not at risk for DCS because they are not ab-sorbing increased levels of nitrogen. They are not immune to barotrauma, however, which can lead to AGE if a pneumothorax occurs. Also, "free-diving blackouts" can occur, in which hyper-ventilation before a dive leads to a hypoxic syncopal event as the blood oxygen level falls during the dive.

11. What can I do to dive safely myself or to advise others how to dive safely?

First and foremost is to be properly trained in the type of diving you are going to do. Second is be familiar with all your equipment. Avoid overexertion during the dive. Avoid excess alcohol the night before the dive, and never dive while drinking alcoholic beverages. Dress appropriately in gear that minimizes temperature extremes. Always dive with a buddy. Review emergency pro-cedures before the dive: hand signals, location of spare regulators, dive profile, and backup plans.

Plot your dive profile within the parameters allowed by tables or your computer. Remember: Any diver can abort any dive for any reason at any time. If you think you might have the bends, contact medical assistance as soon as possible.

BIBLIOGRAPHY

1. Degnen CJ: Barotrauma. In Harwood-Nuss AL, Linden CH, Luten RC, et al (eds): The Clinical Practice of Emergency Medicine, 2nd ed. Philadelphia, Lippincott-Raven, 1996, pp 1479–1480.
2. Degnen CJ: Decompression sickness. In Harwood-Nuss AL, Linden CH, Luten RC, et al (eds): The Clinical Practice of Emergency Medicine, 2nd ed. Philadelphia, Lippincott-Raven, 1996, pp 1480–1482.
3. Dickey IS: Barotrauma. In Rosen P, Barkin RM, et al (eds): Emergency Medicine: Concepts and Clinical Practice, 3rd ed. St. Louis, Mosby, 1992, pp 985–993.
4. Kizer KW: Scuba diving and dysbarism. In Auerbach PS (ed): Wilderness Medicine: Management of Wilderness and Environmental Emergencies, 3rd ed. St. Louis, Mosby, 1995, pp 1176–1208.
5. Linden CH, Renzi FP: Venous air embolism. In Harwood-Nuss AL, Linden CH, Luten RC, et al (eds): The Clinical Practice of Emergency Medicine, 2nd ed. Philadelphia, Lippincott-Raven, 1996, pp 1486–1488.
6. Stewart CE: Barotrauma and diving emergencies. In Stewart CE (ed): Environmental Emergencies. Baltimore, Williams & Wilkins, 1990, pp 336–360.
7. Viner BL: Arterial gas embolism. In Harwood-Nuss AL, Linden CH, Luten RC, et al (eds): The Clinical Practice of Emergency Medicine, 2nd ed. Philadelphia, Lippincott-Raven, 1996, pp 1477–1479.

20. WILDERNESS EMERGENCY MEDICAL SERVICES

Jonathan D. Apfelbaum, M.D.

1. What is the difference between wilderness emergency medical services (EMS) and urban EMS?

The remote location of wilderness EMS from resources, the challenges of terrain, the extended time that a victim may be cared for while awaiting and during a rescue, and the wide spectrum of incidents that may occur. Wilderness EMS is a blend of emergency medicine training and outdoor wilderness skills.

2. How are wilderness emergency medical technicians (WEMTs) different from regular EMTs?

The Department of Transportation develops and updates the EMT curriculum. This is the standard to qualify for the National Registry or individual state exams. Passing such an exam certifies the EMT as a state or National Registry EMT. No national standard for WEMT exists. Based on the recommendations of the Wilderness Medical Society and several other groups, however, a similar curriculum for wilderness care at an EMT level exists. A WEMT course includes 100 hours of class time and 10 hours of emergency department time in an EMT course, plus an additional 48 to 80 hours of training. This added course work focuses on the expanded requirements for prolonged extrication, special equipment, extended patient care, and injuries unique to the backcountry setting.

3. What procedures can be performed by WEMTs?

It depends on their level of training and the system in which they operate.

All prehospital providers are bound by the protocols and standards under which they practice. Different states and health care systems have a variety of policies regarding what health care providers may and may not do given their level of training. All health care providers should know the standard of care for their level of training, what procedures may be performed, and the protocols and policies of their system.

Currently, key elements in WEMT training include technical skills and authority (so long as the WEMT is working in a system with established protocols) to perform the following.

- Airway management, including endotracheal intubation.
- Shock management, including intravenous therapy
- Use of military antishock trousers (MAST), although this is currently experiencing decreased use and popularity.
- Oxygen administration.
- Medication administration, including epinephrine for allergic reactions; antibiotics for certain circumstances (controversial); acetazolamide, nifedipine, and furosemide for altitude sickness; and pain medications for injuries.
- Field rewarming techniques.
- Field reduction of dislocations and splinting.

4. Are the standards for wilderness and mountain rescue teams different around the world?

In the United States, most teams are volunteer, with a wide range of qualifications and skills. In Europe, most teams are full-time professionals, with greater training and subject to more standards. In many parts of the world, especially wild or remote areas, organized and available rescue teams do not exist at all, and expeditions must be self sufficient.

5. What questions must be answered when assembling a team and preparing for a rescue?
- What time of day is it and will it be? (Are you prepared for a night rescue?)
- What are the weather conditions, and are you prepared for them?
- How long ago did the accident occur?
- What are the injuries?
- How many victims?
- How many people are in the victim's party?
- How well prepared are they?
- Does anyone in the party have medical experience or training?
- Do you have a location, or is this a search and rescue?
- Is a "hasty" team (a smaller, less equipped team sent ahead to provide initial care or to search and rescue while the main team prepares and follows) needed? Have they left yet?
- Are all team members prepared?
- Are all team members trained for this type of rescue?
- Who is on the medical team?
- Who is on the evaluation team?
- Is the team equipment organized and divided up adequately?
- How urgent is the situation?
- Is a helicopter needed or available?
- Is the weather adequate for air rescue?
- Will multiple agencies be involved?
- Are communications coordinated between the different agencies?

6. Who is responsible for mountain search and rescue? How is this done?
- Search and rescue (SAR) is the responsibility of national and state parks, sheriffs, or state conservation officers, depending on the state or park. National and state parks do not have a "duty to rescue," however.
- As mentioned in question 4, most rescues are done by volunteer groups.
- 90% of rescues are done by foot.
- 95% of rescues happen without physicians present.
- Only Yosemite and Grand Teton National Parks use helicopters extensively.
- Only Denali National Park uses fixed-wing aircraft extensively and helicopters occasionally.
- Only Yosemite, Grand Teton, and Mount Rainier National Parks have rangers specifically trained in technical rescues, advanced medical care, and helicopter operations.
- Many backcountry and climbing areas are outside parks. Rescues in these areas are by local fire and rescue departments, with or without the benefit of special training or technical skills.

7. What special knowledge is needed for mountain search and rescues?
- Understanding equipment used in SAR operations (ropes, slings, carabiners, harnesses, helmets, litters, litter harnesses, haul systems, and litter patient packaging equipment), including their maintenance and care.
- Basic radio communication.
- Basic helicopter operation and procedures.
- Understanding of search and rescue procedures.
- Knowledge of the Incident Command System and its use in SAR.
- Basic rope handling and knot tying skills.
- Advanced skills as needed for specific circumstances, including water SAR, white-water rescue, avalanche SAR, technical or vertical (rock) techniques, or cave training.

8. What are some examples of circumstances likely to be "extended rescues"?
Mountain, wilderness, rural, white-water, air-sea, cave, and avalanche rescue, as well as expedition and disaster medicine and most search and rescue missions. The terms "extended rescue" and "extended emergency care" refer to medical care and rescue efforts beyond the first, or "golden," hour.

9. What government agencies are responsible for search and rescue?

The Aerospace Rescue and Recovery Service operates the Air Force Rescue Coordination Center (AFRCC). This is the federal agency responsible for coordinating SAR activities in the continental United States. All states have legislation that provides support to local governments during emergencies; however, only 22 of the 50 states have a state agency responsible for coordination and SAR support. AFRCC coordinates efforts with the Civil Air Patrol (CAP), Military Assistance to Safety and Transportation (MAST), and other federal resources. The State SAR Coordinator works with AFRCC as well as with state police, the military, and aeronautical resources. The County Sheriff of the jurisdiction involved works locally with the State SAR Coordinator as well as with local independent SAR groups (often volunteer), fire departments, police, and rescue units.

10. What are the four phases of SAR?
- Locate.
- Access.
- Stabilize.
- Transport.

11. How many SAR missions occur each year in the United States?

Specific numbers are not reported. It is estimated that more than 100,000 SAR missions occur annually.

12. What are factors that may cause someone to need to be rescued?

Any one, or a combination, of the following may produce a situation that results in the need to be rescued.
- Improper clothing or footgear.
- Fatigue.
- Dehydration.
- Hypo- or hyperthermia.
- Overextension of abilities.
- Lack of physical conditioning.
- Inadequate food.
- Inadequate planning.
- Inadequate leadership.
- Itinerary confusion.
- Inadequate recognition of environmental, physical, or mental factors.
- Inadequate preparation for weather conditions.
- Lack of navigational proficiency (getting lost).
- "Invincible" mind-set.

13. Is an EMS provider who is on a trip liable for care rendered during that trip?

Liability in medicine is full of minefields. Basically, the easiest question is, "Is the provider acting as the trip EMS provider or as a person on the trip who happens to be an EMS provider?" If the provider is the latter, then he or she is not duty bound to assist others in need. If he chooses to help, he is generally protected from liability by the Good Samaritan Law. The Good Samaritan Law provides protection for medical personnel assisting within the scope of their skills, voluntarily, at an emergency scene. If an EMS provider is acting as the trip EMS support, the he is liable to provide care and coverage at the accepted standard of care. In addition, because EMTs and almost all EMS providers act under a physician's license, the doctor under whom the EMT is working is also liable for his actions.

14. What are some unique ethical dilemmas associated with wilderness EMS?
- How much risk will you accept for yourself and your team when planning SAR (e.g., going out in a snowstorm looking for a child)?

- If a rescuer becomes injured, who will you treat first? The original victim or the rescuer?
- If a limited amount of supplies is available, who gets treated?
- How will the care affect others in the group (e.g., leaving divers in the water to get a diver with the bends to a hyperbaric chamber)?
- How do the relationships of people in the group affect their choices for care and decisions regarding the group?

More so than in everyday life, a serious emergency in a wilderness area stresses many aspects of our relationships and our decision-making capabilities. From a survivalistic point of view, it is necessary to take care of ourselves and our teammates before we care for the victim. Many potential circumstances can arise, however. There are an unlimited number of responses to this question. One must think about potential circumstances ahead of time and plan appropriate ways to incorporate a productive reaction to insure the survival of ourselves, our team, and our patients and to deliver care effectively.

15. Where can I get more information about wilderness EMS?

The Wilderness Medical Society: P.O. Box 2463, Indianapolis, IN 46206; (317) 631-1745

BIBLIOGRAPHY

1. Cooper DC, LaValla PH, Stoffel RC: Search and rescue. In Auerbach PS (ed): Wilderness Medicine: Management of Wilderness Environmental Emergencies, 3rd ed. St. Louis, Mosby, 1995, pp 506–534.
2. Henry GL, Stein ER: Medical liability and wilderness emergencies. In Auerbach PS (ed): Wilderness Medicine: Management of Wilderness Environmental Emergencies, 3rd ed. St. Louis, Mosby, 1995, pp 1429–1435.
3. Hubbell FR: Wilderness emergency medical and response systems. In Auerbach PS (ed): Wilderness Medicine: Management of Wilderness Environmental Emergencies, 3rd ed. St. Louis, Mosby, 1995, pp 566–579.
4. Iserson KV: Ethics of wilderness medicine. In Auerbach PS (ed): Wilderness Medicine: Management of Wilderness and Environmental Emergencies, 3rd ed. St. Louis, Mosby, 1995, pp 1436–1446.
5. Klainer PH: Prehospital emergency medical services. In Harwood-Nuss AL, Linden CH, Luten RC, et al (eds): The Clinical Practice of Emergency Medicine, 2nd ed. Philadelphia, Lippincott-Raven, 1996, pp 1517–1520.
6. Stewart CE: Environmental emergencies in the wilderness context. In Stewart CE (ed): Environmental Emergencies. Baltimore, Williams & Wilkins, 1990, pp 375–387.

21. WILDERNESS MEDICAL KITS

Thomas G. Burke, M.D.

1. When assisting at the scene of a wilderness accident or taking part in a rescue, what is the most important initial consideration?

Safety. There is a reason why the person has become the patient. Assess the scene for danger before entering. You cannot be of any assistance and, furthermore, will become a burden if you are injured also.

2. What are some of the important considerations when organizing a wilderness medical kit?

The purpose of the trip and the suspected injuries should begin to tailor your needs. It is then essential to know who will be using this kit and if they will be comfortable with its contents. Certain licenses and certificates are no guarantee that their holder will know how to respond in a back country setting. The terrain and environmental conditions expected to be encountered also should help predict what supplies will be needed. The number of people in the party, duration of the trip, and time expected for evacuation and rescue will help determine the quantity of supplies needed and the extent of field treatment that may be necessary. The size, weight, and cost of the kit must be compatible with the trip's budget and goals. Finally, the kit should be stored in a durable, watertight container that is easily recognizable. Everyone on the trip must know where the kit is located at all times.

3. What should every member of the wilderness party have?

Identification	Rain gear
Multipurpose pocket knife	Ace bandage
Nylon cord	Duct tape
Whistle	Bandanna
Lighter or waterproof matches	

4. What equipment and over-the-counter medication should be included in a general wilderness medical kit?

Equipment

Scissors	Resealable plastic bags
Forceps (Tweezers)	Pencil and paper
Thermometer	Penlight
SAM splint	Scalpel
Stethoscope	Rescue mask
Triangular bandage and safety pins	BP cuff

Wound management materials

Gloves
20-ml irrigation syringe and 18-gauge angiocatheter
Povidone-iodine 10% solution
Alcohol pads
Self-adhesive wound closure strips (butterfly or steri-strips)
Tincture of benzoin
Moleskin

Bandaging materials

4 x 4 sterile gauze dressing	Cotton swabs
Nonadherent sterile dressing	Ace bandage
Cloth tape	Microthin adhesive dressing (Tegaderm)
Adhesive bandages	

Over-the-counter medications
Ibuprofen (Motrin)—analgesic
Acetaminophen (Tylenol)—analgesic
Dyphenhydramine (Benadryl)—antihistamine
Pseudephedrine (Pseudofed)—decongestant
Bismuth solution (Pepto Bismol)—for gastrointestinal upset and diarrhea
Antacid (Mylanta)
Decongestant nasal spray (Afrin)—nasal vasoconstrictor
Antifungal cream (Tinactin)
Hydrocortisone cream 1% for allergic skin reaction
Bug repellent
Sunscreen
Antibiotic ointment (Neosporin)—for cleansed wounds
Meclizine (Bonine)—for motion sickness
Antidiarrheal (Imodium AD)

Items such as intravenous fluids, prescription and advanced cardiac life support medications, litters, and specific rescue gear can be added on an individual basis. IMPORTANT: When carrying any medication into the wilderness, you must know how to use it appropriately. You must be aware of the benefits, side effects, dosage, and the allergy history of the patient.

5. What are good sources of information for customized medical kits for specific settings such as high altitude, white water sports, cold exposure, and tropical travel?

The Wilderness Medical Letter, published by the Wilderness Medical Society, has published a series of articles with detailed suggestions for these areas of sport and recreation. They can be found in the medical section of many libraries or obtained from the society: PO Box 2463, Indianapolis, IN 46204; (317) 631-1745.

BIBLIOGRAPHY

1. Fogerty WW (ed): Wilderness Medical Society Practice Guidelines for Wilderness and Environmental Emergencies. Merrillville, IN, ICS Books, 1995.
2. Tilton B (ed): Wilderness Medicine Handbook, 2nd ed. Pitkin, CO, Wilderness Medical Institute, 1997.
3. Zell SC, Goodman PH: Wilderness equipment and medical supplies. In Auerbach PH (ed): Wilderness Medicine: Management of Wilderness and Environmental Emergencies, 3rd ed. St. Louis, Mosby, 1995, pp 413–445.

22. LIGHTNING

Jonathan D. Apfelbaum, M.D.

1. How many people are killed or injured each year by lightning?

Approximately 150 to 250 people are killed each year, and 800 to 1000 are injured.

2. What are some myths regarding lightning strikes?

- Lightning is always fatal. Actually lightning injuries are fatal in about 30% of victims. (See "rules of 70%" in question #4.) Some of these data were collected before advanced resuscitation measures (such as intubation) were developed, so it is projected that lightning is fatal in less than 20% of cases.
- Lightning turns people into "crispy critters" with severe burns. Lightning rarely causes significant burns, so the victim may be found with few, if any, signs of external trauma.
- Lightning never strikes the same place twice. Lightning loves objects such as tall metal towers. For example, the Sears tower and the Empire State Building are hit thousands of times each year.
- Victims of lightning strike remain "electrified." Not so, but the conditions that led the victim to be struck may continue to exist and, as we just learned, lightning can strike the same place twice.
- The bodies of lightning victims can remain in "suspended animation." Just doesn't happen.
- Lightning injuries are like other high-voltage injuries. Although lightning injuries can be fatal, usually far less energy is imparted to the victim than with regular high-voltage exposure. Therefore, usually far less injury occurs with lightning strikes.

3. What are mechanisms of injury from lightning strikes?

- Direct strike. In this case, the electricity is conducted directly through the victim. It carries the highest rates of death and injury.
- Contact. The victim is touching an object that gets struck (e.g., talking on the phone when the wires are struck).
- Side flash or "splash." Lightning jumps from an object and catches the victim in its circuit.
- Step voltage. The lightning strikes the ground and spreads radially. It enters the victim because of the potential difference created by the resistance between the feet, because one is closer to the strike than the other.
- Blunt, or direct, trauma. The victim is thrown by the strike. Injuries result from implosion/explosion forces along the lightning pathway or from debris or muscle contractions. Burns from clothing or jewelry also occur.

4. What are the "rules of 70%"?

- 70% of people struck by lightning will live.
- 70% will have sequelae from their injuries.
- 70% will be single-victim strikes.
- 70% of strikes occur in the afternoon or evening.
- 70% occur in the summer.

5. How is a mass casualty situation with lightning different from other mass casualty incidents?

In most mass casualty incidents (MCIs), victims who appear dead are deemed low priority, and care is directed at the living. In lightning strike, those who are living will probably recover and are unlikely to die. The major cause of death is cardiopulmonary arrest; with early aggressive

CPR, recovery is possible. Therefore, care is initially directed at resuscitating the dead, in reverse of the standard practice with MCI.

6. Why is lightning different from other high-voltage injuries?

The average lightning strike has 10 to 20 million volts, and the figure may be as high as 2 billion volts. The duration of the shock is very brief, however, only 1/10,000th to 1/1,000th of a second, so much less energy is delivered. Lightning is direct current (DC) as opposed to alternating current (AC). The path of lightning tends to stay along the outside of the victim, vaporizing sweat and moisture, causing the classic "feather burns" and blowing off clothes. A small amount of energy may "leak" internally and cause cardiac arrest, seizure, muscular contractions, or neurologic dysfunction, but it does not cause the extensive tissue destruction seen with AC electrical injuries.

7. What is the worst place to be struck by lightning?

The head. Studies have shown that persons who are struck on the head have two to three times the rate of cardiac arrest and are more likely to die. Metal worn in the hair or on the upper body seems to increase the risk.

8. Is it safe to be in a car during a thunderstorm?

Yes. It appears that the lightning travels around the outside of the vehicle before striking the ground.

9. What sort of long-term damage can lightning victims experience?

Eye disorders, including cataracts; hearing problems, since half the victims have their eardrums ruptured; psychiatric disorders, such as anxiety, depression, post-traumatic stress disorder, and the imagined ability to predict lightning strikes or other delusions; and neurologic deficits, such as balance problems, memory difficulties, or impairment of other functions.

10. Why does a lightning strike cause the heart to stop?

The shock acts as a massive DC countershock, which can depolarize the heart and cause asystole. Muscle dysfunction and respiratory arrest can cause secondary hypoxic cardiac arrest as well.

11. Can lightning strike without a storm?

Unfortunately, yes. The so-called "bolt from the blue" can occur many miles from precipitating weather conditions and may be unpredictable. Fortunately, it is very uncommon.

12. What can be done to decrease the chance of a lightning strike?

Stay indoors or in a car. If outdoors, stay away from high areas where you will be one of the tallest points around. Avoid tall trees or singular sheltering objects, because if they are struck, the lightning could "splash." Take shelter in valleys, hollows, or groves of trees. Metal should be removed from the hair and upper body.

13. Am I safe inside during a storm?

Actually, no. Numerous cases of lightning strikes indoors have been documented, usually when the house or phone line is struck (particularly if the person is on the phone at the time). The charge acts as a "contact" strike and incorporates the victim into the strike. It is a good idea to stay off the phone during a storm.

14. If you are not killed and have no external signs of trauma, do you need follow-up and medical evaluation?

Absolutely. The sequelae listed in question 9 are not limited to those who suffer cardiac arrest. All persons unfortunate enough to have been struck by lightning should have a thorough medical evaluation and follow-up.

BIBLIOGRAPHY

1. Brown DFM, Gross PL: Lightning injuries. In Harwood-Nuss AL, Linden CH, Luten RC, et al (eds): The Clinical Practice of Emergency Medicine, 2nd ed. Philadelphia, Lippincott-Raven, 1996, pp 1491–1493.
2. Cooper MA: Lightning injuries. In Rosen P, Barkin RM, et al (eds): Emergency Medicine: Concepts and Clinical Practice, 3rd ed. St. Louis, Mosby, 1992, pp 979–984.
3. Cooper MA, Andrews CJ: Lightning injuries. In Auerbach PS (ed): Wilderness Medicine: Management of Wilderness and Environmental Emergencies, 3rd ed. St. Louis, Mosby, 1995, pp 261–290.
4. Stewart CE: Electrical injuries: Lightning injury. In Stewart CE (ed): Environmental Emergencies. Baltimore, Williams & Wilkins, 1990, pp 297–306.

23. BITES, STINGS, AND ENVENOMATIONS

Jonathan D. Apfelbaum, M.D.

1. You are with a group hiking in the mountains when one member is bitten by a snake. What do you do?

Keep calm. Leave the snake alone. Examine the victim. The questions to be answered are: Was the snake poisonous? Did it envenomate the victim? What sort of injuries does the person have?

2. How can you tell if a snake is poisonous?

There are two types of venomous snakes in the United States: the Crotalidae or pit vipers, and the Elapidae, or coral snakes. Pit vipers include rattlesnakes, copperheads, and cottonmouths. They are marked by triangular heads, a "pit" looking like an extra nostril, and rattles (on the rattlesnake's tail).

The coral snake is a brightly colored red, black, and yellow ringed snake. The color combination is similar to that of the harmless king snake, which mimics its dangerous cousin as a defense mechanism. The coral snake is red, yellow, and black, as in the saying, "Red on yellow, kill a fellow. Red on black, venom lack."

The site of the bite helps in identification as well. If there are two puncture wounds, that is indicative of fangs and a poisonous snake. Keep in mind that a snake may bite several times or miss with a fang, leaving one or more fang marks.

3. What are the signs of pit viper envenomation?

Swelling at the site of the bite, pain greater than what would be expected, weakness, lightheadedness, nausea, redness at the site, bleeding, decreased blood pressure, shock, diaphoresis, tingling or numbing sensation, chills, and taste changes.

4. So I cut a pair of "X's" over the bite and suck out the venom, right?

Wrong. Suction with mechanical snake bite kits (such as the Sawyer's extractor) can be helpful but needs to be used within the first few minutes. Even then it removes only one third of the venom. Cutting and sucking places the patient at risk for tissue injuries from cutting and places the rescuer at risk from bloodborne exposure, without any demonstrated benefit. Indeed, it is associated with a significant incidence of wound infections and increased injuries and is no longer recommended for the emergency care of snake bites.

Proper therapy is to splint the affected extremity, place the limb below the level of the heart, remove rings or other constrictive devices, keep the patient calm, dress the wound, and evacuate to a medical facility, preferably by litter.

5. What is the grading system for Crotalidae bites?

Grade 0 (dry strike): fang marks without systemic or local effects.

Grade 1 (minimal): local swelling only.

Grade 2 (moderate): swelling progressing beyond the area of the bite with systemic effects.

Grade 3 (severe): marked local swelling of the entire limb or region with serious systemic signs and symptoms.

Grade 4 (very severe): severe systemic symptoms with rapid progression, shock, seizures, or altered mental status.

6. How often does a dry strike occur?

A dry strike means that envenomation did not occur, and this happens about 25% of the time.

7. What if the snake was small or a baby rattler?

Doesn't make a difference. Venomous snakes are born with their envenomation apparatus fully formed and potent.

8. What is significant about Gila monster bites?

The Gila monster is one of only two venomous lizards in the world. It and the Mexican beaded lizard both reside in the Southwest. They deliver venom by chewing and dribbling the venom into cuts. They have a very strong jaw and tend to hang on when they bite. The biggest problem is getting the lizard to let go. Recommendations are to place the affected limb down where the lizard can get its feet on the ground and to pry its mouth open with a stick. There are no proven methods to get it to release. Other techniques have included flaming or killing the animal. Injuries usually are related to the bite, although systemic effects similar to those of mild Crotalidae bites have been described. Treatment is supportive.

9. How dangerous is a scorpion sting?

Most scorpions found within the United States are not significantly dangerous. The exception is the Centruroides scorpion found in Arizona, New Mexico, the Grand Canyon, southwest Colorado, and the California side of the Colorado River. Symptoms of non-Centruroides scorpion stings include local reaction with swelling and pain at the site. Centruroides scorpions, which are small and yellow, may produce systemic effects including pain at the site of envenomation with little local swelling, hyperexcitability, increased salivation, tachypnea, muscle twitching, convulsions, spasticity, and respiratory failure. Stings by Centruroides have been reported to be fatal in 25% of patients younger than the age of five and in 1% of adults. The fatality rate has decreased significantly with advances in medical care. Currently, there is an antivenom available only in Arizona.

10. A surfer accidentally steps on a stingray and is stung. What is the treatment?

Stingray, scorpion fish, stonefish, catfish, oldwife fish, rabbitfish, ratfish, stargazer fish, surgeonfish, toadfish, weaverfish, and stinging sharks are all venomous fish. Fortunately, the poisons are unstable in heat and become nontoxic when exposed to increased temperatures. Symptoms include severe pain at the sting site; pain radiating up the limb; numbness at the puncture site; systemic intoxication with paralysis and problems with vision, speech, and gait; malaise; nausea and vomiting; shock; respiratory depression; and death. Treatment is first to address the ABCs, then place the affected extremity in water heated to 42° Celsius (or as hot as can be tolerated without scalding) for 30 to 90 minutes. Stonefish antivenom is available in some parts of the world. In the United States it is available through Sea World in San Diego, California, and Cleveland, Ohio.

11. A child comes running down the beach toward you, screaming that a shell bit her. She appears agitated and ill and seems to be deteriorating in front of you. What stung her? What is the treatment?

The cone shell is an attractive, colorful mollusk found in Hawaii, Mexico, California, and throughout the Indo-Pacific waters. It is a highly venomous creature with a paralytic poison similar to curare. Symptoms start with burning pain at the site of injection, followed by numbness and blue discoloration around the site. The numbness and tingling spread, particularly around the mouth. Double vision, problems in speaking, blurry vision, itching, nausea, vomiting, and muscle weakness may follow. The paralysis may be incomplete, with only muscle weakness, or may be complete. Symptoms may occur in 10 to 30 minutes. Treatment is supportive, although some texts suggest using hot water, as in question 10.

12. What is the treatment for jellyfish stings?

The true "jellyfish" is only one of three classes of Coelenterates, but their stings are all treated the same, as are the stings of sea anemone and fire coral. Vinegar (acetic acid) should be poured over the site for at least 30 minutes. Alcohol is a second choice if acetic acid is not available. The stingers left on the skin can be removed by applying a drying agent, such as talc, baking soda, or sand. Applying shaving cream and shaving the area has also been found to be effective. The tentacles should not be handled because of the risk of EMS personnel being stung as well. There is antivenom available for the deadly box jellyfish, found in Australia.

13. What happens with Hymenoptera (bees, wasps, hornets, and ants) stings?

Two types of reactions occur. The first, and most life threatening, is the allergic, or anaphylactic, reaction. Information on that type of reaction can be found elsewhere in this book. The second is a toxic reaction, from the venom itself. Depending on the number of stings, symptoms can include pain and swelling at the site, nausea, vomiting, diarrhea, lightheadedness, headache, fever, malaise, muscle spasms, swelling elsewhere on the body, syncope, or seizures.

14. How should a bee's stinger be removed?

Care should be taken not to squeeze the stinger, because the venom sac is still attached and this maneuver may inject more venom. Rather, it should be scraped off the victim as soon as possible to minimize the amount of venom injected.

15. What venomous creature kills the most people per year in the United States?

The bee. Between 50 and 100 people per year die of bee stings.

16. Are tick bites significant?

Yes. Ticks are associated with many diseases, such as tick paralysis, Lyme disease, Rocky Mountain spotted fever, tularemia, Colorado tick fever, and Q fever. The most important thing is to remove the tick completely, making sure that the head and mouth parts are disengaged from the skin. This can be done in a number of ways. Grasping the tick close to the skin and pulling with a slow, even pressure is probably the easiest method. Care should be taken not to jerk or twist the tick, which causes the mouth parts to break off.

17. What are the signs of a black widow spider bite?

The initial bite may or may not be felt. After 10 to 60 minutes, systemic symptoms begin. Fever, nausea, vomiting, headache, lightheadedness, diaphoresis, and difficulty in swallowing may all occur. Abdominal muscle spasm with severe pain may mimic an acute surgical emergency. Facial muscle spasm, tearing of the eyes, photophobia, and swollen eyelids may cause the classic "facies latrodectisima." Treatment is supportive.

18. What is the most common spider bite in the United States?

The jumping, or Phidippus, spider. Fortunately, although rather aggressive, it is not significantly venomous. Local wound care is sufficient.

19. Are tarantulas dangerous?

With the exception of some of the South American and Australian species, the mygalomorphs are not particularly dangerous. They have a short-acting mild venom that causes local symptoms and requires only local care. The South American tarantula, banana spider, red-legged orange-kneed tarantula (if you can see that detail, you are too close), and Australian funnel spider are all considered dangerous. Envenomation can produce severe pain, nausea, vomiting, diaphoresis, salivation, muscle spasms, confusion, dyspnea, coma, cardiac arrest, and even death. There is an antivenom available for the South American tarantula and the funnel spider.

20. What are the odds of being bitten by a shark?

One in five million. If you swim with a buddy, it decreases your risk by half.

BIBLIOGRAPHY

1. Boyer Hassen LV, McNally JT: Spider bites. In Auerbach PS (ed): Wilderness Medicine: Management of Wilderness and Environmental Emergencies, 3rd ed. St. Louis, Mosby, 1995, pp 769–786.
2. Connor DA, Selden BS: Scorpion envenomation. In Auerbach PS (ed): Wilderness Medicine: Management of Wilderness and Environmental Emergencies, 3rd ed. St. Louis, Mosby, 1995, pp 831–842.
3. Curry SC: Black widow spider envenomations. In Harwood-Nuss AL, Linden CH, Luten RC, et al (eds): The Clinical Practice of Emergency Medicine, 2nd ed. Philadelphia, Lippincott-Raven, 1996, pp 1446–1448.
4. Curry SC: Scorpion envenomations. In Harwood-Nuss AL, Linden CH, Luten RC, et al (eds): The Clinical Practice of Emergency Medicine, 2nd ed. Philadelphia, Lippincott-Raven, 1996, pp 1465–1467.
5. Dart RC, Sullivan JB: Crotalid snake envenomation. In Harwood-Nuss AL, Linden CH, Luten RC, et al (eds): The Clinical Practice of Emergency Medicine, 2nd ed. Philadelphia, Lippincott-Raven, 1996, pp 1450–1453.
6. Edmonds C: Marine animals that cause trauma. In Edmonds C (ed): Dangerous Marine Creatures: Field Guide for Medical Treatment. Flagstaff, AZ, Best Publishing, 1995, pp 1–54.
7. Edmonds C: Venomous marine animals (stinging). In Edmonds C: Dangerous Marine Creatures: Field Guide for Medical Treatment. Flagstaff, AZ, Best Publishing, 1995, pp 55–162.
8. Gentile DA: Tick-borne diseases. In Auerbach PS (ed): Wilderness Medicine: Management of Wilderness and Environmental Emergencies, 3rd ed. St. Louis, Mosby, 1995, pp 787–812.
9. Iseke RJ: Hymenoptera envenomation. In Harwood-Nuss AL, Linden CH, Luten RC, et al (eds): The Clinical Practice of Emergency Medicine, 2nd ed. Philadelphia, Lippincott-Raven, 1996, pp 1456–1458.
10. Kizer KW: Marine envenomations. In Harwood-Nuss AL, Linden CH, Luten RC, et al (eds): The Clinical Practice of Emergency Medicine, 2nd ed. Philadelphia, Lippincott-Raven, 1996, pp 1461–1465.
11. Minton SA, Bechtel HB: Arthropod envenomation and parasitism. In Auerbach PS (ed): Wilderness Medicine: Management of Wilderness and Environmental Emergencies, 3rd ed. St. Louis, Mosby, 1995, pp 742–768.
12. Stewart CE: Bites and stings. In Stewart CE (ed): Environmental Emergencies. Baltimore, Williams & Wilkins, 1990, pp 160–258.
13. Sullivan JB, Wingert WA, Norris RL: North American venomous reptile bites. In Auerbach PS (ed): Wilderness Medicine: Management of Wilderness and Environmental Emergencies, 3rd ed. St. Louis, Mosby, 1995, pp 680–709.

24. TACTICAL MEDICINE

Randolph N. Royal, NREMT-P, EMT-T

1. What is a tactical medic?

A person assigned to a law enforcement special operations (or SWAT) team. The tactical medic can ultimately reduce mortality and morbidity, reduce line of duty injury and disability costs, and improve the supported agency's posture in liability-prone circumstances. This is done by having preventive medicine strategies in place and good medical care integrated into the tactical operation before an injury occurs.

2. What are the qualifications of a tactical medic?

Tactical medics can be emergency medical technicians (EMTs), paramedics, nurses, and physicians, with the level of qualification being decided by what best meets the team's needs. Many teams use paramedics due to their accessibility, ability to provide advanced airway management, and relatively low cost. EMTs also can be an acceptable alternative in areas in which an advanced life support program cannot be developed. Physicians are highly desirable from a medical standpoint but may lack the field skills of everyday emergency medical services (EMS) providers. Regardless of what level is chosen, the provider must train closely with the tactical team and become an integral part of the team. A medical provider who cannot anticipate the team's actions is a liability to the team; integration and knowledge are essential. Some teams also require the tactical medic to meet the same physical, psychological, and background investigation standards that the tactical officers are required to meet. This is an understandable request since tactical medics are often exposed to the same operationally sensitive material as team members. Many tactical medics are trained through the EMT-tactical (EMT-T) program, a 58-hour training program also known as CONTOMS.

3. Describe the CONTOMS program.

CONTOMS, which stands for counter narcotics tactical operations and medical support, is a cooperative effort between the Department of Defense, Uniformed Services University of the Health Sciences, Department of the Interior, United States Park Police, Special Forces Branch, and the Henry M. Jackson Foundation for the Advancement of Military Medicine. The program was started in 1990 to meet the need for specialized medical training to support tactical law enforcement operations. The goal of CONTOMS is to offer a nationally standardized curriculum, certification process, and quality assurance procedure to meet the needs of EMTs and paramedics who operate as part of a law enforcement tactical team. The program also tracks data to guide the educational efforts so that they meet the dynamic needs of law enforcement and EMS communities.

4. In what types of incidents do tactical medics participate?

All of the activities of his or her team. Tactical law enforcement involves many areas, including hostage takings, barricaded subjects, high-risk service of arrest and search warrants, dignitary protection, and crowd control. These activities take place on street corners, at drug labs, in everyday business, and in housing from the ghetto to affluent neighborhoods. The exact profile of the law enforcement team's missions depends largely on the police department's size, activity level, and demographics of the area the agency serves.

5. Does the tactical medic act as a law enforcement officer?

This varies around the country. On some teams, the medics train and work with the unit for special situations but are specifically designated as medical support; during an incident they will standby at a designated area. As the operation progresses, they will move within sight of or close to the scene and are called in when needed. Other units use the medic as an entry team member but specifically for rapid medical intervention. These medics are not armed but are trained in tactical operations. Finally, some medics are sworn law enforcement officers who are armed typically with a handgun for personal protection during tactical entries. Their main focus is still medical intervention.

6. What is a tactical entry?

A maneuver designed to gain access and enter a possible high-threat incident with little forewarning while being as quick and aggressive as possible to catch a perpetrator off-guard and unarmed. The entry typically is made in a "stack" formation, in which the officers and the medic are lined up in a row. Each officer has a specific duty and responsibility. The medic usually is toward the end of this stack and is carrying a specialized medical pack.

7. Describe the contents of the medical entry pack.

The contents are designed for specialized situations directed toward trauma situations. The pack varies for each team but typically is designed for rapid airway intervention, fluid resuscitation, and emergency wound care. Body substance isolation equipment, such as gloves and masks, also are carried.

8. Explain "cover and concealment."

These terms are used in tactical situations that are important for team safety. In relation to the perpetrator, the officer is "concealed" if he is hidden from view but does not have protection from bullets. An officer under "cover," on the other hand, has the protection of a bulletproof barrier. Bushes are a concealment; a concrete wall is a cover.

9. Describe a "remote assessment."

In a tactical situation, access to a patient may be denied because of a threat, such as a gunman. A remote assessment is done from a place of cover as close as safely possible to the patient. Through the use of binoculars or eyesight a physical exam is done from afar. When possible, verbal information is gathered. Using this information, the medic decides whether a need exists for a tactical entry to extricate the patient to a place of safety for further evaluation and treatment. The risk to team members and the ultimate outcome of the patient are key factors in this decision.

BIBLIOGRAPHY

1. Abbott J, Gifford M: Prehospital Emergency Care: A Guide for Paramedics, 3rd ed. New York, Parthenon Publishing, 1995.

25. HAZARDOUS MATERIALS MEDICINE

Randolph N. Royal, NREMT-P, EMT-T

1. What is a hazardous materials medic?

A paramedic assigned to a hazardous materials (Hazmat) response team who trains and works with the team and is responsible for the team's medical well being and for medical operations at Hazmat incidents.

2. Describe the training of Hazmat medics.

Medics should have a good foundation of regular hazardous materials training and preferably be a certified Hazmat technician as well as maintain their paramedic and advanced cardiac life support certifications. They also should have specific medical training directed at hazardous materials. A number of courses are offered around the country that provide information on advanced medical interventions for these types of incidents and training for the support and rehabilitation of Hazmat teams.

3. What is the Hazmat medic's function on a Hazmat scene?

Although some teams use the medic as part of the Hazmat entry team, it is best that the medic be in a support function with a main concern for the team's safety. The Hazmat medic is a good source for research and information about the medical effects of the chemical that is being dealt with and a ready resource if treatment is needed. The Hazmat medic also should be directly involved in the monitoring of team members in both the preentry and the postentry stages of an incident throughout the duration of the scene. Hazmat medics may be called upon to treat victims of a chemical exposure with specific antidotes that fall within their training.

4. How does the medic monitor Hazmat team members?

Typically the medic will evaluate the initial vital signs, including the pulse, blood pressure, and respirations. They will document the member's body temperature and weight and evaluate the person's overall appearance and condition. This is done before the member puts on protective clothing and enters an area and again upon exiting the area. The information gathered is compared and evaluated and a determination is made by the Hazmat medic on whether the member can reenter the working area or whether the member will need to undergo rehabilitation and rest before reentry. The medic will also keep track of the entry team member's time inside the protective suits, time in the work area, and their self-contained breathing apparatus (SCBA) air pressure and usage. This information is given to the incident commander. (See figure, top of following page.)

5. Where should exposed patients be treated?

It depends on the chemical that is involved, but a scene typically will be set up with a specific structure. The "hot zone" is the actual contaminated area, and entry into this area is limited to members in proper protective clothing who need to enter the area for reconnaissance and mitigation. The size of the hot zone is based on the chemical and its particular hazards. The hot zone has only one entry/exit point. The "warm zone" is the area were team support services are located. Patients will exit the hot zone and will enter the decontamination area located in the warm zone. Once the patients have been decontaminated, the Hazmat medic will evaluate them and treatment can start. If transport is needed, the patient will be moved to a transport vehicle in the outer perimeter known as the cold zone.

Entry Monitoring Flow Sheet

Team Member _____ Date _____ Incident # _____
Incident _____
Chemical Identification _____

Entry #1	Entry #2	Entry #3
Time In _____	Time In _____	Time In _____
Time Out _____	Time Out _____	Time Out _____
SCBA In _____	SCBA In _____	SCBA In _____
SCBA Out _____	SCBA Out _____	SCBA Out _____
In Out 5 Minute	In Out 5 Minute	In Out 5 Minute
BP___ ___ ___	___ ___ ___	___ ___ ___
P ___ ___ ___	___ ___ ___	___ ___ ___
R ___ ___ ___	___ ___ ___	___ ___ ___
Temp___ ___ ___	___ ___ ___	___ ___ ___
Wgt ___ ___ ___	___ ___ ___	___ ___ ___

Example of Monitoring Flow Sheet.

6. Should decontamination be done before medical intervention?

Rescuer safety must be the number one priority. A person who is not properly decontaminated will only complicate the situation, possibly leading to a larger area of contamination and a greater number of injuries. The decontamination process usually involves gross decontamination in contained areas, the removal of clothes, and multiple showers. In some cases, properly protected team members may have to help a patient completely through this process, up to delivery to the Hazmat medic.

7. Are there specific medications that can be given to help exposed patients?

The following medications can be used by a trained Hazmat medic:

1. Cyanide poisoning kits that contain amyl nitrate, sodium nitrite, and sodium thiosulfate.

2. Atropine in large doses for organophosphate (insecticide) and carbamate poisoning.

3. Methylene blue for treatment of methemoglobinemia as a result of nitrate and nitrate exposures.

4. Calcium gluconate for hydrofluoric acid incidents.

5. Pralidoxime for organophosphate poisoning.

6. Tetracaine for chemical exposure to the eyes.

8. Are Hazmat team members involved with long-term medical monitoring?

The Hazmat medic can help coordinate annual physicals for team members, document potential exposures, and keep track of pertinent medical information for each member. It is a good idea to keep a medical record on each member. This up-to-date information should be kept on the Hazmat response vehicle in case a member needs evaluation at a medical facility.

BIBLIOGRAPHY

1. Bronstein AC: Emergency Care for Hazardous Materials Exposure. St. Louis, Mosby, 1988.
2. Stutz DR, Ulin S: Hazardous Materials Injuries: A Handbook for Pre-Hospital Care, 3rd ed. Beltsville, MD, Bradford Communications Corporation, 1992.

26. HIGH-ANGLE RESCUE

Randolph N. Royal, NREMT-P, EMT-T

1. What kind of medical care usually takes place during high-angle rescue (HAR)?

As in any medical emergency, care varies widely based on the patient's injuries. Mechanism of injury, weather, life hazards, access, and extrication circumstances all enter into how a patient can be managed most effectively. HAR involves everything from rescuing stranded victims with no injuries to fall victims with multisystem trauma. Just as the entrapped victim of a motor vehicle accident will receive care based on access, length of extrication, severity of injuries, and other factors, the same considerations come into play when planning for the care of the HAR victim. For instance, certain decisions are required when considering the care of a person who has fallen from the roof of a two-story building and has received multiple fractures, a possible head injury, and internal injuries and requires transport to a trauma center 12 minutes away. However, when the victim is half a mile up a rocky trail at the bottom of a steep 200-foot slope, just gaining access to the patient is a challenge and planning for efficient care presents an entirely different set of problems.

2. What type of medical equipment is used in HAR?

When the patient is in an area that requires extended off-trail hiking or climbing, the amount of equipment that can be carried will be limited. It is impractical and unsafe to carry a complete advanced life support (ALS) medical kit, personal safety equipment, and rescue equipment required to perform HAR. Therefore, the paramedic on a rescue tam, in conjunction with a physician advisor, must determine what types of problems are likely to be encountered. In general, a kit should include splints and bandages, angiocatheters, fluids and drip sets for intravenous therapy, blood pressure cuff, a stethoscope, warm and cold packs, a pocket mask, and limited medications. Saline or heparin locks can help to avoid having an IV bag and tubing hanging from the litter during extrication through brush and trees.

3. Why is no advanced airway or other ALS resuscitation equipment necessary?

As in any EMS situation, safety of the rescuers is top priority. Most HARs preclude the use of bag-valve-masks (BVM) or doing chest compressions due to terrain. It is accepted standard of care to stop cardiopulmonary resuscitation while moving a patient up or down stairs; extricating a patient down a rock face or steep trail is equally ineffective and, if attempted, places the rescuers at undue risk. A victim who might survive injuries that were sustained in close proximity to a trauma center may not survive the same injuries if they were received in a more remote area.

4. What medications are useful?

- Morphine and diazepam (Valium) for the management of pain and seizures.
- Droperidol (Inapsine) for combative head injuries.
- Epinephrine for allergic reactions to bites and stings and naloxone (Narcan) if you are going to use morphine.

5. Is there medical training outside the traditional EMT-P (paramedic) curriculum that would be beneficial?

Advanced training for orthopedic injuries, such as for the reduction of fractures and dislocations, would be helpful in rescues requiring lengthy extrications. Use of helicopters to extricate victims from remote areas will reduce transport times, and the HAR paramedic should be familiar with procedures for safe air operations. Wilderness medical courses that stress the care of exposure and the considerations necessary for lengthy rescues would also be good preparation.

6. Is all of this necessary for a paramedic, even a HAR paramedic, who works in a large metropolitan area?

Most urban centers are surrounded by and contain areas of unpopulated and undeveloped land. As the population continues to grow, more people are moving outdoors for recreation. Even the rescue of an uninjured climber can take one to two hours, and the complications increase exponentially if the victim is injured. These types of injuries can occur even in the largest cities.

BIBLIOGRAPHY

1. Abbott J, Gifford M: Prehospital Emergency Care: A Guide for Paramedics, 3rd ed. New York, Parthenon Publishing, 1995.

XI. Clinical Care

27. DECISION-MAKING AND CRITICAL INTERPRETATION OF VITAL SIGNS

David Bobes, EMT-P, and Vincent J. Markovchick, M.D.

1. Why is knowledge of vital signs important?

The accurate taking of, and critical interpretation of, vital signs is paramount in determining patient status and triage.

2. What are vital signs?

Besides being the measurements of heart rate, blood pressure, respiratory rate, and temperature, vital signs are the patient's declaration of bodily function during or after insult or illness. Remember that *vital* means "contributing to, or essential for life." Vital signs alone can often determine the patient's status with or without a proper history, mechanism of injury, or the patient's own verbalization of a chief complaint.

3. How is a patient's temperature taken in the field without a thermometer?

Determining an exact temperature in the field is impractical when managing a critical patient. The important factor is to touch the patient. Skin temperature and characteristics can reveal the patient's perfusion status. For example, a patient who has cool moist skin could be volemic or in cardiogenic shock. The patient who feels warm and dry could be in septic or neurogenic shock. When transporting patients who receive blood products during transport, it is essential to have an accurate thermometer to monitor possible allergic reactions.

4. Why should mental status be discussed in a chapter on vital signs?

Mental status is the culmination of the function of organs in the body. The brain is very sensitive to disruption of its environment. Mental status changes should serve as a red flag to the prehospital provider. Once any changes are noted, the provider should rapidly secure the cause of the alteration, whether medical or traumatic.

5. What are some of the mental status changes to look for?

Lethargy, confusion, agitation, syncope, question repetition, unconsciousness, and others.

6. What are normal vital signs?

Average Vital Signs by Age

AGE	PULSE	RESPIRATIONS	BLOOD PRESSURE
1 year	80–140	30–40	82/44
5 years	70–116	20–26	90/52
10 years	70–116	15–20	100/60
Adult	60–100	12–20	120/80

7. Are there any age-specific problems with vital signs?

Yes. Children have a greater cardiac reserve than adults and are less likely to exhibit expected vital sign changes until compensation is nearly exhausted. On the other end of the spectrum, manifestations of vital sign changes takes longer for the geriatric patient and even may never occur.

8. How do medications affect vital signs?

Especially in the elderly, many medications, such as antihypertensives, beta-blockers, calcium channel blockers, and antiarrhythmics, may inhibit certain mechanisms of response within the body. It is important that the provider appreciates the actions of prescription medications and anticipates their effect on the body.

9. When are normal vital signs not normal?

When the patient is beyond the stage of compensation for his or her illness or injury, e.g., a blunt trauma patient with splenic involvement that is no longer tachycardic, or the acute asthmatic that no longer presents tachypneic and now has a "normal" respiratory rate. This period represents a time of imminent precipitous decompensation to the patient. The prehospital provider must recognize the patient at risk and intervene immediately and aggressively.

10. What are some of the vital sign abnormalities to look for?

Tachycardias that have no apparent explanation, traumatic bradycardias, hypertension, hypotension, and orthostatic vital sign changes in the suspected hypovolemic patient. Orthostatic vital signs are not to be attempted on a *known* hypotensive patient or a patient with suspected vertebral fracture. Diaphoresis, pallor, and cyanosis all testify toward the signs and symptoms of shock. Tachypnea, hyperpnea, and sudden unexplainable mental status changes all require further investigation. All vital sign changes from the accepted normal limits require an explanation.

11. When should vital signs be included in the physical exam?

As soon as practical. Baseline functions should be recorded, and abnormal vital sign findings should be an indication for serial assessments to determine if intervention is achieving the desired effect. However, vital sign acquisition should never take the place of critical intervention skills when they are indicated.

12. What is the fifth vital sign?

Pulse oximetry. If the emergency medical services provider has the capability of pulse oximetry, it should be used in patients who display abnormal vital signs, appear seriously ill/injured, or have respiratory complaints of dyspnea or chest pain. Nevertheless, a pulse oximeter reading alone does not offer satisfactory data to determine critical intervention. For example, a reading of 82% in the emphysemic patient that has no respiratory distress may not be an indication for intubation. However, the normally healthy adolescent with a pulse oximeter reading of 93%, a stab wound to the chest, and complaints of shortness of breath may need aggressive airway intervention. Pulse oximetry does possess unique qualities of which the provider must be aware. The unit cannot distinguish hypovolemia. The reading only indicates if the remaining volume is adequately oxygenated. Vasoconstriction for a multitude of reasons will give a false reading, especially in hypothermic patients. Carboxyhemoglobin will not register on the oximeter unit; therefore, it is important to treat patients who are symptomatic after CO exposure. Patients wearing fingernail polish will not register a true reading. Pulse oximetry should not replace judgment; it is just another tool to aid data collection. It is crucial to look at all information to develop appropriate treatment intervention.

13. What other considerations are important?

Vital signs are a matter of interpretation. If the findings are questionable, they should be repeated immediately; if they are abnormal, they should be repeated as soon as possible. Blood pressures of suspicion should be taken in the opposite arm. Inconsequential vital sign changes may be a response to stimuli and should return to normal with minimal intervention in a brief time (i.e., a sympathetic nervous system response after a minor traffic accident resulting in a brief tachycardia, or a hyperventilating patient after an emotional plight). If the findings do not return to normal, the provider must offer an explanation. Equipment failure is another consideration that cannot be ruled out in the field.

14. What effect does improper sphygmomanometer cuff size have on blood pressure readings?

If the cuff is too small it will give a falsely elevated reading, and if it is too large it will give a falsely low reading.

15. Are there any absolute "dont's" concerning vital signs?

Don't ever estimate vital signs! The acquisition of vital signs is a simple act that requires little time. The importance of an accurate set of vital signs must not be underestimated. There are no excuses to allow for patient vulnerability.

BIBLIOGRAPHY

1. American College of Surgeons Committee on Trauma: Advanced Trauma Life Support, 5th ed. Chicago, IL, ACS, 1993.
2. Bates B: A Guide to Physical Examination and History Taking, 6th ed. Philadelphia, J.B. Lippincott, 1995.
3. Berk WB: Emergency Medicine Handbook, 2nd ed. Detroit, MI, Detroit Receiving Hospital/University Health Center, 1992.
4. Campbell JE: Basic Trauma Life Support, 2nd ed. Englewood Cliffs, NJ, Prentice-Hall, 1988.
5. Marokovchick VJ, Pons PT, Wolfe RE (eds): Emergency Medicine Secrets. Philadelphia, Hanley & Belfus, 1993.
6. Rosen P, et al (eds): Emergency Medicine: Concepts and Clinical Practice, 4th ed. St. Louis, Mosby, 1997.
7. U.S. Department of Transportation: Emergency Medical Care: A Manual for the Paramedic in the Field. Washington, DC, U.S. Government Printing Office, 1983.

28. THE PREHOSPITAL PHYSICAL ASSESSMENT

Susan Bobes, M.D., and David Bobes, EMT-P

1. What do soccer and the prehospital assessment have in common?
Nobody wants to touch the object in play with their hands.

2. What is the purpose of the physical exam?
The goal of doing a "hands-on" physical exam is to identify immediately any potentially life-threatening illness or injury. It also helps to provide an objective database on which to establish treatment priorities. A good physical exam plus a well-taken history are the essential elements in making an initial diagnosis.

3. How is the physical examination performed?
It is important to remember that prehospital providers function as the eyes, ears, and hands of the physician. Critical to the task is performance of inspection, palpation, and auscultation of the patient in an organized format.

4. What are the primary components of initial patient evaluation?
The first steps in physical assessment of an injured or ill patient are easily remembered as:
A Airway and ventilation
B Breathing and oxygenation
C Circulation/hemorrhage control
D Disability or neurologic status
E Exposure
These steps should be rapidly assessed in every patient in an organized manner.

5. When should intervention supersede completion of the assessment?
When a life threat is identified during initial assessment, management should begin immediately. Only critical intervention skills should be performed. For example, if a patient has an obstructed upper airway, this should be corrected immediately by suction, insertion of a nasal or oral airway, or intubation. Once this intervention has been accomplished, the initial survey of the patient should continue until completed.

6. How do vital signs fit into the physical exam?
Initial vital signs (i.e., pulse, blood pressure, and respiratory rate) are essential in evaluating the breathing and circulation portions of the initial assessment.

7. What do I do when my initial survey is finished?
If no life threats are identified in the initial survey, a more thorough examination can ensue. This includes a hands-on head-to-toe assessment.

8. Do I always have to complete a head-to-toe exam?
No. When a patient is able to talk and give a chief complaint, it may be appropriate to do a focused exam. A focused exam is only appropriate for minor injuries or illnesses. An example would be a patient with an isolated ankle injury from sports play. If the history or the mechanism of injury suggests that there could be underlying injury or illness, however, a more detailed exam should be performed.

9. What is the purpose of a detailed exam?

The detailed exam is performed to identify potential signs of disease that might otherwise go undetected. It should be accomplished in a concise, organized manner so that nothing is missed or forgotten. This is where inspection, palpation, and auscultation come into play. Physical exposure of the patient is key to completing inspection. Missing a stab wound sure could be embarrassing, not to mention life threatening. Palpation is important to determine possible injury that could be masked by something more painful. Auscultation of the lungs could differentiate between upper and lower airway obstruction.

10. How does the physical assessment differ for the critical patient?

Good question. In the serious medical or critically injured patient, the completion of the secondary exam may not be possible. Management of the life threat takes priority. Time should not be squandered on scene completing the detailed exam once the patient at risk has been identified. Completion of the detailed exam should occur en route to the hospital after the life threats have been stabilized.

11. When is the physical assessment unreliable?

In any patient who has altered mental status or a distracting painful injury (e.g., femur fracture or who has ingested drugs or alcohol).

12. What other tools do I have to help with physical assessment?

For the trauma patient, accurate assessment of the mechanism of injury may predict potential patient injury. Mechanism alone should determine the level of resuscitation in the patient who is unable to provide a chief complaint or indicate a pain response. A complete history including environmental factors (i.e., temperature, surrounding hazards, medicines) is also invaluable in complementing the prehospital exam.

13. Is making a diagnosis that important?

Absolutely not. A diagnosis is nice, but the most important principles are that a thorough history and physical are performed and that appropriate patient intervention is accomplished. If the diagnosis is not obvious, presupposition of the patient's condition should not be conveyed to the receiving facility. This information could mislead triage or delay making a definitive diagnosis.

14. When does physical assessment stop?

Never. Constant reassessment is a crucial element in determining the patient's ongoing status. Diligent appraisal of the ABCs should avert potential mishaps. Changes in the patient's condition should be relayed to the receiving facility. A high index of suspicion is essential to providing quality prehospital care.

BIBLIOGRAPHY

1. American College of Surgeons Committee on Trauma: Advanced Trauma Life Support, 5th ed. Chicago, IL, ACS, 1993.
2. Bates B: A Guide to Physical Examination and History Taking, 6th ed. Philadelphia, J.B. Lippincott, 1995.
3. Campbell JE: Basic Trauma Life Support, 2nd ed. Englewood Cliffs, NJ, Prentice-Hall, 1988.
4. Markovchick VJ, Pons PT, Wolfe RE: Emergency Medicine Secrets. Philadelphia, Hanley & Belfus, 1993.
5. Rosen P, et al (eds): Emergency Medicine: Concepts and Clinical Practice, 4th ed. St. Louis, Mosby, 1997.
6. U.S. Department of Transportation: Emergency Medical Care: A Manual for the Paramedic in the Field. Washington, DC, U.S. Government Printing Office, 1983.

29. ELECTROCARDIOGRAM INTERPRETATION

Jedd Roe, M.D., and Michael Taigman, EMT-P

1. What is an electrocardiogram?
An electrocardiogram (ECG) is a graphical recording of cardiac electrical activity.

2. Is ECG interpretation best done in the emergency department?
Yes and no. The emergency department has the advantage of a controlled environment and ready access to 12-lead ECGs, but many abnormal heart rhythms cause serious symptoms, can be recognized on a cardiac monitor, and require immediate prehospital management. The important point is not to get so wrapped up in analyzing the ECG that the patient's symptoms are ignored. Patient assessment remains the foundation on which rhythm management must be based.

3. Electrical activity of the heart sounds complex—where do I start?
At the beginning. Most cardiac tissue is composed of muscle fibers, which, when stimulated by an electrical impulse in a process called depolarization, contract in an organized fashion. This electrical impulse comes from the second type of cardiac tissue, which is a specialized group of cells called pacemakers. These cells have two special properties. First they initiate depolarization, and then they automatically begin recharging so that depolarization can be induced again. The electrical impulse generated by pacemaker cells is conducted through the heart by a specialized conduction system, and the integrity of this system is important for producing a coordinated contraction of the atria and ventricles.

4. Where does electrical activity begin?
A normal cardiac impulse originates at the sinoatrial (SA) node located in the right atrium. The SA node usually discharges at a rate of 60–100 times per minute, and the impulse is conducted down a series of internodal pathways to the atrioventricular (AV) node, which lies near the junction of the atria with the ventricles. Here the impulse is delayed to allow the atria to contract and augment ventricular filling with blood. This delay usually lasts 0.12–0.20 seconds, and conduction proceeds into the ventricular septum via the bundle of His. This bundle divides into right and left bundle branches that conduct the impulse rapidly to the muscle fibers of the ventricles by a series of Purkinje fibers embedded within the ventricular walls. The result is ventricular contraction.

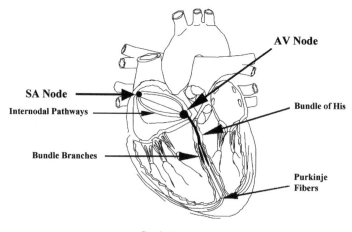

Conducting system.

5. Is the SA node the only pacemaker site?

No. The SA node is the usual pacemaker because it has the highest discharge rate at 60–100 beats per minute (bpm) and thus discharges before the other pacemaker sites can recharge. Other sites, which take over when the SA node fails, include ectopic (distinct from the SA node) atrial sites (40–60 bpm), AV node (junctional) pacemaker (40–60 bpm), and ventricular sites (30–40 bpm). The rates specified for these pacemakers are the inherent rates of the cells, but the sympathetic and parasympathetic (through the vagus nerve) nervous systems may act on the SA and AV nodes to accelerate and slow down cardiac rate, respectively. Drugs and some disease processes also may alter a pacemaker's rate.

6. What does an ECG do?

The ECG is a tracing on a monitor or graph paper as a graph that shows cardiac electrical voltage (y-axis) vs. time (x-axis). The graph paper is comprised of 1-mm squares. As the paper travels through the machine at 25 mm/sec, each square represents 0.04 sec. Voltage is measured in millimeters. Each portion of the tracing corresponds to physiologic electrical activity of the heart.

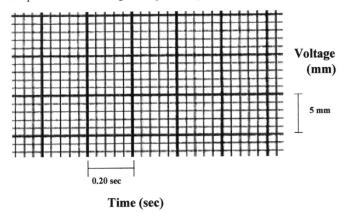

Electrocardiogram paper.

7. What does one physiologic cycle of cardiac activity look like?

The cycle begins with atrial contraction, which is represented by the P wave of the ECG cycle (see figure). The QRS complex occurs with ventricular depolarization, and the T wave follows as an expression of the recharging of the ventricles (repolarization). The QRS is the largest complex and, thus, the easiest starting point. It is defined relative to the baseline. The Q wave is the first negative (downward) deflection from the baseline and may not be present in all tracings. The R wave is the first positive (upward) deflection from baseline, and the S wave is defined as the first negative deflection below baseline following the R wave. If there is a second positive deflection after the R wave, it is described as an R′ wave (R prime). Like the Q wave, the S wave may not be noted in all cases.

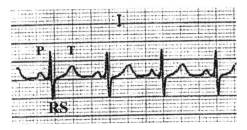

The electrocardiogram cycle.

8. Do the atria also repolarize?

Yes. However, repolarization occurs during ventricular depolarization, and the tracing of atrial repolarization is usually obscured by the higher ventricular depolarization voltages.

9. What other portions of the ECG cycle are important?

The P–R interval is defined as the time from the onset of the P wave to the beginning of the QRS complex (see figure). This interval describes the time delay between atrial and ventricular contraction, and if conduction is slowed by disease or drugs, the P–R interval will be prolonged beyond the normal value of 0.20 seconds. The QRS interval is measured from the first deflection from baseline (a Q wave or R wave) to the end of the S wave (or R' wave). A normal QRS complex is less than 0.12 seconds in duration, and when conduction is pathologically delayed by disease of the septal conducting system, the QRS complex widens beyond 0.12 seconds. The last important interval is the ST segment, which is the segment between the end of the QRS complex and the beginning of the T wave. Elevation of the ST segment is a crucial sign in diagnosing such entities as myocardial infarction or pericarditis. Depression of the ST segment can be seen with ischemia of myocardial muscle, drugs (e.g., digoxin), and thickening of the ventricular wall, which commonly results from chronic hypertension.

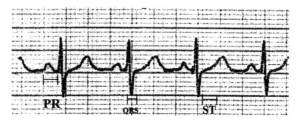

The intervals and ST segment.

10. How do I obtain an ECG from the patient?

First, electrodes are attached to the skin. These patches or metal pads function as receivers transmitting electrical data from the patient to the cardiac monitor through attached cables. The standard monitoring leads are I, II, and III, and electrodes are attached to the right arm, left arm, and left leg. As a wave of positive charges (depolarization) approaches a positive electrode, an upward deflection is recorded, and a downward deflection results as the electrical activity moves away from a positive electrode. The standard leads are represented as follows:

Lead	Positive Electrode	Negative Electrode
I	Left arm	Right arm
II	Left leg	Right arm
III	Left leg	Left arm

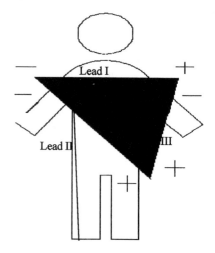

Because of the different electrode positions, each lead gives a view of the heart's electrical activity from a different perspective. In addition, 12-lead ECGs use the limb leads as a common negative electrode and place positive electrodes at 6 sites across the anterior chest. These precordial leads are numbered V_1–V_6, and enable closer examination of the septum and left ventricle.

The standard limb leads. The monitor records electrical activity as it moves toward the positive electrode.

11. Can I get information similar to that from the precordial leads of a 12-lead ECG by using a standard field monitor?

Yes. The addition of modified chest leads (MCLs) to the standard leads offers useful analogs to the precordial leads for the prehospital environment. MCL_1 is one of the most commonly used, and in this case the positive electrode is placed in the fourth intercostal space (level of the male nipple), just right of the sternum, and the left arm acts as the negative electrode. This lead may be particularly useful for identifying P waves and determining whether a rhythm is of ventricular or supraventricular origin.

12. What is axis?

Axis is a term that describes the direction in which depolarization spreads through heart muscle. For reference purposes, the direction of electrical current in lead I is labeled 0°, whereas in lead II the direction is 45° and in lead III 90°. Patterns noted in these leads demonstrate the alteration of axis in certain disease states:

1. **Normal axis.** The QRS complexes are seen to be positive in leads I, II, and III.

2. **Left axis deviation.** The QRS complex is positive in lead I and negative in leads II and III. This pattern is sometimes seen in the setting of myocardial ischemia or enlargement of the ventricular wall due to chronic hypertension.

3. **Right axis deviation.** This pattern generates a negative QRS complex in lead I, whereas the QRS complex of lead III is positive. Right axis deviation is seen in some patients with chronic lung disease and enlargement of the right ventricle.

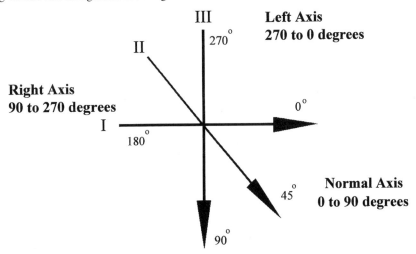

Direction of arrow indicates direction toward positive electrode.

13. What is the most important part of ECG interpretation?

Stay organized. Choose a format for ECG analysis, and use it in exactly the same way for every tracing that you examine.

14. Is there an easy way to organize ECG interpretation?

I like to simplify the process as much as possible. Ask yourself the following questions:

1. What is the rate?
2. Is the rhythm regular or irregular? If it is irregular, is a pattern present?
3. Is the QRS complex wide (> 0.12 sec) or narrow (normal)?
4. Do you see P waves, and are they related to the QRS complexes?

Answering these questions usually allows you to diagnose the abnormal heart rhythms (dysrhythmias) that require prehospital management.

15. How do I calculate rate?

Two methods are commonly used. Most ECG paper has marks on the top every three seconds. Therefore, the rate can be approximated by counting the number of QRS complexes in a 6-second period and multiplying by 10. A more inexact method is to find an apex of a QRS complex aligned with a solid line on the graph paper and to count the big (5 mm) boxes before the identical point of the following QRS. The rate is obtained by dividing the number of boxes into 300.

$\downarrow$ **Time between the hashmarks (arrows) is 6 sec** $\downarrow$

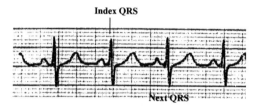

Method 1—Find three hashmarks. Count the number of QRS complexes they contain, and multiply by 10.

Index QRS

Next QRS

Method 2—Count the number of big boxes between the QRS complexes and divide into 300.

Rate calculation.

16. How do I determine whether a rhythm is regular?

First, the pulse corresponds exactly to each QRS complex, and the time between impulses is the same. Rhythm is easiest to measure by comparing the distance between neighboring R waves (R–R interval) at multiple different points of the ECG recording. One also may analyze the distance between P waves. Regular rhythms may originate from all pacemaker sites. When a normal P wave is associated with each QRS complex, the rhythm originates at the SA node and is called a normal sinus rhythm.

17. What if I see an irregular rhythm?

Try to determine whether there is any pattern to the irregularity. Some heart blocks may show irregular patterns that repeat predictably (regularly). Premature beats are the most common cause of irregular rhythms. They may arise from ectopic foci in the atria, junction (AV node), or ventricles. Premature atrial contractions (PACs) show a P wave with a different shape from the normal P wave originating from the SA node. The remainder of the conduction proceeds as usual, giving a normal QRS complex. A premature junctional complex (PJC) originates near the AV node, and conduction moves in two directions, down to the ventricles and up the atria. Because conduction normally goes down the septum and ventricles, the QRS complex is normal, but conduction is reversed through the atria, showing an inverted P wave. Ectopic beats originating from the ventricles, premature ventricular contractions (PVCs), are common. A widened, slurred QRS

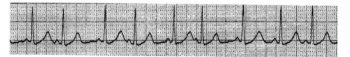

PACS—Note changing P wave morphology

Premature atrial contractions.

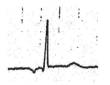

PJC showing inverted P wave

Premature junctional contractions.

complex is seen, which may vary in shape and axis depending on whether the focus is high or low in the ventricle. Typically, a long compensatory pause follows a PVC, as the regular atrial impulse finds the ventricles in an absolute refractory period and conduction stops. The next atrial impulse generally proceeds as usual.

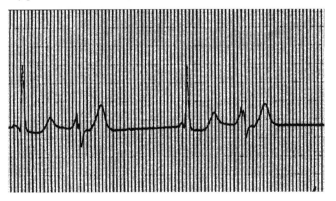

Premature ventricular contraction with compensatory pause.

18. What is the significance of QRS width?

When the normal conducting system from the AV node through the bundle of His to the bundle branches and Purkinje fibers of the right and left side is used and intact, ventricular contraction follows in an organized fashion and produces a normal QRS (duration < 0.12 sec). Impulses may arise in the ventricles below this conducting system. Thus, electrical activity flows more slowly from one working muscle fiber to another. The result is a widened QRS complex (duration > 0.12 sec). This type of QRS morphology also may be seen with sinus or atrial pacemakers when conduction down the bundle of His or individual ventricular conduction bundles is delayed. For example, the typical finding of a right bundle-branch block (RBBB) is a P wave associated with a widened QRS complex showing an RSR′ morphology in lead MCL$_1$, whereas a left bundle-branch block (LBBB) shows an upright widened QRS complex in MCL$_6$.

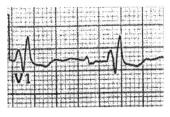

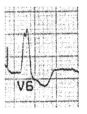

RBBB—Showing RSR′ pattern in V$_1$ (MCL$_1$)

LBBB—Upright QRS complex in V$_6$ (MCL$_6$)

Right and left bundle-branch blocks.

19. Are all P waves the same?

No. We have already seen that differently shaped P waves may occur with PACs. P waves from the SA node are positive when viewed in leads I, II, and III, whereas P waves originating close to the AV node are inverted and seen immediately before or after the QRS complex (e.g., PJCs). Atrial flutter shows sawtooth-shaped P waves with a fast rate of 300 between them. Usually a variable number of P waves precedes each QRS complex, because some are blocked from proceeding; the result is an irregular rhythm. A close relative to atrial flutter is atrial fibrillation, and the pattern can often switch from one to the other. With atrial fibrillation, no organized atrial activity is seen—only a chaotic, disorganized pattern of electrical activity along the baseline between QRS complexes. Ventricular complexes are generated in an irregular fashion because of the chaotic activity in the atria.

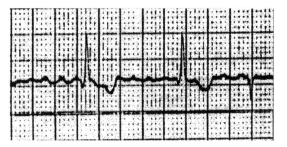

Atrial Fibrillation—Note chaotic baseline

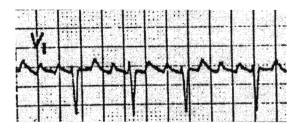

Atrial Flutter—With sawtooth P waves

Atrial fibrillation and atrial flutter.

20. Are all P waves followed by QRS complexes?

Under normal circumstances, yes. Each QRS is preceded by a P wave, and the P–R interval is constant (< 0.20 seconds). In pathologic settings, these characteristics do not hold. A fixed relationship between the QRS and P wave may coexist with a prolonged P–R interval (> 0.20 sec), as seen with first-degree atrioventricular (AV) block. Fortunately, this condition is usually benign, and no specific care is indicated. In other settings, one may see more P waves than QRS complexes. These P waves may be blocked in a regular fashion (e.g., 3 P waves:1 QRS), an irregular manner (ratio varies), or completely blocked, with P waves occurring independently of ventricular depolarization.

21. What dysrhythmias are important in terms of prehospital management?

The easiest dysrhythmia to recognize is asystole, which occurs when no electrical activity is present. The patient is pulseless and unresponsive. One must take care to ensure that the monitor, cable, and electrodes are properly applied. This goal is easily accomplished by verifying the presence of asystole in a second lead.

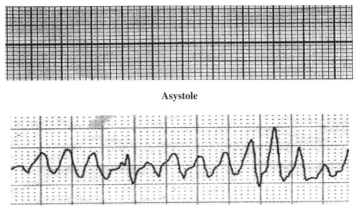

Asystole

Ventricular Fibrillation

Asystole and ventricular fibrillation.

22. What is ventricular fibrillation?

Ventricular fibrillation is defined as chaotic, uncoordinated electrical activity of ventricular muscle fibers. There is no cardiac output, and the patient becomes pulseless and unresponsive. A tracing of ventricular fibrillation demonstrates irregular, chaotic ventricular waves of varying amplitudes (see figure in question 20). Initially the amplitude changes are coarser or greater in magnitude, but with time the changes become finer as the rhythm progresses to asystole. Care must be taken not to confuse this rhythm with artifact seen with patient movement, loose connections, or defective electrodes.

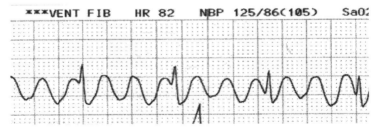

Is it real? Or is it artifact? In this case the patient was moving an arm.

23. What bradycardic rhythms are concerning?

Almost any bradycardic rhythm should be examined closely. Sinus bradycardia shows a regular pattern with positive P waves in lead II associated with each ventricular complex. Although this rhythm may be normal in athletes and younger people at rest, treatment should be considered when accompanied by symptoms suggesting cardiac disease.

24. Can bradycardias arise from other sites?

Yes. If the SA node fails as a pacemaker, automaticity occurs at other (escape) pacemaker sites. After a pause in the underlying rhythm, the escape pacemaker begins an impulse as a protective mechanism against cardiac arrest. If the AV node is the pacemaker site, junctional bradycardia may be seen. This rhythm is generally regular with a normal QRS complex; if P waves are seen, they are inverted in lead II and appear immediately before or after the QRS complex. Another escape rhythm is bradycardia of ventricular origin, also referred to as an idioventricular rhythm. The rhythm is usually regular with a widened QRS complex (> 0.12 sec). Usually, P waves are not present, and hemodynamic compromise frequently results.

25. What are heart blocks?

Cardiac disease may slow conduction through the AV node. The consequence of blocking or partially blocking these impulses is called heart block or, more accurately, atrioventricular (AV) block. AV block usually is classified into three types. First-degree AV block is seen in patients with sinus rhythms who manifest a pronged P–R interval (> 0.20 sec).

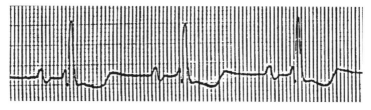

First-degree atrioventricular block.

In second-degree AV block, conduction of a P wave impulse does not occur consistently. The first type of second-degree AV block is a variable block (also known as Wenckebach or Mobitz type I) in which the rhythm demonstrated shows P waves associated with each QRS complex, but the P–R interval progressively increases. Eventually, conduction of the P wave is completely blocked, and a P wave is seen without a following QRS complex. Because the site of blockade is at the AV node, normal QRS complexes are seen, and there is little risk of progression to the more serious AV blocks.

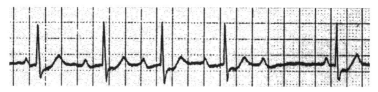

Second-degree variable atrioventricular block.

In contrast, the second type of second-degree AV block, known as fixed AV block or Mobitz type II, presents with a constant ratio of P waves to each QRS complex. The P–R intervals are constant; with 3:1 conduction, for example, two P waves are completely blocked before the third successfully conducts its impulse down the remainder of the conducting system. The site of block may be anywhere in the AV node or septum. The higher up the block, the narrower the QRS complex. Blocks lower in the conducting system are associated with a widened QRS complex and a higher risk that the block will progress to complete AV block or asystole.

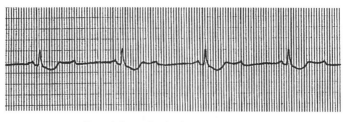

Second-degree fixed atrioventricular block.

Third-degree AV block or complete AV block shows atrioventricular dissociation. In other words, both P waves and QRS complexes are present but show no relationship to one another and P–R interval measurements vary in a random nature. This situation often is unstable, because the patient is bradycardic and often shows signs of hypoperfusion.

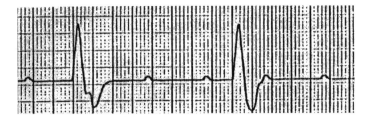

Third-degree (complete) atrioventricular block.

26. What strategy do you use for tachycardic rhythms?

Two important questions influence future management of the rhythm:
1. Is the rhythm regular or irregular?
2. Is the QRS complex wide or narrow?

Irregular tachycardias should make one look for patterns suggestive of atrial fibrillation or flutter, ectopic beats, or tachycardias arising from ectopic foci. Regular tachycardias may arise from the same pacemakers as bradycardic rhythms and have the same characteristics as the slower rhythms from these sites. For example, sinus tachycardia shows the same P wave morphology as sinus bradycardia and a consistent relationship of the P wave to the QRS complex but has a rate over 100 bpm (but usually < 150 bpm). The same is true for tachycardias from junctional or ventricular pacemakers.

27. I see a regular narrow complex tachycardia. What does that tell me?

Because the QRS complex is narrow, the impulse originates from a pacemaker at the AV node or higher in the conduction system (supraventricular). Because the rate is fast, usually over 160 bpm, the P waves of atrial depolarization are obscured by the QRS complexes. Vagal maneuvers may slow the rate so that underlying P wave morphology (sinus, flutter waves, no P waves) may be appreciated.

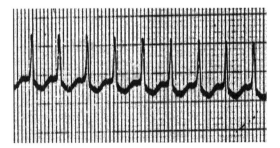

Narrow complex tachycardia.

28. So a regular, wide complex tachycardia means that the impulse originates below the AV node?

Yes, no, maybe! Certainly tachycardia arising from a pacemaker below the AV node can produce regular tachycardia with a QRS complex greater than 0.12 sec duration (see figure). The problem is that a wide complex tachycardia also may arise from a pacemaker above the AV node if a conduction abnormality exists. Most commonly, such conduction abnormalities involve a bundle-branch block or an accessory pathway. An accessory pathway is a conduction pathway between the atria and ventricles in addition to the normal conduction system. If block is present at the AV node, conduction may proceed earlier than expected back to the atria through the accessory pathway. This type of retrograde conduction is responsible for producing wide complex tachycardias of supraventricular origin.

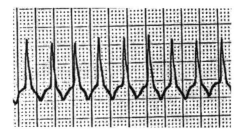

Wide complex tachycardia.

29. How can I differentiate between ventricular and supraventricular rhythms?

First, ventricular tachycardia is more common, particularly in people over the age of 50 and people with a history of cardiac disease. It is commonly thought that patients with ventricular tachycardia appear more ill (e.g., lower blood pressure or altered mentation), but this is not necessarily the case. ECG criteria that may be helpful in distinguishing ventricular tachycardia include a QRS complex greater than 0.14 sec duration and atrioventricular (AV) dissociation, in which P waves may be seen that bear no relationship to the QRS complex.

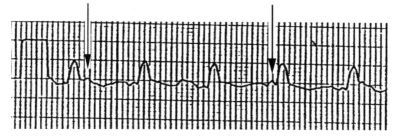

Atrioventricular dissociation. Arrows show P waves that bear no relationship to the QRS complexes.

A fusion beat may be seen when an impulse from the atria arrives at the septal conduction system at the same time as a ventricular impulse, and the resulting QRS complex is a combination of the bizarre, wide ventricular QRS complex and the normal, narrow QRS complex.

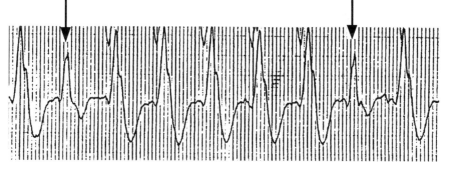

Arrows indicate fusion beats.

Unfortunately, both of these ECG characteristics may not be present in every case. It may then be necessary to examine the QRS morphology in MCL_1 and MCL_6. If the QRS complex shows an R wave greater than 0.03 sec duration or a deep slurred S wave, a ventricular origin is suggested. In MCL_6, a QR or QS complex is suggestive of a ventricular rhythm. In addition, if the axis points toward the right shoulder, as shown by negative QRS complexes in leads I, II, and III, chances are greater that the wide complex tachycardia is ventricular. If MCL_6 is a primarily negative complex, chances are that the patient is in ventricular rather than supraventricular tachycardia.

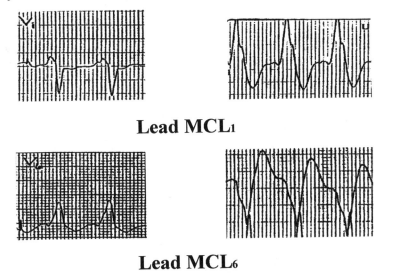

Lead MCL₁

Lead MCL₆

Examples of QRS morphology suggesting ventricular tachycardia.

In contrast, rhythms of supraventricular origin usually demonstrate QRS complexes with a duration of 0.12–0.14 sec and often show an RS complex in one of the MCL leads. The R–S interval is not over 0.10 sec in any MCL lead, and there is no evidence of AV dissociation. Morphology criteria suggestive of ventricular origin are absent.

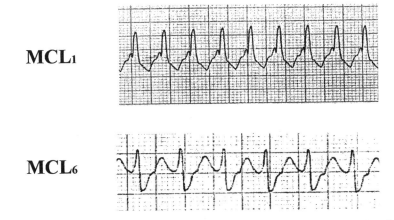

MCL₁

MCL₆

Supraventricular rhythm. Note the absence of morphology criteria suggestive of ventricular origin.

30. Is it important to distinguish between supraventricular and ventricular tachycardia in the field?

No. It is more important to have an effective management strategy for wide complex tachycardia. Effective management, which is examined in more detail in chapter 30, should be based on the probability that a rhythm is ventricular and the need to treat the most emergent cause first.

31. What are artificial pacemakers?

An artificial pacemaker is usually implanted under the skin just below the clavicle. An easily palpable battery is connected to electrode wires that are passed through the subclavian vein to be embedded in the right ventricle. The pacemaker has a sensing device to detect whether the heart is producing an impulse. If no impulse is detected in the required time, the pacemaker fires initiating contraction in the right ventricle. On the ECG, the initial pacemaker impulse is detected as a spike ("pacer spike") that is immediately followed by a wide QRS complex because the impulse began in the right ventricle. Some patients have an atrioventricular pacemaker that demonstrates two pacer spikes on the ECG. One corresponds to atrial contraction, and the other stimulates the ventricles.

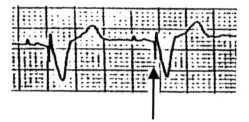

Arrow points to pacer spike.

32. Is a 12-lead ECG useful in the field?

Yes and no. Newer field monitors have the capability of producing a 12-lead ECG. The most useful application of a 12-lead ECG is in the diagnosis of myocardial infarction or ischemia. With the advent of thrombolytic therapy for myocardial infarction, many emergency medical service systems are evaluating this management strategy for field use, and a 12-lead ECG is required to determine whether eligibility criteria for thrombolytics are met. Although the usefulness of thrombolytics in the field is controversial (especially in metropolitan areas with short transport times), a 12-lead ECG still may have a role to play. One of the barriers to administration of thrombolytics in the emergency department is the time that it takes to obtain a 12-lead ECG. If the patient arrives at the emergency department with a 12-lead ECG, thrombolytic therapy may be initiated more rapidly. Most systems find that the use of modified chest leads gives all of the information necessary for field management of myocardial infarction.

33. Can I diagnose myocardial infarction without a 12-lead ECG monitor?

With modified chest and standard limb leads, a paramedic may diagnose the presence of myocardial infarction (MI) or ischemia and its location. The most specific criterion for MI is the presence of ST segment elevation. Its presence in leads II or III suggests an inferior wall MI,

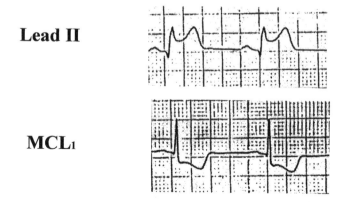

Lead II

MCL_1

Inferior wall myocardial infarction. Note reciprocal change in MCL_1.

whereas elevation in MCL_1–MCL_4 occurs with MI of the anterior wall. Lateral wall MI is suggested by ST elevation in leads I, MCL_5, and MCL_6. In addition, reciprocal changes in the form of ST depression are often seen in the side opposite the infarction. For example, with an inferior wall MI, ST elevation will be seen in leads II and III, whereas ST depression will be noted on the anterior MCL leads.

Lead II

MCL4

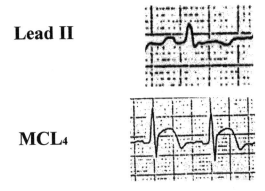

Anterior wall myocardial infarction with reciprocal change in lead II.

BIBLIOGRAPHY

1. Atkins JM: Basic rhythm interpretation. In Pons P, Cason D (eds): Paramedic Field Care: A Complaint Based Approach. St. Louis, Mosby, 1997, pp 181–209.
2. Dubin D: Rapid Interpretation of EKGs, 3rd ed. Tampa, FL, Cover Publishing, 1983.
3. Yealy DM, Delbridge TR: Dysrhythmias. In Rosen P, Barkin R (eds): Emergency Medicine: Concepts and Clinical Practice, 4th ed. St. Louis, Mosby, 1998, pp 1583–1630.

30. ARRHYTHMIAS

Paul Davidson, M.D.

1. What are the first questions to ask in approaching a patient with arrhythmia?
1. Is the patient clinically and hemodynamically stable?
2. Is the rate fast or slow?
3. Are the complexes wide or narrow?
4. Is the rhythm regular or irregular?

2. What is clinical instability?
Physical signs of poor cardiac output such as pulmonary edema, chest pain, obtundation, and diaphoresis.

3. What is hemodynamic instability?
Definitions differ according to various authors, but certainly a systolic blood pressure < 90 mmHg or the absence of a radial pulse are concerning signs.

4. Define a narrow complex tachycardia.
A rhythm that is narrow (< 3 boxes wide or 0.12 sec) and fast (> 100 bpm).

5. Name the common causes of regular narrow complex tachycardia.
Sinus tachycardia, atrial flutter, junctional tachycardia, atrial tachycardias, and reciprocating tachycardias, such as atrioventricular (AV) node reentry tachycardia and Wolff-Parkinson-White syndrome in orthodromic reciprocating tachycardia.

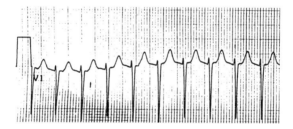

Atrioventricular node reentry tachycardia. Note the absent ("buried") P wave.

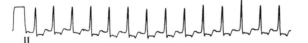

Wolff-Parkinson-White syndrome, going "down the node and up the pathway." Note the inverted P waves.

6. Now name the common causes of irregular narrow complex tachycardia.
Atrial fibrillation, atrial flutter with variable block, and multifocal atrial tachycardia.

Atrial fibrillation. Note the irregularly irregular rhythm.

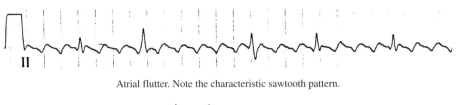

Atrial flutter. Note the characteristic sawtooth pattern.

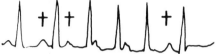

Multifocal atrial tachycardia. Note at least three different P-wave morphologies.

7. Why is it important to establish regularity vs. irregularity?

Because irregular rhythms (and some regular rhythms) are not treatable with adenosine. Patients with an irregular narrow complex rhythm who are stable should be transported. If they are unstable, you should contact the base and prepare to cardiovert the patient.

8. How do you make the diagnosis of atrial fibrillation with a rapid ventricular response?

Sometimes it is obvious from the rhythm strip, and at other times the rhythm strip may look like a regular supraventricular tachycardia (SVT). The diagnosis is easy if you palpate a pulse and simultaneously look at the monitor or auscultate the heart. Atrial fibrillation is the only rhythm that results in an irregularly irregular pulse with varying intensity and a pulse deficit (fewer beats are palpated than are visible on the monitor or heard with the stethoscope).

9. How should a stable narrow complex tachycardia be treated?

Assuming that you have ruled out sinus tachycardia and atrial flutter, use adenosine, 6 mg by rapid IV push, preferably in an antecubital or external jugular vein, followed by a bolus of saline flush.

10. What if adenosine, 6 mg IV, does not work?

Try adenosine, 12 mg by rapid IV push. The success rate of converting paroxysmal SVT is about 60% with 6 mg and over 90% with 12 mg.

11. Why not give 12 mg as the initial bolus?

This is a good idea that more clinicians are using, because 6 mg of adenosine often fails to convert paroxysmal SVT.

12. How does adenosine work?

Adenosine puts the AV node in a "headlock" for about 6 seconds and therefore terminates any arrhythmia that uses the AV node as part of its circuit (i.e., AV node reentry tachycardia or Wolff-Parkinson-White in orthodromic reciprocating tachycardia). It will not convert sinus tachycardia, atrial flutter, or atrial fibrillation.

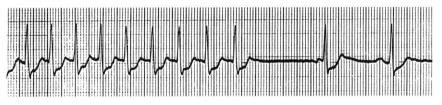

Atrioventricular node reentry tachycardia terminated with adenosine.

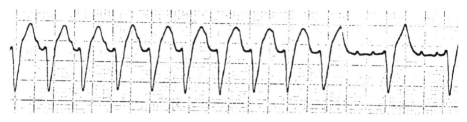

Adenosine uncovering atrial flutter as the cause of tachycardia.

13. What are the three possible outcomes after you push adenosine?
1. Termination of the tachycardia
2. Unmasking of underlying atrial activity (such as atrial flutter)
3. No effect at all. The tachycardia actually laughs at you.

14. What prescription drugs interact with adenosine?
Dipyridamole (Persantine) and carbamazepine (Tegretol) enhance the effect of adenosine, whereas theophylline negates the effects of adenosine.

15. In what group of patients is adenosine relatively contraindicated?
Adenosine causes prolonged bronchospasm in asthmatic patients; in a few cases, it has precipitated respiratory arrest requiring intubation.

16. What if adenosine does not work and the patient is still stable?
Initiate transport and consider IV verapamil, 2.5–5 mg by IV push.

17. What is a wide complex tachycardia?
A rhythm that is wide (i.e., 12 sec or 3 boxes) and fast (i.e., > 100 bpm).

18. What big decision must you make in patients with wide complex tachycardia?
Distinguishing between ventricular tachycardia and SVT with aberrancy.

19. What does *aberrancy* mean?
Abnormal conduction of the electrical impulse from the atria to the ventricles. Examples of aberrancy include right bundle-branch block, left bundle-branch block, or conduction down an accessory pathway, as seen in Wolff-Parkinson-White syndrome.

20. What should you assume that a wide complex tachycardia is?
Assume that it is ventricular tachycardia, which is 6 times more common than SVT with aberrancy.

21. With what must you *never* treat a wide complex tachycardia?
Verapamil or other calcium channel blockers, because they cause cardiovascular collapse in patients with VT.

22. Is the medical history of any value with wide complex tachycardia?
Yes—if the patient has had a myocardial infarction, there is a 98% chance that it is VT.

23. Can you distinguish VT from SVT with aberrancy by vital signs?
No. Both may have stable or unstable vital signs, depending on the patient.

24. Can the heart rate help to distinguish VT from SVT with aberrancy?
No. There is too much overlap between the two.

25. How can you distinguish VT from SVT with aberrancy on a rhythm strip?

A few simple rules make the diagnosis of VT on a rhythm strip:

1. If the width of the complexes is greater then $3\frac{1}{2}$ boxes, it is VT.

2. Atrioventricular dissociation, which is seen as P waves marching through the QRS complexes, is present with VT.

3. A P wave may capture the ventricle at precisely the correct instant, leading to a "capture beat," which looks like a typical PQRST complex in the middle of the wide complex tachycardia.

4. A fusion beat may be seen, which results when the ventricle is stimulated from itself and from the atrium at the same time. Its width is therefore less than a beat originating from the ventricle.

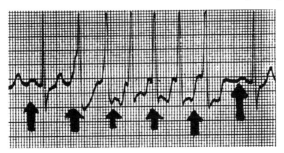

Ventricular tachycardia with visible P waves (evidence of atrioventricular dissociation).

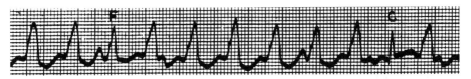

Ventricular tachycardia with a capture beat (C) and fusion beat (F). (From American Heart Association: Textbook of Advanced Cardiac Life Support. Dallas, TX, American Heart Association, with permission.)

26. Are all of the mental gyrations of attempting to distinguish VT from SVT with aberrancy worth the effort?

No. Simply assume that it is VT and treat accordingly.

27. What is the first drug to give a patient with stable wide complex tachycardia? Why?

Lidocaine, 1.5 mg/kg IV, because VT is 6 times more common than SVT with aberrancy. Give up to 3 mg/kg of lidocaine if needed.

28. What should you do if lidocaine does not work and the patient is still stable?

Adenosine, 6 mg by IV push and then 12 mg IV, if needed.

29. What should you do next if adenosine does not work and the patient is still stable?

Simply transport with continuous cardiac and patient monitoring.

30. What if the patient becomes unstable en route?

Synchronized cardioversion is the next step.

31. Besides VT and SVT with aberrancy, what else can cause wide complex tachycardia?

Hyperkalemia, torsades de pointes, and tricyclic antidepressant poisoning should be considered.

32. A patient with stable VT suddenly loses pulses and becomes obtunded. What do you do?

Immediately countershock the patient with 200 joules. If the patient fails to convert, countershock with 300 joules and then 360 joules, if needed. If the patient is still pulseless, start CPR, hyperventilate with 100% oxygen, intubate, and give IV epinephrine (See advanced cardiac life support [ACLS] protocols for dosing.) The ACLS algorithm takes a "drug-shock, drug shock" approach with lidocaine, 3 mg/kg total, and bretylium, 10 mg/kg total.

33. What is the rationale for this treatment approach?

Most successful resuscitations depend on early defibrillation. Epinephrine restores coronary artery perfusion and increases the odds that countershock will restore spontaneous circulation. The use of lidocaine and bretylium in pulseless VT is listed as probably helpful by ACLS, despite the fact that neither medication has been proved to help defibrillate patients.

34. What controversy surrounds the dosing of epinephrine?

ACLS guidelines changed in 1992 to accommodate different dosing regimens. Some physicians argue that the 1-mg dosage (which was extrapolated from animal experiments) is too low and that 0.1 mg/kg is a more appropriate dosage. Another group proposes that an escalating dosage of epinephrine should be used.

35. Is there any practical advantage to giving high-dose epinephrine to patients in cardiac arrest?

No data prove that high-dose epinephrine improves survival or neurologic recovery compared with standard-dose epinephrine. Until such data become available, high-dose epinephrine should not be used routinely.

36. What is asystole? Under what circumstances is it reversible?

Asystole is most often a flat-line confirmation of death rather than a dysrhythmia to be treated. Rarely it results from heightened vagal tone or complete heart block and is potentially reversible.

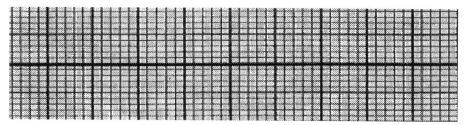

Asystole.

37. When is it necessary to confirm asystole in two leads?

The ACLS authors made this recommendation on the basis of one case report of a patient who was actually in ventricular fibrillation in two of the three leads, although the third lead showed asystole. The author of the case report surmised that ventricular fibrillation may have a vector (direction) and that all cases of asystole should be confirmed in two leads. Others say that this theory is hogwash and that the better reason to confirm asystole in two leads is to be sure that the monitoring equipment and leads are attached properly. You will find many more cases in which leads have fallen off than in which patients have ventricular fibrillation with a vector.

38. Should transcutaneous pacing be tried in all cases of asystole?

Absolutely not. Prehospital research has proved that the chance of reestablishing spontaneous circulation with pacing is very low if the period of asystole is more than 5 minutes. Save pacing for the rare patient who deteriorates from a perfusing rhythm to asystole in front of you.

39. What drugs are recommended for asystole?

After the patient is intubated and IV access is obtained, epinephrine and atropine may be given to help restore circulation, although the likelihood of their success is about the same as the likelihood of Rush Limbaugh joining the Democratic party. Intravenous theophylline has been successful in a few anecdotal cases, but more rigorous study failed to support the incredible success of earlier reports. If the patient remains asystolic after intubation, oxygenation, and ACLS drugs, seriously consider pronouncing the patient dead in the field, thus avoiding needless increased costs to the family.

40. Define absolute and relative bradycardia.

Absolute bradycardia is less than 60 bpm. Relative bradycardia refers to a heart rate above 60 in patients with low cardiac output who may benefit from an increased rate. Both absolute and relative bradycardia may need to be treated according to the ACLS algorithm.

41. When is a pulse of 40–59 bpm considered normal?

In a well-conditioned athlete, this is a normal resting pulse.

42. Bradycardia should be treated under what three circumstances?

1. Symptoms. The simple fact that a patient has a heart rate of 50 does not mean that you should start waving the atropine needle!
2. Mobitz 2 second-degree heart block.
3. Third-degree heart block.

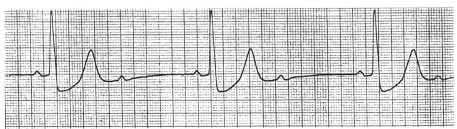

Mobitz type 2 atrioventricular block leading to bracycardia.

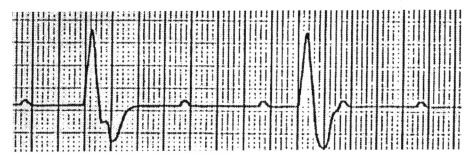

Complete (third-degree) heart block.

43. What is the first-line drug for bradycardia? How does it work?

Atropine exerts a strong anticholinergic effect on the AV node, thus blocking the bradycardic effect of the vagus nerve.

44. When does atropine have no effect at all?

Atropine does not work in heart transplant patients, in whom the vagus nerve has been cut. Epinephrine is the drug of choice in transplant patients. Atropine may worsen bradycardias that result from heart block below the AV node, which seems paradoxical. However, atropine is still a first-line drug for bradycardia. If the ventricular rate decreases after a dose, be prepared to use epinephrine.

45. Why is isoproterenol potentially dangerous for bradycardia?

Isoproterenol has earned a "potentially harmful" designation in the ACLS guidelines because it increases myocardial oxygen demand without increasing myocardial oxygen supply. It is a powerful chronotrope and is used to treat bradycardias, but one must be cautious because it may exacerbate myocardial ischemia. Conversely, epinephrine increases myocardial oxygen demand *and* supply and is a more balanced chronotrope. Dopamine and dobutamine are also acceptable.

46. A patient in third-degree heart block has a few premature ventricular contractions (PVCs). Should lidocaine be given?

No. Lidocaine suppresses the ventricular pacemakers that keep the patient alive.

47. What should I know about transcutaneous pacing?

Arrange the pads just left of the sternum in front and the spine in back. Most patients will capture with less than 70 milliamps. Capture may not occur in patients with big chests, chronic obstructive pulmonary disease, dilated cardiomyopathies, and pleural or pericardial effusions. It is proven therapy for bradycardia, as opposed to drugs that may have downsides, such as atropine and isoproterenol. Benzodiazepines are often required concomitantly because the electric shocks can be painful.

48. What is torsades de pointes?

It literally means "twisting of the points," which describes the spindle appearance of this unique type of polymorphic ventricular tachycardia.

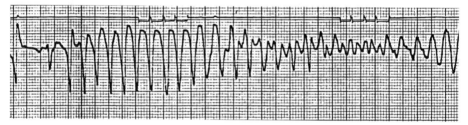

Torsades de pointes.

49. What causes a patient to go into torsades?

Antiarrhythmic drugs (quinidine, procainamide, disopyramide, sotalol), antihistamines (benadryl, hismanal, seldane), electrolyte disturbances (hypokalemia, hypomagnesemia), and ischemia.

50. How does torsades differ from garden variety monomorphic VT?

Torsades is often intermittent and fast (> 300 bpm), and every beat looks different from the beat before it (i.e., polymorphic). It is associated with a long QT interval on the rhythm strip.

51. How does treatment differ for torsades and monomorphic VT?

The primary treatment of torsades involves speeding the rhythm with dopamine, isoproterenol, and/or overdrive pacing at the hospital with a transvenous pacer. By speeding the sinus rate, the QT interval therefore shortens and the propensity of the heart to go back into the torsades "spindle" is diminished. Magnesium sulfate, 2 gm IV, is also an effective treatment for torsades and seems to work even in patients who are not hypomagnesemic. Lidocaine is ineffective, and IV procainamide and other class IA antiarrhythmics are absolutely contraindicated because they prolong the QT interval even further.

52. What if a patient has a long spindle of torsades and becomes unstable?

Defibrillate the patient with 200 joules. Multiple shocks may be required before the patient can be stabilized.

53. What do you do about PVCs? Do they always require therapy?

No. They are common in adult medical patients.

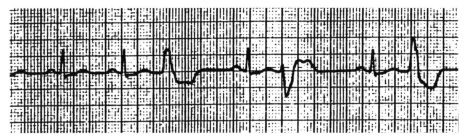

Multifocal premature ventricular contractions. (From American Heart Association: Textbook of Advanced Cardiac Life Support. Dallas, TX, American Heart Association, 1990, with permission.)

54. What are the four guidelines for giving lidocaine to treat PVCs?

1. Greater than 6 PVCs per minute
2. Multifocal PVCs
3. Couplets, triplets
4. Bigeminy, trigeminy

BIBLIOGRAPHY

1. American Heart Association: Textbook of Advanced Cardiac Life Support. Dallas, TX, American Heart Association, 1990.
2. Harken AH: Cardiac dysrhythmias. Sci Am I(3):1–8, 1996.
3. Lowenstein SR, Halperin B, Reiter MJ: Paroxysmal supraventricular tachycardias. J Emerg Med 14:39–51, 1996.
4. Wagner GS: Marriot's Practical Electrocardiography, 9th ed. Baltimore, Williams & Wilkins, 1994.

31. CARDIAC ARREST

Julie Seaman, M.D.

1. What is the approximate survival rate for out-of-hospital cardiac arrest when the patient is pulseless on EMS arrival?
One to two percent.

2. What is the survival rate in patients who arrest in the presence of EMS personnel?
Ten to fifteen percent. So this is clearly one disease process for which EMS presence and intervention have been shown to make a definite impact.

3. What intervention has been shown to improve survival in cardiac arrest?
Defibrillation! The patient's prognosis diminishes exponentially for every minute that defibrillation is delayed.

4. When performing precordial compression during cardiopulmonary resuscitation (CPR), what percentage of cardiac output is typically achieved?
Thirty percent of normal cardiac output.

5. How can I remember all the steps for treatment of ventricular fibrillation or pulseless ventricular tachycardia?
There is a mnemonic that goes as follows that describes the various steps in the treatment algorithm: **Shock** (200 J), **Shock** (200–300 J), **Shock** (360 J), **Everybody** (epinephrine), **Shock** (360 J; always shock 30–60 sec after each medicine is administered), **Little** (lidocaine), **Shock**, **Big** (bretylium), **Shock**, **Mega** (magnesium), **Shock**, **Pro** (procainamide), **Shock**.

6. What are the adult doses of cardiac drugs?
- Epinephrine—1 mg IV push every 3–5 minutes. If these initial doses don't work, epinephrine can then be given in intermediate doses (2–5 mg), high doses (0.1 mg/kg), or escalating doses (1 mg, 3 mg, 5 mg).
- Lidocaine—1.0–1.5 mg/kg IV push every 3–5 min to a maximum of 3 mg/kg.
- Bretylium—5 mg/kg IV push. Repeat in 5 min at 10 mg/kg.
- Procainamide—30 mg/min to a maximum of 17 mg/kg.
- Atropine—1 mg IV push every 3–5 min to a maximum of 0.03–0.04 mg/kg.
- Adenosine—6 mg IV push, then 12 mg IV push.

7. How is advanced cardiac life support (ACLS) modified for pediatric cardiac arrests?
- Defibrillation voltage is less—2 J/kg, then 4 J/kg, 4 J/kg, and so forth.
- Epinephrine dose is 0.01 mg/kg (which is 0.1 ml/kg of a 1:10,000 solution; remember that a 1:1000 solution has 1 mg epinephrine in 1 ml of solution and a 1:10,000 solution has 1 mg of epinephrine in 10 ml of solution).
- Lidocaine and bretylium doses remain the same.
- Atropine dose is 0.02 mg/kg (minimum 0.1 mg, maximum 0.5 mg in a child and 1 mg in an adolescent).
- Adenosine dose is 0.1 mg/kg (maximum 6 mg) and then dose is doubled, as in adults.

8. Is it common to injure children while performing CPR?
No, but it does happen. In one study of more than 200 children, 7% sustained injury, 3% sustained significant injury (pneumothorax, gastric perforation, retroperitoneal hemorrhage, epicardial hematoma), and 0.5% sustained rib fractures.

9. **What is the most common cause of pediatric arrest?**

Respiratory arrest. So the first step in managing any pediatric arrest is to establish an airway and ventilate the patient.

10. **How does one determine the correct endotracheal tube size for a child?**

(Age/4) + 4 is a formula that provides one way to determine endotracheal tube size. Another is to look at the size of the child's pinkie.

11. **What is the current evidence for use of high-dose epinephrine?**

Epinephrine increases systemic pressures, myocardial perfusion, and cerebrally directed flow. Currently, there is no evidence that high doses of epinephrine improve survival to hospital discharge. Although the subject is controversial, current recommendations are to use standard 1-mg doses of epinephrine. If initial doses have no effect, in selected cases one may advance to higher doses of epinephrine.

12. **When should one consider giving bicarbonate in an arrest?**

In a patient with known or suspected renal failure, hyperkalemia is a common cause of arrest. In this situation, empiric sodium bicarbonate may be life saving.

13. **How does hypothermia alter ACLS?**

- The severely hypothermic patient (< 28°C) is unresponsive to defibrillation or cardiac medications. If the patient has a pulse, even a bradycardic pulse, CPR should not be performed. If the patient does not have a pulse but has rhythm on the monitor, CPR should be initiated. Defibrillation and ACLS medications should be withheld until the patient has an adequate temperature for response, however.
- A hypothermic patient is very susceptible to induced arrhythmias. Therefore, all unnecessary movement and stimulation should be avoided. The patient should be covered with blankets. Heated blankets, warm water, and all other rewarming modalities should be withheld until hospital arrival and evaluation.

14. **Does lightning or electrical injury alter ACLS?**

Death from lightning is nearly always the result of respiratory arrest or cardiac dysrhythmias. Unlike ischemic cardiac arrest, the heart often recovers spontaneously from lightning-induced asystole. If respiratory arrest is not prolonged, survival after cardiac arrest is possible. Lightning produces enough energy to short-circuit the central and autonomic nervous systems as well as the cardiac conduction system. Indeed, the cause of respiratory arrest is usually electrical injury to the brain stem.

15. **How does the management of traumatic arrest differ from that of cardiac arrest?**

Rather than myocardial ischemia, these patients suffer from injuries such as cardiac tamponade, tension hemopneumothorax, aortic rupture, myocardial lacerations, and hypovolemic shock. Standard ACLS measures will be of little of no benefit. Treatment must be directed at rapid transport and appropriate trauma intervention.

16. **What is the most commonly found injury in those patients who present in traumatic arrest but survive to hospital discharge?**

Pericardial tamponade, most often secondary to a stab wound of the heart.

17. **In what situations would out-of-hospital declaration of death be appropriate?**

- Asystole confirmed and unresponsive to ACLS.
- Obvious death (decay, rigor mortis, decapitation).
- Frozen body with asystole on the monitor.

BIBLIOGRAPHY

1. Bush CM, Jones JS, et al: Pediatric injuries from cardiopulmonary resuscitation. Ann Emerg Med 28(1):40–44, 1996.
2. Rainer TH, Robertson CE: Adrenaline, cardiac arrest, and evidence based medicine. J Accid Emerg Med 13(4):234–237, 1996.
3. Schwab RA, Steele MT, et al: The emergencies of summer: Optimum management of injuries caused by heat, water, bolts and venom. Emerg Med Rep 18(13):125–127, 1997.

32. ALTERED MENTAL STATUS

W. Peter Vellman, M.D.

1. What does "altered mental status" mean?

A state of abnormal mentation. It also has been referred to as altered state of consciousness, clouded consciousness, acute confusional state, or deliria. Altered mental status describes the state of awareness between normal consciousness and coma. Consciousness is described as the state of awareness of the self and the environment. Coma is the opposite of consciousness or the total absence of awareness of self and environment even when the subject is externally stimulated. Altered mental status almost always combines a generalized reduction or alteration in the content of consciousness (a cortical function) with at least some reduction in total arousal (a brainstem function). This usually involves a defect in attention. The patient may not think clearly or quickly and can be easily distracted. Orientation, memory, and the ability to interpret stimuli may be faulty.

2. What can cause altered mental status?

There are a variety of structural and metabolic causes. One mnemonic for remembering them is AEIOU TIPS, which stands for the following:

A   Alcohols (and other drugs)
E   Epilepsy, endocrine (all types), exocrine (liver)
I   Insulin (low or high blood sugar)
O   Opiates, oxygen
U   Uremia
T   Trauma, temperature extremes
I   Infection (sepsis, meningitis)
P   Poisons, Psychiatric
S   Shock, stroke, space occupying lesions

The prehospital provider should commit to memory this mnemonic, which will allow a rapid and routine differential diagnosis for the causes of altered mental status and also will help to understand and simplify treatment.

3. What historical features are important?

After understanding the causes of altered mental status, the prehospital provider can direct the questions of the history to family members or bystanders (e.g., did the patient sustain a head injury, ingest alcohol or other toxins, is the patient an insulin-dependent diabetic). Because the patient has an alteration in mentation, a history taken from the patient may be unreliable. It is therefore important to use other sources, including family members, bystanders, police officers, or observing the patient for medi-alert tags or bracelets. It is useful to determine how long the patient has had mental status changes and whether the change was abrupt or gradual. In patients with chronic dementia or organic brain syndromes it is important to determine how their current mental status differs from their baseline mental status.

4. Are there physical findings that may be important?

Yes. The physical exam is very important and may yield valuable clues as to the underlying cause. A standard evaluation including the ABCs should be undertaken initially and any supportive measures instituted immediately. Primary and secondary surveys and periodic reassessment of the patient should be performed to determine any further change in mental status.

5. What should I look for in a patient who has ingested alcohol?

Alcohol alone can cause an abnormal mental status, which initially may be manifested as stimulation or agitation. This may be followed by a depressant effect on the central nervous system, including a blunting of motor coordination and reflexes. Further elevation in blood alcohol can lead to coma and respiratory arrest.

It is of utmost importance, however, to determine if the patient has other causes of altered mental status, including head injury or the ingestion of other toxins or poisons. It should be assumed that a patient has altered mental status from alcohol alone only after other treatable causes such as hypoglycemia or narcotic overdose have been ruled out.

In children it is important to consider the possibility of hypoglycemia caused by alcohol. In the naive drinker, particularly with a thin body habitus, the glycogen stores may be rapidly depleted during alcohol intoxication with a subsequent sudden drop in serum glucose. These patients are at particular risk for irreversible brain damage secondary to prolonged hypoglycemia if not recognized and treated.

6. How is a seizure patient with altered mental status evaluated?

Patients with a known seizure disorder who have abnormal mentation may be in a postictal state as a result of a recent seizure. These patients will typically be confused and combative. Other physical findings that may support the diagnosis of a recent seizure should be sought, including tongue or lip biting or incontinence of bowel or bladder. One should observe for medi-alert tags. Patients with a seizure disorder have a higher incidence of intracranial hemorrhage. The postictal period is variable and can last briefly to several days. Patients may require physical restraining during this period.

During seizure activity there is a switch from aerobic to anaerobic metabolism as a result of increased muscle activity and decreased or absent ventilation. Therefore, seizure activity will result in a metabolic acidosis reflected as a depression in serum CO_2. This can be measured from venous blood (red top) but will correct fairly rapidly after the seizure activity has stopped. It is important, therefore, to draw blood at the time an intravenous line is established.

7. How are diabetic patients evaluated?

Patients who are insulin dependent or take oral medications for diabetes are predisposed to two problems: hypoglycemia and hyperglycemia. Overmedication or intentional overdose of glucose-lowering drugs may result in hypoglycemia, which generally is manifested by a fairly sudden change in mentation associated with tachycardia and diaphoresis. These are sympathomimetic responses to sudden hypoglycemia. Neurologic manifestations may include paresthesias, cranial nerve palsy, transient hemiplegia, clonus, diplopia, and decerebrate posturing. Patients with hypoglycemia and fever should always be evaluated for a possible source of infection. Hypoglycemia may occur in chronic alcoholics with liver disease, acute alcohol intoxication in inexperienced drinkers, and in patients with insulin-producing pancreatic tumors.

Hyperglycemia results from a relative or absolute insulin deficiency and manifests in one of two disease states: diabetic ketoacidosis (type I or insulin-dependent diabetes) or hyperosmolar nonketotic hyperglycemia (type II or adult-onset diabetes). Diabetic ketoacidosis is associated with Kussmaul respirations, dehydration, and a fruity (ketotic) odor to the breath. Nonketotic hyperosmolar states are associated with dehydration and hyperosmolality without ketoacidosis and are more likely than DKA to cause significant mental status changes primarily as decreased level of consciousness.

8. If opiate ingestion is suspected, how should the patient be treated?

The opiate syndrome is classically associated with depressed mentation, a blunted affect, and pinpoint pupils. Respiratory depression and respiratory arrest can be associated with opiate use. There is additive central nervous system depressant effect with opiates and drugs such as alcohol, barbiturates, and benzodiazepines. Many opiate preparations are available for use as analgesics, cough suppressants, and antidiarrheals. It is important for the prehospital provider to recognize these medications.

Commonly Prescribed Opiate Preparations

GENERIC NAME	TRADE NAME
Codeine	Tylenol #3
Meperidine	Demerol
Hydrocodone	Vicodin, Lorcet, Lortab
Oxycodone	Percodan, Percocet, Tylox
Hydromorphone	Dilaudid
Propoxyphene	Darvocet, Darvon
Diphenoxylate	Lomotil

Opiates are popular street drugs that come in a variety of preparations containing heroin, methadone, morphine, opium, and codeine. They may come in a variety of strengths and purity. It is not unusual for an emergency department to experience a sudden increase in the number of opiate overdoses based on the arrival of a particularly potent batch of drugs. The effects of opiates are rapidly reversed with the use of naloxone (Narcan), which should be administered for suspected opiate overdoses in 2-mg intravenous increments. Some opiates, particularly propoxyphene and diphenoxylate may require higher doses for satisfactory reversal. If there is an effect from naloxone administration and the patient's condition suddenly deteriorates, more naloxone should be administered. Absence of a response to naloxone may imply that there is a concomitant overdose with other central nervous system depressants that are not reversed by naloxone, such as barbiturates or benzodiazepines.

9. How can one determine if someone has altered mentation because of uremia or liver failure?

The alteration in mentation in a uremic patient occurs because of the increasing blood urea nitrogen and the subsequent changes in serum osmolality. Advanced uremic patients may develop a condition called uremic frost in which a high concentration of urea in sweat yields a "frosty" appearance to the skin as the sweat dries. The skin of a uremic patient may also get a sallow, yellow color resulting from an accumulation of carotene-like pigments. Patients with advanced liver disease may develop a flapping tremor or asterxis, a precoma condition that results in a nonrhythmic lapse in voluntary sustained posture of the extremities, head, and trunk. The patient also may be jaundiced and may have a distended abdomen secondary to ascites or liver enlargement.

Uremia or liver failure generally will be suspected because of the past medical history or findings suggesting the underlying illness, such as a renal dialysis shunt in the forearm or jaundice.

10. What should the examination include if the patient has a head injury?

In addition to all of the usual signs and symptoms of a head injury, every examination must include an evaluation of (1) the patient's mental status, (2) pupillary response to light stimulation, and (3) the best motor and verbal response in order to calculate the Glasgow Coma Score. One must always keep in mind the potential for cervical spine injury in patients who have sustained a head injury. Mental status changes from head injury can vary from agitation and combativeness to vacillating levels of consciousness and ultimately to coma.

11. How can temperature extremes change mentation?

The exact mechanism of cerebral dysfunction associated with temperature extremes is unknown; some well-recognized patterns exist. As the core body temperature decreases, cerebral blood flow decreases and mental status changes occur that resemble alcohol intoxication: slurred speech, motor incoordination, mental confusion, and lethargy. These changes can occur at body temperatures below 32°C (90°F). As body temperatures drop below 30°C (86°F), coma, dilated nonreactive pupils, and cardiac arrhythmias may occur.

Elevation in body temperature can result in several distinct syndromes. Mental status changes are not usually associated with heat cramps or heat exhaustion. Heatstroke, however, is a true medical emergency associated with widespread organ (including neurologic) dysfunction and may occur at a body temperature of 41.1°C (106°F) or greater. The neurologic changes in heatstroke may include hallucinations, irritable or bizarre behavior, combativeness, pupillary abnormalities, posturing, hemi- or quadriplegia, status epilepticus, or coma. Sweating may or may not be present.

Children with moderate to high fevers may exhibit altered mentation that may take the form of acute confusion, hallucination, and nightmares. These symptoms are temperature-dependent and do not necessarily imply serious disease. Febrile seizures can be a cause of altered mentation and may require a special evaluation to exclude serious underlying pathology.

12. What infectious processes can result in altered mentation?
Meningitis, encephalitis, and other conditions.

Meningitis is a viral or bacterial infection of the meninges that initially will manifest as headache with fever and signs of meningeal irritation (stiff neck). The mental status may be normal but, as the disease progresses, the patient may have a progressive decrease in level of consciousness.

Encephalitis is an infection that involves the brain parenchyma; it usually affects the temporal lobe but can involve other areas of the brain. With encephalitis comes a rather abrupt onset of an acute confusional state associated with agitation and disorientation that may progress to lethargy, ataxia, seizures, and coma. Patients with encephalitis may occasionally appear to be acutely psychotic. They may require physical and/or chemical restraints. Such patients can be a difficult diagnostic dilemma, but the presence of a fever will usually lead the clinician to the correct diagnosis.

Brain abscesses may also result in confusion and are generally associated with headache and fever. Other symptoms may include focal neurologic deficits and seizures.

13. How does one approach the patient with a suspected poisoning?
The astute prehospital provider will have the standard toxic syndromes committed to memory (see Chapter 41). These toxidromes include sympathomimetic, narcotic, cholinergic, anticholinergic, and other syndromes. All patients with a suspected poisoning should first be detoxified. The attendant should be cautioned against potential self-contamination during the initial evaluation and treatment phase. Careful attention should be paid to the ABCs as well as initial treatment, including establishing an IV and administering oxygen. The patient should be placed on a cardiac monitor and transported expediently to the nearest treatment facility.

14. Can a stroke result in altered mentation?
Yes but not always. Stroke is a broad general term that refers to an intracranial vascular event, which may include an ischemic event such as a transient ischemic attack or an actual infarction of brain tissue. It generally is due to an embolus or a thrombus blocking one of the cerebral blood vessels. Stroke also may refer to a hemorrhagic event in which there is bleeding into the parenchyma of the brain. A stroke can be associated with normal mentation but abnormal motor function, which may render the patient with slurred speech or an inability to express thoughts or enunciate words clearly. Such a state may appear to be mental confusion even when the patient has normal mentation.

15. Can shock result in altered mentation?
Yes.

16. How low does the blood pressure need to be before mental status changes occur?
Physiologic mechanisms help to maintain cerebral blood flow if the systolic blood pressure drops. There is a critical point, however, beyond which the cerebral blood flow starts to decrease.

This is usually heralded by generalized signs of poor perfusion, which may include decreased level of consciousness, poor capillary refill, and cool clammy skin. The signs are usually associated with other physiologic changes, including increased heart and respiratory rates, diminished peripheral pulses, and decreased urine output.

The exact blood pressure at which cerebral blood flow decreases and altered mental status changes occur can vary. The point at which this happens may depend on underlying disease states such as atherosclerotic peripheral vascular disease and other factors. It is generally felt that a systolic blood pressure less than 80–90 mm Hg will result in altered mental status.

17. How does one distinguish functional versus organic causes of altered mental status?

Making the distinction can be very difficult. Mental confusion associated with disorientation to person, place, and time and impaired language and memory may imply an underlying organic disorder. Patients with purely functional, or psychiatric, disorders will usually be oriented and may display abnormality of thought, content, perception, and judgment, which may take the form of delusions, paranoid ideations, thoughts of suicide or homicide, or delusions of grandeur. Hallucinations may occur with both organic and functional disorders; however, auditory hallucinations are more common with psychiatric illnesses and visual hallucinations may be more common with organic disorders.

18. What terms should be used to describe altered mentation?

Because altered mentation can take many forms, it is an art form to be able to accurately describe the mental status changes that may occur. You should be as descriptive as possible and try to avoid confusing terms. For example, stating that the patient was oriented to person and place but disoriented to time is preferable to saying that the patient was confused. You can also use modifiers to accepted medical terminology, i.e., the patient was lethargic, but did respond appropriately when aroused.

19. How can mental status changes be evaluated in young children?

The task is difficult at best. Normal mentation is usually implied by normal behavior and the child's response to its environment. Therefore, a child who seems to be aware of his surroundings and aware of his parents, is consolable by parental holding, makes normal eye contact and follows objects with his eyes, and sits, stands, and walks appropriately for his or her age may be considered to have a normal mental function. Deviations from normal behavior or response to external stimuli and their environment may imply abnormal mentation.

20. Are there special problems in elderly patients?

Yes. Sudden mental status changes in an otherwise healthy adult older than 40 are strongly suggestive of an underlying organic disorder. Elderly patients are also subjected to mental status changes that can occur with aging, such as Alzheimer's disease or senile dementia. The possibility of several diagnoses can make the evaluation of mental status quite difficult. It is important to determine what the baseline mental status was prior to the onset of new symptoms. It may be helpful to have a family member describe new or recent alterations in behavior or mentation that have occurred.

21. What medicolegal implications are there for treating patients with altered mental status?

It is important to determine if a patient who is refusing care has normal decision-making capacity. The prehospital provider must determine quickly if the patient has normal thought process, orientation, and is making decisions that prudent lay persons would make with regard to their health care. A series of questions should be asked that include basic orientation questions, whether the person understands what the underlying condition involves, and what the consequences of the medical condition may be. When treating someone with altered mental status, the implied consent laws should prevail. If the prehospital provider determines that the patient does not have normal decision-making capacity, the provider should act in the best interest of the patient irrespective of the patient's expressed wishes. This may involve soliciting help from law enforcement and physically or chemically restraining the patient. Careful documentation of why the patient is deemed to have abnormal decision-making capacity should be included in the medical record.

22. Of what should the field treatment for someone with altered mental status consist?
Evaluate the ABCs and treat any life-threatening emergencies. All patients should be placed on oxygen and a cardiac monitor and have an IV line established. Blood should be drawn for at least a red top tube. Always consider the reversible causes of altered mental status, particularly hypoglycemia and narcotic poisoning. If there is any suspicion for hypoglycemia, $D_{50}W$ should be administered. Naloxone should be given. Regardless of their response to treatment, all patients should be transferred to a hospital emergency department for further evaluation.

BIBLIOGRAPHY

1. Hurst JW: Medicine for the Practicing Physician, 3rd ed. Newton, MA, Butterworth, 1992.
2. Plum F: The Diagnosis of Stupor and Coma. Philadelphia, FA Davis, 1980.
3. Tintintalli J (ed): Emergency Medicine: A Comprehensive Study Guide, 4th ed. New York, McGraw-Hill, 1996.

33. SEIZURES

Kim M. Feldhaus, M.D.

1. What is a seizure? Why should I know about them?

A seizure results from excessive and disorderly neuronal discharges in the cerebral cortex. An estimated 6.4% of the general population will experience at least one nonfebrile seizure within their lifetime, and they are among the most common prehospital chief complaints. You will definitely treat patients with seizures!

2. Are there different types of seizures?

Yes, seizures can be generalized (involving the entire body) or partial (focal or just part of the body). Primary generalized seizures result from excessive disorderly neuronal discharge, which begins simultaneously in both sides of the cerebral cortex. Generalized seizures include grand mal and petit mal seizures. All patients with grand mal seizures will have bilateral tonic-clonic activity and a loss of consciousness. Partial, or focal, seizures begin in a focal area of the brain. They may spread and become generalized, or they may stay as focal. Patients who experience a focal seizure may remain conscious.

3. What is the "ictus"?

The ictus is the period when the seizure occurs. Thus, preictal describes the period before a seizure, and postictal is the period after the seizure. Patients who have partial seizures may have a preictal forewarning, or an aura, that the seizure is about to begin. Patients whose seizures are generalized from the beginning do not have this aura.

4. What is a Jacksonian march?

As a focal seizure spreads across the cerebral cortex, you may see what started out as focal tonic-clonic activity spread to other parts of the body. For example, the tonic-clonic activity may begin in a patient's arm and then spread to his face, other arm, and legs. This is the Jacksonian march.

5. Define a febrile seizure.

A generalized seizure occurring in a child 3 months to 5 years old associated with a fever (often more than 102° Fahrenheit) but not an intracranial source of infection is classified as a febrile seizure.

6. Can anyone have a seizure?

Yes, any individual may have a seizure when placed under the right stress, such as hypoxia, fever, low blood sugar, or an intracranial catastrophe.

7. Define idiopathic epilepsy.

An individual with idiopathic epilepsy, or an epileptic, is an individual with a potential to have a seizure under circumstances that would not induce seizures in most individuals.

8. List the differential diagnosis of seizures.

Seizures may be confused with syncope, classic migraines, vertigo, drug reactions such as dystonia, decerebrate posturing, and complex migraines. Syncopal episodes are frequently confused with seizures because the patient may have some jerking muscular movements for a few seconds when he passes out.

9. Define status epilepticus.

Status epilepticus is a condition in which a seizure lasts more than 30 minutes, or in which recurrent (generally four or more) seizures occur without a return to baseline mentation between seizures.

10. Name the most common metabolic cause of seizures.

Hypoglycemia is the most common metabolic cause of seizures. Hyponatremia is a less common cause. Any patient who is diabetic, who has a history of hypoglycemia, or who has altered mentation upon your arrival should be treated with glucose.

11. Name the common drugs used to treat seizures.

Phenytoin (Dilantin), carbamazepine (Tegretol), valproate or valproic acid (Depakote), and phenobarbital are commonly prescribed for patients with generalized seizures.

12. You are called to see a patient who has just had a seizure. What questions would you ask the witnesses regarding what they saw?

Did the patient lose consciousness? Did he injure himself as he fell? How long did the seizure last? What did the event look like? How did the individual act when the event was over? Is there any history of recent head trauma or fevers? Remember, all patients with grand mal seizures will have a loss of consciousness, may injure themselves as they fall, and are commonly confused after the event. Generalized seizures may be manifested as generalized tonic, clonic, or tonic-clonic activity. Focal seizures will not result in a loss of consciousness. They may involve only one limb or the face, and they may then spread.

13. How do I distinguish a syncopal episode from a seizure?

Patients with syncope usually do not have violent shaking of the extremities, although they may have a few twitching movements of the extremities. Tongue-biting, incontinence, and postevent confusion or amnesia are not associated with syncopal events but are common with seizures.

14. How do I distinguish pseudoseizures (psychogenic seizures) from true seizures?

Pseudoseizures are often longer than true seizures, and rarely will the patient have a postictal period. Patients can often recall events that occurred during their "seizure," have not been incontinent, and do not usually incur physical damage during the event. Patients with pseudoseizures have no alterations on their electroencephalograph tracing during the "seizure."

15. You are evaluating a patient who has had a generalized tonic-clonic seizure. What might you find on physical exam?

Altered mental status (postictal confusion), intraoral trauma or tongue lacerations, and signs of incontinence. Perform a complete exam to try to determine an underlying cause of the seizure. Check carefully for signs of general or head trauma, look for evidence of alcohol or drug use, and be sure to perform a complete neurologic exam.

16. List the intracranial, infectious, metabolic, and toxic causes of seizures.

Intracranial causes include brain tumor, subdural hematoma, subarachnoid hemorrhage, stroke, and intracranial bleeding. Infections, including meningitis and encephalitis, can cause seizures. Common metabolic causes include hypoglycemia and hyponatremia. Overdoses of various drugs such as tricyclic antidepressants, cocaine, amphetamines, antihistamines, theophylline, and isoniazid are commonly associated with seizures. Withdrawal from alcohol causes seizures quite frequently; however, acute intoxication with alcohol has also been associated with seizures.

17. What are the two most common causes of recurrent seizures?

Noncompliance with antiepileptic medication and withdrawal from alcohol.

18. An 8-month pregnant patient has just had a seizure. You should be especially concerned about what condition?

Eclampsia. The differential diagnosis of a patient who has a seizure in her third trimester of pregnancy must include eclampsia. This condition is manifested by hypertension, proteinuria, and seizures. The treatment is emergent delivery of the fetus and placenta.

19. What is the approach to a patient with a seizure?

As always, start with the ABCs. Most patients do not require active airway management (i.e., intubation) unless the seizure is prolonged or they are unable to control their airway because of severe postictal depression of mentation. Supplemental oxygen is important and should be routinely used. Begin an IV line in order to have access should another seizure occur. (Note: Dilantin will crystallize in dextrose-containing solutions. If possible, avoid these solutions and use normal saline or lactated Ringer's.)

20. Are spinal precautions necessary in all seizure patients?

Cervical spine immobilization is recommended for all seizure patients in a few EMS systems; however, this may not be necessary in patients with a simple uncomplicated seizure. Certainly, seizures associated with motor vehicle accidents, falls from a significant height, or extensive facial trauma warrant caution and immobilization.

21. How do I stop a seizure?

Most seizures are brief and self limited and will have stopped spontaneously before or shortly after your arrival. If the patient is still seizing or has a recurrent seizure, benzodiazepines are the drug of choice for use in the prehospital arena. Diazepam (Valium) has traditionally been used. Dosage is 5–10 mg IV push for an adult. Also, don't forget to check the blood sugar.

22. Your patient begins to have a seizure and you are unable to establish an IV line. What do you do?

Diazepam may be administered per rectum, through an endotracheal tube or through an intraosseous line. The dosage is the same, 5–10 mg (or 0.1 mg/kg for a child).

23. Is an Advanced Life Support response required for all seizure patients?

Most EMS systems require an Advanced Life Support team to respond to patients with a complaint of seizure, and in many systems protocols require IV access in all patients. Recent evidence suggests, however, that this level of care may not be needed for patients who are conscious with normal or rapidly improving neurologic conditions and normal vital signs and who have no serious concomitant illness or injury.

24. Do all seizure patients need to be transported to an emergency department?

Most seizure patients should be transported. Patients with a known prior seizure disorder who have a short postictal period and a normal mental status may refuse transport, however, and should be instructed to follow up with their primary care physician and not drive an automobile until cleared by their doctor.

25. Why is it important to draw a red-top tube of blood on any patient who has had a seizure?

A transient anion-gap acidosis secondary to lactic acidosis will occur in all patients who have had a true major motor or grand mal seizure. Since this acidosis may resolve 20–30 minutes following the seizure, electrolyte studies done on blood drawn after arrival at the ED may be normal or nondiagnostic. Electrolyte studies that are normal on field blood drawn within 10–15 minutes of the "seizure" will rule out a grand mal seizure and save the patient a very expensive seizure workup.

BIBLIOGRAPHY

1. Abarbanell NR: Prehospital seizure management: Triage criteria for the advanced life support rescue team. Am J Emerg Med 11:210–212, 1993.
2. American College of Emergency Physicians: Clinical policy for the initial approach to patients presenting with a chief complaint of seizure, who are not in status epilepticus. Ann Emerg Med 22:875–881, 1993.
3. Bledsoe BE: Nervous system emergencies. In Bledsoe BE (ed): Paramedic Emergency Care, 2nd ed. Englewood Cliffs, NJ, Prentice-Hall, 1994, pp 738–767.
4. Jagoda A, Riggio S: Seizures. In Harwood A (ed): The Clinical Practice of Emergency Medicine, 2nd ed. Philadelphia, Lippincott-Raven, 1996, pp 889–894.
5. Kirby S, Sadler RM: Injury and death as a result of seizure. Epilepsia 36:25–28, 1995.
6. McArthur CL, Rooke CT: Are spinal precautions necessary in all seizure patients? Am J Emerg Med 13:512–513, 1995.
7. Pons PT: Prehospital considerations in the pregnant patient. Emerg Med Clin North Am 12:1–7, 1994.

34. FEVER

Kim M. Feldhaus, M.D.

1. A patient with a temperature of 104° Fahrenheit has a fever. True or false?

Maybe! A fever is defined as an elevation of body temperature that occurs because the body's internal thermostat has been reset at a higher level. This is most commonly caused by infections. Elevations of body temperature that are not caused by "resetting" the thermostat occur when the body's heat production exceeds heat loss. This is not defined as a fever; rather, the term applied is hyperthermia.

2. How does the body regulate temperature?

The brain's hypothalamus regulates heat production (by increasing metabolism and shivering) and heat loss (by varying the blood flow to the skin and by sweating). It directly measures the blood temperature and has an intrinsic set point of about 98.6° Fahrenheit (37° Celsius).

3. What is the main source of heat production in the body?

The primary source of heat production is metabolism of food into energy. The basal metabolic rate can be increased or decreased depending on the body's needs. Heat is also produced during physical exercise.

4. Explain the four ways that the body loses heat.

Most heat is lost through *radiation* of heat from exposed skin. *Evaporation* of sweat also allows for heat loss; the effectiveness of this method depends on the humidity of the ambient air. *Convection* is a third process of heat loss; wind blowing across exposed skin will "pull" heat from the body. Heat loss through convection is increased when the skin or clothing is damp. Heat loss may also occur through *conduction*—a direct transfer of heat from one's body to another object or substance. Conduction is responsible for a significant percent of heat loss when a person is immersed in water.

5. Why is it important to know the anatomic site where the temperature was measured?

Rectal and tympanic membrane temperatures reflect the temperature in the body's core. In general, a rectal temperature is about 1° Fahrenheit (0.6° Celsius) higher than oral temperature. Thus, a normal rectal temperature is 99.6°F (37.6°C). Conversely, temperatures taken in a patient's axilla will be about 1°F (0.5°C) lower than oral temperatures. An axillary temperature of 98.6°F is equivalent to an oral temperature of about 99.6°F. Axillary temperatures may take 5–7 minutes to obtain and are quite unreliable. In general, they should not be used in the prehospital environment.

6. How does an infection cause a fever?

Infectious agents (viruses, bacteria, or fungi) cause the release of chemicals known as pyrogens. These pyrogens result in an elevation of the hypothalamic set point above the usual set point of 98.6°F.

7. What other conditions (besides infection) result in an elevation of temperature?

Strokes and tumors can affect the hypothalamus directly, resulting in dysfunction of the temperature regulatory system. Sympathomimetic drugs such as amphetamines or cocaine can result in increased heat production, as can the adrenergic state associated with drug or alcohol withdrawal. If the body is unable to lose this heat, an elevated temperature occurs. High environmental temperatures, high humidity, or extreme physical activity on a hot day can overwhelm the body's ability to lose excess heat.

8. In a patient with a history of fever, what questions should be asked?

How old is the patient? When did the fever start? How high is the fever? Any recent travel? Associated symptoms? Other chronic medical conditions? What antifever or antipyretic medications have been taken? When? What dose?

9. What patients are at special risk from a fever?

Fever in infants and children should always prompt concern. Any fever in a child younger than 3 months old is abnormal and may indicate a life-threatening emergency such as meningitis. All these children should be evaluated by a physician. Elderly patients may develop serious infections without a fever; the presence of a fever in this population requires a full medical evaluation. Fever in immunocompromised hosts, including patients with diabetes, AIDS, or cancer, may be the harbinger of serious illness.

10. Explain the effect that elevated temperature may have on the other vital signs.

A patient's heart rate is increased approximately 10 beats per minute for every 1°C (1.8°F) rise in temperature. The respiratory rate also increases as the temperature increases. Hypotension in the setting of a fever is an ominous sign and generally indicates a serious infectious process or sepsis.

11. What is the most important exam finding to assess in febrile patients?

The most important observation to make is how well the patient is tolerating the fever. Does he or she look toxic? What is the mental status? In children, note whether they are playful, smiling, alert, and interactive with you and their caregivers.

12. What are purpura, and what is their importance?

Purpura are purple or maroon blotches on the skin that do not blanch with pressure. Purpura are often associated with meningitis. Other serious infections may result in a variety of rashes. Always perform a careful skin exam when evaluating a febrile patient.

13. Define sepsis and bacteremia.

Bacteremia occurs when bacteria invade the blood stream. These bacteria may release toxins that cause vasodilatation, hypotension, and shock. Sepsis refers to the life-threatening shock that may result from bacteremia. All septic patients are bacteremic, but not all bacteremic patients are septic.

14. You are treating a 62-year-old diabetic female who has a heart rate of 112, blood pressure of 88/64, and a respiratory rate of 28. She is slightly confused, and her skin feels warm and dry to the touch. What would be appropriate field treatment?

Given the patient's age and past medical history of diabetes, she is at risk of developing a serious bacterial infection and all its consequences. Hypotension and altered mentation should be of concern; presume she is septic until proven otherwise. Field treatment will include glucose, fluid support for hypotension, and transportation to the emergency department for prompt antibiotic therapy.

15. What is a febrile seizure? What are its characteristics? Who is at risk?

A febrile seizure is a generalized tonic-clonic seizure that may occur in children (usually between 6 months and 5 years old) when they have a rapidly rising temperature. Children who have had one febrile seizure are at increased risk of having a second seizure, either during the current infectious state or during a future febrile illness. Febrile seizures usually are brief, single seizures with short postictal periods. Children who present in status epilepticus or who are afebrile upon your evaluation should have other causes considered.

16. List appropriate field treatments for elevated temperature.

Patients with elevated temperature are often dehydrated, and intravenous administration of fluids is critical. Oxygen should be given to all tachypneic patients as well as to those in respiratory distress, and cardiac monitoring should be considered. Field measures to lower temperature should be begun for patients with a temperature of more than 104° Fahrenheit.

17. Describe appropriate methods to lower a patient's temperature.

Undress the patient as much as possible and place him or her in a cool environment. Sponging with tepid lukewarm water is very effective. Avoid ice-water baths; if the patient's skin is cooled too quickly, shivering will result and will lead to increased heat production.

BIBLIOGRAPHY

1. Bledsoe BE: Environmental emergencies. In Bledsoe BE (ed): Paramedic Emergency Care, 2nd ed. Englewood Cliffs, NJ, Prentice-Hall, 1994.
2. Dierking BH, Everidge JM, Ramenofsky ML: Initial prehospital assessment of the pediatric patient. J Emerg Med Serv 13:59, 1988.
3. Goodykoontz C: Fever. In Pons PT (ed): Prehospital Field Care: A Complaint-Based Approach. St. Louis, Mosby, 1997.
4. Thomas H, Folstad S: Fever. In Harwood-Nuss A (ed): The Clinical Practice of Emergency Medicine, 2nd ed. Philadelphia, Lippincott-Raven, 1996.
5. Zukin DD, Grisham JE: The febrile child. In Rosen P, et al (eds): Emergency Medicine: Concepts and Clinical Practice, 3rd ed. St. Louis, Mosby, 1992.

35. CHEST PAIN

Scott Branney, M.D.

1. How big a problem is chest pain?

Big! More than 650,000 people die of coronary artery disease each year, with almost two thirds of these involving sudden cardiac death outside the hospital. Another 1.3 million people have nonfatal heart attacks each year, resulting in more than 1.5 million coronary care unit admissions per year. Pulmonary embolism is the third most common cause of death in the United States, at nearly 650,000 deaths per year. More important, studies have suggested that the diagnosis is missed almost 400,000 times per year. Finally, although not as common, untreated aortic dissection has a mortality of 25% at one day, 50% at one week, and 90% at one year.

2. What problems exist in diagnosing chest pain?

There are two means by which the signals that communicate chest "pain" are transmitted. *Somatic pain* arises in the chest wall and is carried by very specific afferent nerves to the spinal cord. This permits very specific mapping of the painful stimulus. On the other hand, *visceral pain* arises in the heart and lungs as well as the esophagus and stomach. These organs are sparsely innervated, and signals enter the spinal cord at multiple levels, resulting in very poor specificity for where the pain originated. As such, pain from unimportant causes can be identical to the pain from life-threatening causes.

3. What's the best approach to sort out these diseases?

There are two basic concepts to help evaluate chest pain. First, focus on identifying life-threatening causes: myocardial infarction, angina, pulmonary embolus, aortic dissection, pneumothorax, or pneumomediastinum. Second, if there is any doubt, always treat the patient according to the worst possible scenario that the history and physical findings could represent. The most important tool for evaluating chest pain is a good history, with physical examination coming in a distant second.

4. What are the important elements in the history of the patient's chest pain?

Certain key elements should be noted: When did the pain start? How did it start? What does it feel like? Where do you feel the pain? Do you feel it anywhere else? Does anything make the pain better or worse? Does it change with movement? Respiration? Are there any other symptoms (nausea, vomiting, shortness of breath, syncope, cough)? Beyond a history of the current chest pain, a past medical history including risk factors for chest pain, medications, and pertinent family history can be useful.

5. What in the history would suggest coronary artery disease?

Classically, the pain is described as dull or pressurelike and is retrosternal or felt in the left chest. In general, the pain crescendos, with a duration of 10 minutes or less for angina. Pain that radiates to neck or arms is three to four times more likely to represent a myocardial infarction (MI) as is pain that is associated with diaphoresis, nausea, or shortness of breath. Dyspnea is the sole complaint in approximately 15% of patients having an MI and is an associated symptom in 50%. The five cardiac risk factors that should be assessed in every patient are a history of tobacco use, family history (MI in mother < age 55, father/brothers < age 45), diabetes mellitus, hypertension, and hypercholesterolemia. Without an electrocardiogram, it may be impossible to differentiate unstable angina from an acute myocardial infarction.

6. What about pain described as heartburn or "like gas pains"?

This is a common description, and while it may represent indigestion, it can also describe cardiac ischemia. One study noted that of patients with "pressurelike" chest pain, 24% had infarctions and another 30% had anginal pain. They also noted that of patients describing "burning or indigestion," 23% had infarcts and 21% had unstable angina. There are numerous instances of patients with indigestion who have some relief after belching or a bowel movement but go on to be diagnosed with coronary artery disease. It has also been reported that 7–10% of patients with acute myocardial infarction had complete relief of their pain with antacids alone.

7. What should be noted in the physical exam for coronary artery disease?

Probably the most important physical finding is, how does the patient look? A patient who is anxious and diaphoretic with a sense of impending doom may well have a significant problem. It is also very important to identify signs of cardiogenic shock (pale, cool, clammy, rales, hypotension, mental status change, jugular venous distention). These patients are best evaluated at a facility that can perform cardiac catheterization.

8. What about treatment?

All patients should receive oxygen as the basis of therapy. (Document whether it helps.) Sublingual nitroglycerin (either spray or tablet) acts as a direct coronary artery dilator and will often provide significant relief from the pain of angina but may show little effect with an MI.

9. What about pulmonary embolism?

More than 95% of cases of pulmonary embolism (PE) will present as one of three syndromes. (1) Pulmonary infarction with acute onset of pleuritic chest pain, dyspnea, and hemoptysis. (2) Acute cor pulmonale with acute dyspnea, cyanosis, right ventricular failure, and hypotension. (3) Unexplained dyspnea. These symptoms are very nonspecific and can be difficult to sort out, particularly if the patient has pre-existing pulmonary disease. Only a few patients (approximately 20%) will present with the classic findings of pleuritic chest pain, dyspnea, and hemoptysis.

10. What risk factors predispose one to development of PE?

Commonly described risk factors include a history of deep vein thrombosis, injury or surgery to the lower extremities, immobility, obesity, tobacco and birth control pill use, history of coagulation disorders, and increasing age.

11. What signs or symptoms suggest PE?

The major problem in diagnosing PE is that there are very few specific signs or symptoms. A high index of suspicion for the disease is important. Common symptoms include dyspnea (84%), pleuritic chest pain (74%), apprehension (63%), and cough (50%). Syncope is more common with massive PE. The most frequent sign of PE is tachypnea (85%), while tachycardia, localized rales, and fever occur in about 50% of patients.

12. Who is at risk for spontaneous (nontraumatic) aortic dissection?

Aortic dissection primarily occurs in individuals 50 to 70 years old. While relatively rare before age 40, it does occur in select populations. Hypertension is the most common risk factor, occurring in 70–90% of patients. The risk factors for patients younger than age 40 include connective tissue diseases (Marfan's and Ehlers-Danlos syndromes), congenital abnormalities (bicuspid aortic valve and aortic coarctation), chromosomal abnormalities (Turner's syndrome), and pregnancy (half of all female cases younger than age 40).

13. How does the pain differ from coronary artery disease or PE?

The pain of aortic dissection is commonly described by the patient as "ripping" or "tearing." The pain often migrates, moving down the back as the dissection spreads. This occurs in up to

70% of patients. The pain is usually maximal in intensity right from the start rather than progressive, like ischemic pain. Only rarely (10%) does painless dissection occur. The pain is unlikely to improve with narcotic therapy.

14. What other signs or symptoms are associated with aortic dissection?
Patients may have one of three patterns of neurologic findings: (1) stroke, (2) ischemic peripheral neuropathy (with an ischemic limb), or (3) paraparesis or paraplegia if the blood supply to the spinal cord is impaired. Patients may often appear "shocky" (clammy, cool, diaphoretic), although the blood pressure may be normal to elevated. Reduced peripheral pulses or unequal pulses when comparing limbs is very suggestive of dissection.

15. Besides trauma, what else causes pneumothorax?
Pneumothoraces occur spontaneously, most commonly in males age 20 to 40 who are taller than average. Other causes include asthma, tobacco use (emphysema), and barotrauma (diving accidents). Patients commonly describe chest pain (in 90%) that is pleuritic (sharp and worse on inspiration). Dyspnea also occurs in up to 80% of patients.

16. How should pneumothoraces be treated in the field?
If the patient is hemodynamically stable, high-flow oxygen should be administered via a nonrebreather mask. If patients are starting to show signs of tension pneumothorax (altered mentation, hypotension, absent breath sounds, and tachycardia), needle thoracostomy is indicated.

17. How else can barotrauma occur?
One of the more common methods is coughing or forced exhalation against a closed glottis, such as when smoking crack or marijuana. This can result in either pneumothorax or pneumomediastinum. Commonly, patients complain of sharp pleuritic substernal chest pain. They may have evidence of subcutaneous emphysema moving up into the neck. The classic physical finding is "Hamman's crunch," which is a crunchy sound heard over the area of the heart.

18. Are there any other causes of pneumomediastinum?
Esophageal rupture can also result in pneumomediastinum. This is often referred to as Boerhaave's syndrome. It commonly occurs in male patients 50 to 70 years of age, often with a significant alcohol use history. Prior forceful emesis followed by severe chest pain, dyspnea, and subcutaneous emphysema is the classic presentation. Pleuritic chest pain and an acute abdomen are suggestive of esophageal rupture.

19. What type of chest pain is associated with cocaine use?
Chest pain is the most common cocaine-related medical problem, affecting about 64,000 patients per year. Cocaine can cause significant coronary artery vasospasm (potentiated by tobacco use), as well as causing accelerated atherosclerosis. True myocardial infarction occurs in 6–10% of cocaine chest pain. For the most part, cocaine chest pain is treated as you would treat any other ischemic chest pain. Those patients with significant anxiety, elevated blood pressure, or increased heart rate should be treated with benzodiazepines as a first-line agent. This reduces both the cardiac and central nervous system toxicity of cocaine.

20. What about chest pain in patients with sickle cell disease?
The acute chest syndrome is a common complication of sickle cell disease. It is characterized by pleuritic chest pain, rales, and fever. It can be very difficult to distinguish from pneumonia. Therapy includes aggressive oxygen therapy via nonrebreather mask as well as volume resuscitation with IV crystalloids.

21. How does the approach to chest pain differ with children?
Chest pain in children is not uncommon, with nearly 650,000 visits per year. Compared with adults, chest pain is more often chronic, with 30% of children having had it 6 months or more in

one series. Fortunately, serious causes of chest pain are relatively rare, accounting for only about 5% of cases in most series.

CONTROVERSY

22. What is the role of the 12-lead electrocardiogram in the prehospital environment?

Pro. Several studies have shown that paramedics are capable of obtaining prehospital electrocardiograms (EKGs) of good quality, and that adding EKG data to the paramedic's clinical assessment improves sensitivity for the detection of angina and MI (from 60% to 90%). It has also been shown that prehospital 12-lead EKGs correlate well with EKGs done at the emergency department (ED) and may speed the diagnosis of ischemic heart disease. At least one study has shown significant reductions in the time between arrival at the ED and receipt of thrombolytic therapy when prehospital EKGs are transmitted to the ED physicians.

Con. Although it has been shown that prehospital personnel can obtain EKGs and that it increases their sensitivity for detecting ischemia, it has not yet been shown to improve patient care. Most studies suggest that prehospital personnel overcall ischemia. They do identify most patients with ischemia but also transport other patients without ischemia as well. So much of the diagnosis of ischemia is dependent on history that a negative EKG in the field (or in the ED) cannot be used reliably to decide which patients do not have ischemic heart disease. Performing an EKG in the field may delay the patient's arrival at the ED.

23. Should thrombolytic therapy be initiated in the field?

Pro. Time is myocardium. It has been shown that the early administration of thrombolytic therapy leads to better outcomes and fewer complications. Several European studies have shown that giving thrombolytics in the field reduces the time to thrombolytic therapy by 40 to 50 minutes without significant complications.

Con. No United States study to date has shown improved outcome when thrombolytic therapy is given in the field. While time to thrombolytic therapy is important, the major time delay comes from symptomatic patients not accessing emergency medical care, not from delays in receiving thrombolytic therapy. One US study also showed that of patients classified as having an MI by virtue of their prehospital EKG, only 51% actually did so. Initiating thrombolytics in such patients exposes them to possible bleeding complications.

BIBLIOGRAPHY

1. Brouwer MA, Martin JS, Maynard C: Influence of early prehospital thrombolytic therapy on mortality and event-free survival. Am J Cardiol 78:497–502, 1996.
2. Grijseels EW, Bouten MJ, Lenderink T: Pre-hospital thrombolytic therapy with alteplase or streptokinase. Practical applications, complications, and long term results. Eur Heart J 16:1833–1838, 1995.
3. Hollander JE: The management of cocaine-associated myocardial ischemia. N Engl J Med 333:1267–1272, 1995.
4. Karagounis L, Ipsen SK, Jessop MR, et al: Impact of field-transmitted electrocardiography on time to in-hospital thrombolytic therapy in acute myocardial infarction. Am J Cardiol 66:786–791, 1990.
5. Manganelli D, Palla A, Donnamaria V: Clinical features of pulmonary embolism: Doubts and certainties. Chest 107:25s–32s, 1995.

36. ABDOMINAL PAIN

Christina Johnson, M.D.

1. What are important types of abdominal pain?

Visceral pain results from spasm or stretch of the muscle wall of a hollow organ, distention of the capsule of a solid organ, or inflammation or ischemia to an abdominal organ. The patient experiences visceral pain as a dull, poorly localized pain. **Parietal pain**, in contrast, occurs when there is inflammation of the parietal pleura, as with peritonitis. Parietal pain is localized over the area of peritoneal inflammation and tends to be sharper and more severe. Both visceral pain and parietal pain may be referred to other regions of the body. For instance, gallbladder pain may radiate to the infrascapular region, and left diaphragmatic pain can radiate to the left shoulder. **Neurogenic abdominal pain** occurs in cases of thoracic herpes zoster, arthritis or discitis, and postoperative neuropathy. Here the pain follows a dermatomal or peripheral distribution and tends to be sharp and carefully defined.

2. Define the term "acute abdomen."

This is a term used by surgeons and emergency physicians to describe abdominal conditions that may require surgical exploration. Examples of such conditions include a perforated appendix, perforated gastric or duodenal ulcer, strangled bowel, ruptured intraperitoneal abscess, ruptured spleen or liver, and ruptured ectopic pregnancy. A patient with an acute abdomen usually has secondary peritonitis and may present with a rigid abdominal wall or rebound tenderness upon examination. A patient with an acute abdomen usually prefers to lie still and may complain about bumps in the road during the ambulance ride to the hospital.

3. What is key information to elicit from the patient's history?

The time of onset of abdominal pain can be important to the clinician's assessment of the nature of the patient's pain. Pain that begins suddenly and is severe usually implicates a serious cause. The distribution and character of the pain may define likely injured or diseased organs. Pain that begins in the periumbilical region and progresses to the right lower quadrant is typical of appendicitis. In contrast, pain that is periumbilical and radiates to the back is more likely to be due to pancreatitis. Pain that is increased by deep inspiration is due to irritation of the diaphragm, as in cholecystitis.

Precipitating and alleviating factors also provide clues to diagnosis. For example, epigastric pain that is exacerbated by drinking coffee or an empty stomach may be due to gastritis or an ulcer, whereas one would expect these conditions to improve with eating food. Associated symptoms also can be important to the diagnosis. Fever and chills are present in cases of infection, while nausea, vomiting, and anorexia are nonspecific symptoms. Vomiting that follows the onset of abdominal pain may indicate intestinal obstruction, pancreatitis, appendicitis, or cholecystitis. Hematemesis, melena, and hematochezia point to intestinal bleeding, which limits the differential diagnosis of abdominal pain considerably. Menstrual history, presence of dysuria or hematuria, and abnormal pattern of bowel movements also should be elicited. Finally, a history of previous similar pain and previous abdominal surgeries may help in diagnosing and managing the patient's abdominal pain.

4. What are cardiovascular causes of abdominal pain?

Weakening of the wall of the abdominal aorta leads to formation of an aneurysm. Aneurysms may enlarge, leak, or rupture, leading to significant abdominal and back pain. Arterial insufficiency in the abdomen can lead to intestinal ischemia and/or infarct. Some patients with myocardial ischemia or infarct experience pain that localizes or radiates to the epigastrium.

5. What are some gastrointestinal causes of abdominal pain?

Causes of Pain	Description
Gastritis	Inflammation of the stomach lining associated with excess gastric acid production and gastric irritants such as nonsteroidal anti-inflammatory agents and alcohol
Gastric or duodenal ulcer	Erosion of the mucosal lining of the stomach or, more commonly, the duodenum
Cholelithiasis	Formation of gallstones that may become obstructed and cause pain
Cholecystitis	Infection within the gallbladder or biliary tree
Bowel obstruction	Usually caused by adhesions from prior surgery
Appendicitis	Infection of the appendix, an appendage of the large intestine
Diverticulitis	Inflammation of diverticuli of the large bowel, seen in older patients
Pancreatitis	Inflammation of the pancreas, which may be caused by obstruction of biliary gallstones, medications, or alcohol
Hepatitis	Inflammation of the liver caused by viral infection, alcohol, or medications

6. What are some examples of common genitourinary causes of abdominal pain?

Causes of Pain	Descriptions
Nephrolithiasis	Renal stones, particularly if they obstruct the lumen of the ureter, can cause pain that is referred to the abdomen, back, or groin
Pelvic inflammatory disease	Sexually transmitted diseases that are untreated may progress to infect the Fallopian tubes and can lead to tuboovarian abscess
Ovarian torsion	Twisting of the ovary with resultant ischemia
Ectopic pregnancy	A pregnancy located anywhere except its usual location within the uterus
Ruptured ovarian cyst	Leads to peritonitis as the cyst fluid irritates the parietal peritoneum diffusely
Cystitis	Infection of the bladder; usually with associated symptoms of dysuria and urinary frequency and urgency
Testicular torsion	Pain may radiate up to the abdomen
Epididymitis	Infection of the epididymis that causes pain that may radiate superiorly to the abdomen

7. Some diseases of organs that do not reside within the abdomen can cause abdominal pain. What are some examples of such diseases?

As mentioned above, myocardial ischemia and infarct can lead to pain that is experienced in the epigastrium. Lower lobe pneumonia can cause inflammation of the diaphragm and lead to pleuritic abdominal pain. Patients with diabetic ketoacidosis frequently complain of abdominal pain; the reasons for this are unclear.

8. What are key points of the prehospital physical examination in a patient with abdominal pain?

One must start with a general assessment of the patient. Is the patient diaphoretic and writhing in pain, or is the patient calmly conversing about the nature of his or her pain? Next comes assessment of the patient's vital signs. Is the patient tachycardic, as are most patients with an acute abdomen? Is the patient hypotensive? Causes of hypotension include gastrointestinal or vascular hemorrhage, sepsis, ruptured ectopic pregnancy, pancreatitis, and a vagal response to pain. Does the patient have a tactile fever? Further examination includes auscultation of the lungs and visual inspection, auscultation and palpation of the abdomen. Is the abdomen distended? Are bowel sounds present? Is the abdomen soft or rigid? Always palpate away from the region of greatest abdominal pain first to obtain a reliable exam.

9. How does the patient with colicky pain present?

Patients with gallbladder or renal stones may present with colicky pain. They tend to writhe about and appear restless in their attempts to find comfortable positions.

10. What are some peritoneal signs?

Peritoneal signs, or signs of peritoneal inflammation, include rebound tenderness (pain that is severe with releasing pressure from the patient's abdomen), pain with movement of the patient's stretcher or tapping the patient's heel, and pain that causes abdominal wall rigidity when palpated.

11. If a patient with abdominal pain vomits en route to the hospital, should the emesis be saved?

Yes, if there is a question of blood or bile in the emesis. It can be tested for blood and observed for bile at the hospital.

12. What are the priorities of prehospital management of the patient with abdominal pain?

The patient should be placed in a position of comfort. In the case of a hypotensive patient that position should be supine. A patient who is nauseated should be placed in the left lateral decubitus position and an emesis basin placed nearby. Given that bleeding and/or infarction of vital structures are possible in a patient with abdominal pain, oxygen should be provided. Intravenous fluid administration is appropriate in the prehospital phase, with the amount to be given dependent on the degree of abnormality in the patient's vital signs. Any patient older than 40 may need a cardiac monitor en route to the hospital. Patients with abdominal pain should be prohibited from taking anything by mouth prior to their arrival in the emergency department (ED).

13. Is it appropriate to give patients medication to relieve their abdominal pain en route to the hospital?

No. While doing so may relieve the patient's discomfort, it will make diagnosing the patient's conditions much more difficult and therefore likely to delay definitive treatment.

14. What should the prehospital provider do if a patient with abdominal pain refuses to be transported to the hospital?

Because it is difficult to diagnose the cause of a patient's abdominal pain in the field, it is equally difficult to reassure the patient about the nature of his or her abdominal pain. All patients with abdominal pain should be transported to the hospital for further evaluation and treatment as indicated. If the patient is competent and understands the risks of refusing further care, including potential catastrophic complications, a case can be made for allowing him or her to refuse care *against medical advice* and in consultation with the base station physician.

15. If the patient is transported to the hospital for further evaluation of abdominal pain, what sort of procedures can he or she expect?

In addition to a complete physical examination, including a rectal examination and in women a pelvic examination, the patient may have blood drawn for a complete blood count, pregnancy test if indicated, and liver function tests—amylase or electrolytes depending upon the nature of the pain. Urinalysis is often performed. Ultrasonography, abdominal plain film radiographs, or computed tomograms may be ordered. Any patient with an acute abdomen will require surgical consultation. Despite such a thorough evaluation, the most common ED diagnosis of abdominal pain is "abdominal pain of unknown cause." In such a case the patient is admitted to the hospital or is scheduled for close follow-up.

16. In what ways might an elderly patient with abdominal pain differ from a younger patient?
In general, the elderly patient poses a higher risk for serious conditions and is more likely to have a subtle presentation. Older patients are less likely to (1) manifest fevers when they have infections, (2) present with typical symptoms such as nausea, vomiting, diarrhea, or even pain, and (3) demonstrate peritoneal signs despite having peritonitis. However, they are more likely to delay seeking medical care for their abdominal complaints. They may not manifest abnormal vital signs (e.g., tachycardia) as a younger patient would with an acute abdomen.

17. What are the most common diagnoses of abdominal pain in children?
In decreasing frequency: abdominal pain of unknown cause, gastroenteritis, appendicitis, constipation, urinary tract infection, viral illness, streptococcal pharyngitis, pharyngitis, pneumonia, and otitis.

18. How do the symptoms and signs of abdominal pain differ in pregnant patients?
Almost all pregnant patients experience some degree of abdominal pain during pregnancy. Symptoms such as nausea and vomiting may be due to pregnancy alone or to some other cause. Urinary frequency and urgency are common but may be a result of compression of the bladder by the uterus rather than urinary tract infection. As the uterus enlarges it displaces the abdominal contents and may distort the usual sites of parietal and referred pain. For example, a pregnant patient with appendicitis may complain of right upper quadrant pain because the appendix is displaced superiorly. Pregnant patients have heart rates that are faster than baseline, making interpretation of the severity of alterations in vital signs difficult.

BIBLIOGRAPHY

1. Brewer RJ, Golden GT, Hitch DC, et al: Abdominal pain: An analysis of 1,000 consecutive cases in a university hospital emergency room. Am J Surg 131:219–223, 1976.
2. Burkhart C: Guidelines for rapid assessment of abdominal pain indicative of acute surgical abdomen. Nurse Pract 17:39–49, 1992.
3. Farrell MK: Abdominal pain. Pediatrics 74(suppl):955–957, 1984.
4. Fontanarosa PB: Acute abdominal pain: Exploring the gut-level causes. J Emerg Med Serv 14:28, 1989.
5. Mason JD: The evaluation of acute abdominal pain in children. Emerg Med Clin North Am 14:629–643, 1996.
6. Nathan L, Huddleston JF: Acute abdominal pain in pregnancy. Obstet Gynecol Clin North Am 22:55–68, 1995.
7. Podgorny G: Abdominal pain and analgesia. Ann Emerg Med 10:547, 1981.
8. Sanson TG, O'Keefe KP: Evaluation of abdominal pain in the elderly. Emerg Med Clin North Am 14:615–627, 1996.
9. Silen W: Cope's Early Diagnosis of the Acute Abdomen, 19th ed. New York, Oxford University Press, 1996.
10. Way LW: Abdominal pain. In Sleisenger MH, Fordtran JS (eds): Gastrointestinal Disease, 4th ed. Philadelphia, W.B. Saunders, 1989.

37. EXTREMITY PAIN AND TRAUMA

Susan A. Egaas, M.D.

1. Who gets painful extremity problems?

People of all ages. The age of the patient and the mechanism of injury will help determine what injury you see. The most important piece of history is whether there has been trauma to the affected extremity. Pediatric patients often fall onto an outstretched hand (sometimes referred to as a FOOSH) and will fracture the radius and ulna or, more proximally, the distal humerus. Older patients will often fracture the hip in a fall from a standing position or in falling only a few feet because they have fragile bones secondary to osteoporosis.

2. How can I tell if a hip is fractured?

The only way to tell for certain is by x-ray evaluation, but the clinical exam can be suggestive. Most elderly patients fracture the hip at the femoral neck, and the leg will appear shortened and externally rotated. The patient usually will not be able to bear weight and will have severe pain. Some patients will be able to ambulate. Occasionally, the pain will be referred to the knee, and knee pain will be the only complaint. Always suspect a fracture in an elderly patient with hip complaints.

3. What are the "five P's" used in examining patients with a painful extremity?

Pulselessness, Pain, Paresthesia, Pallor, and Paralysis.

You can check these five clinical signs to determine if there is evidence of limb ischemia. A good pulse obviously indicates perfusion. If the limb is cool and pale, it may not be perfused. Paresthesia (a tingling sensation) may reflect ischemia and nerve damage. Severe nerve ischemia over a prolonged period of time may result in paralysis of the muscle. All these signs may be evident in compartment syndrome or in a patient with another reason for compromised blood flow, such as an embolus occluding an artery.

4. What is compartment syndrome?

Damage to muscle within a closed compartment causes swelling, which effectively pinches off the arterial blood supply. This is most common after a complex tibia fracture but can occur in nontraumatic situations or in another muscle compartment such as the hand or forearm when subjected to crush injuries. A fracture does not have to be present for the patient to have compartment syndrome.

5. How do I suspect compartment syndrome?

First is the history of a fracture, crush injury, or compression of the extremity. The physical exam reveals a tense and tight feeling to the muscles of the involved compartment of the extremity, along with pain with movement of the distal part of the extremity and tenderness on palpation.

6. What else can cause compromised arterial blood flow?

Arterial occlusion of a limb will present as a pulseless extremity. As the ischemic time progresses, the limb will become pale, cool, and insensate. Arterial occlusion can happen as a result of trauma (e.g., a gunshot wound), emboli from a blood clot in the heart, or clotting of a partially occluded artery (similar to an acute myocardial infarction). These lesions may be reversed if treated in time.

7. What if the vein is occluded?

Occlusion of a deep vein in the leg or pelvis is a DVT (deep venous thrombosis). Occlusion of a deep vein leads to swelling and pain, and sometimes you may palpate a fibrotic cord in the extremity. A clot can break off and travel to the heart and out into the pulmonary circulation, causing a pulmonary embolus. A patient with a possible DVT needs a formal medical evaluation to establish the diagnosis. Most often ultrasound is used to make this diagnosis. A DVT requires treatment with anticoagulants (i.e., heparin) to prevent propagation of the clot.

8. What about shoulder or other dislocations?

An anterior shoulder dislocation is the most common dislocation. It is usually caused by a fall onto the inside of the upper arm, which is abducted and externally rotated. The patient may have a history of multiple previous dislocations. Any dislocation may be associated with a fracture. Always check for distal pulses and sensation and splint the affected area in the position that you find the patient. Do not attempt to relocate the joint in the field, but rather transport the patient in a position of comfort.

9. What is nursemaid's elbow?

This is a layman's term for subluxation of the radial head at the elbow in a small child. This occurs between the ages of 1 and 5. The mechanism of injury is usually pulling of the extended and pronated arm, which can occur when lifting a child by the arm. The child often is crying and will not use the affected extremity. There is no obvious deformity and no neurovascular compromise.

10. Why do patients with sickle cell disease get bone pain?

During a vaso-occlusive crisis, the patient may have severe constant bone pain due to the abnormal blood cells occluding small nutrient blood vessels to the bone, thus causing ischemia.

11. What causes a red and warm joint?

There are multiple possibilities; you will usually not be able to diagnose these in the field. A joint that has a bacterial infection is the most serious emergency because the infection can destroy tissue and cartilage, leaving a crippled joint if untreated. More commonly seen is *gout*, a type of arthritis caused by uric acid crystals forming in the joint space. This often affects the big toe and may be so painful that even the weight of a bed sheet makes the patient cringe. It is difficult to tell gout from an infected joint by exam, and diagnosis requires aspirating fluid from the joint space. Certain types of chronic arthritis cause inflammation in joints, which can be warm and red, but the history should allow you to diagnose a chronic rather than an acute problem.

12. What joint problems do hemophiliacs get?

Hemophiliacs can bleed into both muscle and joint spaces with relatively minor trauma. The severity of the bleeding depends on the severity of the disease. Patients with a very low level of clotting factors will usually be diagnosed at a young age. Others have severely deformed joints secondary to multiple bleeding episodes.

BIBLIOGRAPHY

1. Bennett J, et al (eds): Cecil Textbook of Medicine, 20th ed. Philadelphia, W.B. Saunders, 1996.
2. Tintinalli J, et al (eds): Emergency Medicine—A Comprehensive Study Guide, 4th ed. New York, McGraw-Hill, 1996.

38. DYSPNEA

Vincent J. Markovchick, M.D., and Paul Murphy, EMT

1. What is dyspnea?
Dyspnea is the subjective perception of shortness of breath.

2. How do I assess a patient who is dyspneic?
Visually determine the mental status, skin color, presence of nasal alar flaring, and use of accessory muscles and respiratory rate, and assess the A and B of the ABCs. Is there any evidence of upper airway obstruction? Are breath sounds present and equal? Are there any abnormal sounds (i.e., wheezing, rales, rhonchi)? What is the oxygen saturation on room air (if a pulse oximeter is available)? Ominous findings revealing that the patient is becoming tired include an altered mental status, 2 to 3-word dyspnea, or combativeness (from hypoxia) manifested by pulling off the oxygen mask or refusing the nebulizer.

3. What should be done concomitantly with this assessment?
Stop and stabilize when an abnormality is determined. Examples include placing all patients with dyspnea on oxygen. Suctioning of secretions, placement of a nasopharyngeal airway, and intubation for upper airway obstruction may be needed. Administration of bronchodilators such as albuterol via nebulizer is indicated for wheezing.

4. Why should I place all dyspneic patients on oxygen?
All such patients should be presumed to be hypoxic, and supplemental oxygen may improve this. In addition, if a patient should deteriorate and sustain a respiratory arrest, preoxygenation will provide more time in which to establish an airway or intubate the patient prior to the patient's O_2 saturation falling to a dangerously low level.

5. What conditions may cause dyspnea and pleuritic chest pain?
Pulmonary embolus, pneumothorax, pneumonia, and pleurisy.

6. What conditions may cause dyspnea and diffuse wheezing?
Bronchiolitis (in children younger than 2 years), acute bronchial asthma, anaphylaxis, chronic obstructive pulmonary disease (COPD) or emphysema, congestive heart failure (CHF), and bronchitis.

7. How do I distinguish between COPD and CHF?
Do a chest x-ray. Unless you have this available in your ambulance, it is impossible to make this determination with certainty in the field.

8. Why is morphine contraindicated in a patient with COPD?
Morphine may suppress the respiratory drive and may cause hypoventilation, carbon dioxide retention, and respiratory failure.

9. If I can't use morphine to treat a patient whose wheezing may be due to CHF, what should I use?
Sublingual nitroglycerin will reduce afterload without suppressing the respiratory drive. Administration of albuterol may improve bronchial constriction secondary to concomitant COPD, asthma, or bronchitis.

10. Define asthma.

Asthma is bronchiolar constriction caused by intrinsic or extrinsic factors, manifested by dyspnea and diffuse wheezing.

11. How should I treat asthma?

Oxygen (100%) and the administration of inhaled beta$_2$-agonists such as albuterol. They may be given continuously or in-line to intubated patients.

12. When is a normal vital sign very abnormal in an asthmatic?

A "normal" respiratory rate of 14 to 18 is an ominous sign in a patient with diffuse wheezing and indicates respiratory failure and impending respiratory arrest. A respiratory rate of more than 24 indicates that the patient still has the capacity to perform the work of breathing necessary to maintain adequate oxygenation.

13. What is hyperventilation syndrome?

Very deep and rapid respirations secondary to acute anxiety and emotional upset.

14. What are the symptoms of hyperventilation syndrome, and why do they occur?

The patient will have a rapid respiratory rate associated with numbness and tingling, first apparent around the mouth and lips, which is followed by carpopedal spasm or tetany. These occur because hyperventilation dramatically decreases the pCO_2 in the blood, which causes respiratory alkalosis and hypocalcemia.

15. I've heard that patients who are hyperventilating can be treated with rebreathing into a bag or mask.

Absolutely not, since patients who are hypoxic or severely acidotic from other causes will also present with tachypnea and sometimes deep breathing or increased tidal volume. If this is treated with rebreathing techniques, it may further decrease the O_2 level in the blood and lead to disastrous consequences.

16. If rebreathing into a paper bag is dangerous, how do I manage a patient who appears to have hyperventilation syndrome?

First, you must rule out other causes of dyspnea and hyperventilation. A calm and reassuring approach and an attempt to "talk them down" to decrease the depth and rate of breathing is most often successful and always safe. Other causes of hyperventilation such as diabetic ketoacidosis or hypoxia will not improve; all these patients should be treated with O_2 by mask or nasal cannula.

17. How do I suspect the diagnosis of pneumonia?

The presenting signs and symptoms of pneumonia, which is pus in the alveoli of the lungs, include productive cough with green-yellow sputum, dyspnea, tachypnea, fever, chills, pleuritic chest pain, localized rales, and flaring of the nasal alae with inspiration. All such patients should be treated with high-flow O_2.

18. What is a pulmonary embolus?

Pulmonary embolus (PE) is a blood clot that originates in the veins of the lower extremities or pelvis, breaks off, and is carried to the right ventricle and to the lungs via the pulmonary artery.

19. How do I make the diagnosis of PE?

The diagnosis can't be made in the field; it is a difficult diagnosis to make even with the aid of sophisticated diagnostic imaging techniques. It should be suspected in any patient with pleuritic chest pain, dyspnea, tachypnea, and tachycardia.

20. What patients are at highest risk for development of PE?
The elderly (i.e., older than age 70), postpartum women, women taking birth control pills, anyone who has prolonged immobility (e.g., bed rest or long leg cast), and patients with cancer or hypercoagulable states (e.g., protein C or S deficiency).

21. What is the treatment?
High-flow O_2 via a nonrebreather mask, cardiac monitoring, transport for ED evaluation, and treatment in the ED with heparin and possibly thrombolytics.

22. What is HAPE?
*H*igh *A*ltitude *P*ulmonary *E*dema, which occurs in susceptible individuals who travel to locations above 8000 feet elevation. It may become life threatening and resolves with administration of O_2 and rapid descent (often of as little as 1000 feet) to a lower altitude.

23. Which vital sign taken in the field is most likely to be inaccurate and why?
The respiratory rate is often estimated rather than counted over 20 to 30 seconds, since EMTs are action oriented and sometimes do not take the time necessary to determine the respiratory rate accurately in patients who do not complain of dyspnea or who look dyspneic.

24. Why is estimating the respiratory rate a dangerous practice?
Some very sick patients may be overlooked, particularly those with metabolic acidosis secondary to sepsis or toxic ingestions, since many of these patients have no complaints of dyspnea and do not appear to be in respiratory distress.

25. What's the message of this chapter?
COUNT the respiratory rate and administer O_2 to every dyspneic patient.

BIBLIOGRAPHY

1. Guerra W: Asthma and chronic obstructive pulmonary disease. In Markovchick V, et al (eds): Emergency Medicine Secrets. Philadelphia, Hanley & Belfus, 1993, pp 82–85.
2. Murphy M: Breathing and ventilation. In Markovchick V, et al (eds): Emergency Medicine Secrets. Philadelphia, Hanley & Belfus, 1993, pp 79–81.
3. Parsons PE: Deep venous thrombosis and pulmonary embolism. In Markovchick V, et al (eds): Emergency Medicine Secrets. Philadelphia, Hanley & Belfus, 1993, pp 89–92.

39. VOMITING AND DIARRHEA

Susan A. Egaas, M.D.

1. What should I note in the history for a patient with vomiting?

Emesis (vomiting) is seen in a variety of medical conditions, including gastrointestinal (GI) problems. Thus, it is important to start with very general questions. Inquire about abdominal pain, diarrhea, and fever. Note exactly how the emesis appears. Is it bloody, or does it look like coffee grounds? Bilious vomiting (yellow bile-stained fluid) in children must be differentiated from the normal regurgitation of milk or formula associated with burping. In a distal small bowel or large bowel obstruction, the patient will eventually vomit feculent material. Always ask about trauma, because a head injury can cause vomiting. Other neurologic complaints such as headache or seizures may indicate the possibility of a neurologic cause. Always ask for a medication list; this can suggest a toxic ingestion (e.g., aminophylline) or metabolic problems (e.g., diabetic ketoacidosis). Never forget that myocardial ischemia can present with nausea and vomiting with or without chest pain. This is frequently seen in inferior-wall myocardial infarction.

2. What is important in the physical exam?

Carefully evaluate the vital signs. A fever may indicate an infectious cause. Orthostatic changes in blood pressure and pulse are indicative of extensive fluid loss and dehydration. A careful inspection of the abdomen may reveal surgical scars. Previous abdominal surgery is a risk factor for bowel obstruction. A rigid abdomen may be caused by an intra-abdominal catastrophe requiring surgical intervention. Observe the emesis for the presence of bile, blood, or fecal odor.

3. What are the complications of vomiting?

In addition to dehydration, the patient is at risk for electrolyte abnormalities and esophageal or gastric tears leading to perforation or bleeding.

4. What about the airway?

Don't forget the ABCs just because the patient primarily has a GI complaint. It is imperative to evaluate the airway of any patient with vomiting because he is at risk for aspiration and subsequent pneumonia. If a patient is intoxicated or has an altered mental status, he is more likely to aspirate. It is particularly important to be aware of possible aspiration in any patient immobilized supine on a backboard in a cervical collar. These patients will aspirate if they do not have a gag reflex and may require advanced airway maneuvers such as intubation.

5. Should a patient who is intoxicated and vomits be intubated to protect his airway?

No. Intoxication and vomiting by themselves are not good indications for intubating a patient unless the patient cannot be positioned on the left side with the head down (e.g., after trauma); the patient does not have a gag reflex; or the patient is clearly hypoventilating (i.e., he has a respiratory rate less than 10 per minute that does not increase with stimulation).

6. What drug ingestions can cause vomiting?

Many different medications can cause vomiting. Some common overdoses that cause nausea and vomiting include acetaminophen and iron (particularly frequent in children), digoxin, and theophylline.

7. What does it mean when a patient vomits "coffee grounds"?

This is a common description of the emesis in a patient who has previously bled into the stomach. The stomach acid changes the color and appearance of the blood. Treatment is the same as for any patient who vomits bright red blood. Two large-bore peripheral IV lines should be quickly inserted and a bolus of IV fluids (20 ml/kg of normal saline or lactated Ringer's) given if the patient is hypotensive or tachycardic.

8. What are the symptoms of food poisoning?

Different types of food poisoning will cause different syndromes. Many bacterial causes of food poisoning cause either primarily vomiting or primarily diarrhea. Onset of symptoms after ingestion of the offending agent may be shortly after the meal (only 1 to 2 hours), or it may take days for symptoms to appear, depending on the exact cause. It can be difficult to make a diagnosis of food poisoning unless multiple patients report symptoms after ingestion of a common meal.

9. What is important about the medical history in diarrhea?

Always ask about the frequency and amount of diarrhea, because the severity of symptoms may suggest associated dehydration. It is important to note whether the diarrhea is bloody because this may indicate infection, inflammatory bowel disease, or gut ischemia. A history of black, tarry, foul-smelling stool suggests melena, which is the result of upper GI bleeding (usually from the stomach or duodenum). The blood darkens with exposure to stomach acid; it acts as a cathartic and travels rapidly through the bowel. Recent travel to another country is often associated with infectious diarrhea.

10. Is there anything different about kids with vomiting and diarrhea?

Children with multiple episodes of vomiting or diarrhea are more likely to become dehydrated and to appear ill or lethargic because they have a smaller volume of body fluids than adults and are unable to tolerate fluid losses. True projectile vomiting in an infant requires medical evaluation for pyloric stenosis, a congenital defect needing surgical repair. Bilious emesis is never normal in infants and should always be evaluated in an emergency facility for the possible presence of an obstructive intestinal lesion. Children with violent coughing spells may vomit after they stop coughing, as in pertussis (whooping cough) or asthma.

11. What about geriatric patients with prolonged or multiple episodes of vomiting or diarrhea?

Like children, elderly adults often have fewer physiologic reserves than normal adults and are more prone to dehydration. Severely dehydrated patients may appear confused or even comatose.

12. When should I administer an antiemetic in the field?

There is no need for the routine administration of an antiemetic except for intractable, persistent, severe retching that may cause rupture of the esophagus (Boerhaave's syndrome).

13. What antiemetic should I administer?

Droperidol (Inapsine), 1.25–2.5 mg slow IV push, is an excellent and safe antiemetic if there are no contraindications such as pregnancy, neuroleptic malignant syndrome, or Parkinson's disease.

BIBLIOGRAPHY

1. Rosen P, et al (eds): Emergency Medicine: Concepts and Clinical Practice, 4th ed. St. Louis, Mosby, 1998.
2. Strange G, et al (eds): Pediatric Emergency Medicine: A Comprehensive Study Guide, 3rd ed. New York, McGraw-Hill, 1996.

40. GASTROINTESTINAL HEMORRHAGE

Michael Stackpool, M.D.

1. How serious a problem is abdominal bleeding?

Five percent of hospital admissions from the emergency department (ED) are for gastrointestinal (GI) bleeding. Although most bleeding stops spontaneously, 8–10% of admitted patients will die of hemorrhage.

2. Who is Treitz, and why should I care about his ligament?

Wenzel Treitz was an Austrian physician for whom the suspensory ligament of the duodenum is named. This ligament crosses the intestine between the second and third parts of the duodenum. It is the border between upper and lower GI bleeding. Bleeding distal to the ligament of Treitz rarely refluxes back into the stomach.

3. Are there any clues to the site of bleeding?

The anatomic site of bleeding cannot always be identified, even in the ED or with invasive procedures. Nonetheless, there are some indicators. *Hematemesis* is the vomiting of frank blood or of partially digested blood, also called "coffee grounds" because of its appearance. It indicates bleeding from the upper GI tract. Black, tarry, or liquid stool with a characteristic odor is melena. *Melena* is also due to upper GI bleeding but signals that more than 100 ml of acute blood or 500 ml of blood over 24 hours have been lost. *Hematochezia* is the passage of bright red blood per rectum. Usually, this is from a lower GI source. In the setting of a severe and brisk upper GI bleed, however, hematochezia may occur. In this event, there should be clear signs of volume depletion and hypovolemic shock. Painful bleeding tends to be from peptic ulcer disease or erosive gastritis, while painless bleeding tends to be from diverticulitis or cancer.

4. What questions should I ask in the history?

It is important to know when the bleeding started and how long it has lasted, where it is from (i.e., emesis or bloody stools), how often it has occurred, and whether it is painful or painless. Any prior episodes of bleeding, any complications, past procedures (endoscopy, colonoscopy, or surgery), and the need for blood transfusions are also important pieces of information. Ask if the patient has any predisposing diseases such as peptic ulcers, hepatitis, diverticulosis, cancer, or inflammatory bowel disease. Many medicines can erode the stomach and intestine wall. Particularly troublesome are the nonsteroidal anti-inflammatory drugs (NSAIDs) and aspirin, but be sure to ask about coumadin or "blood thinners" and steroid use. Abdominal surgery, hypertension, and hiatal hernias predispose to GI bleeding. Alcohol may be the most pervasive and erosive GI irritant and is commonly associated with severe and repeated GI bleeds. Finally, always ask about associated symptoms. The stress of illness and loss of blood can overly tax a weak heart and may result in myocardial infarction. Chest pain, syncope, and signs of shock should be taken very seriously.

5. Are there any age-related differences in GI hemorrhage?

There are differences at the extremes of age. The elderly have fewer reserves and often have existing illnesses. They are at greater risk for severe complications and death. They also tend to more often have cancer, ischemia, and diverticular disease as the reason for bleeding. In young patients, shock can be delayed. Children and adolescents can lose a surprising amount of blood before changes in their vital signs are evident. They also tend to have much more benign reasons for bleeding. Intussusception and Meckel's diverticulum are unique to the pediatric population.

6. What is the prehospital management of GI hemorrhage?

As always, it begins with the ABCs. The airway must be protected from aspiration of blood or stomach contents. If the patient is obtunded or in shock, emergent intubation is indicated. Otherwise, administer oxygen by nasal cannula in stable patients or by non-rebreather mask if any vital sign is abnormal. Two large-bore (14–16 gauge) IV lines should be started and normal saline rapidly infused. In pediatric cases, IV fluids should be watched carefully and limited to 10 ml/lb (20 ml/kg). All patients warrant cardiac monitoring. Obtaining initial and repeat vital signs is crucial to follow the patient's progress and response to initial resuscitation.

7. Is there any way to estimate the severity of blood loss?

As noted previously, melena implies the rapid loss of greater than 100 ml of blood or more over 24 hours. The loss of 1000 ml can result in near syncope or syncope, tachycardia, weakness, or dizziness. The classic signs of shock are a rough guide to the severity of bleeding. Supine tachycardia suggests blood loss of 20% or more. Supine hypotension is a later finding. The patient's mental status can also reveal the extent of bleeding. Confusion, agitation, or obtundation are associated with blood loss approaching 40% of blood volume. The loss of 2000 ml of blood (40% of circulating blood) can result in death. Ten percent will die from this level of bleeding without emergent therapy.

BIBLIOGRAPHY

1. Bono MJ: Lower gastrointestinal tract bleeding. Emerg Med Clin North Am 14:547–555, 1996.
2. Harwood-Nuss A (ed): The Clinical Practice of Emergency Medicine, 2nd ed. Philadelphia, Lippincott-Raven, 1996.
3. McGuirk TD: Upper gastrointestinal tract bleeding. Emerg Med Clin North Am 14:523–545, 1996.

41. OVERDOSE AND POISONING

Michael Stackpool, M.D.

1. How big a problem is exposure to toxins?

The American Association of Poison Control Centers recorded a record 2,155,952 cases of human poison exposure in 1996. This represents 9.3 cases of exposure for every 1000 persons. More than 90% of these occurred in the home, and 85% were accidental. The vast majority of these cases resulted in no or only minor illness. In more than 90% of cases, there was only one substance involved, while in 5% of cases, more than one patient was exposed to the same toxin. Surprisingly, more than half of all exposures (52.8%) are in children younger than 6 years old. Despite this disproportion, of the 726 reported deaths from poisonings, only 4% of victims were younger than 6 years old. Although suicidal intent was present in only 7.6% of cases, it accounted for 79% of the deaths recorded.

2. What are the most common substances?

Cleaning substances are the most commonly identified substances followed by analgesic medicine, cosmetic and personal care products, plants, cough and cold preparations, and pesticides.

3. What are the most dangerous substances?

The five categories with the largest number of fatalities are analgesics (including narcotics), antidepressants, stimulants and street drugs, cardiovascular drugs, and alcohols. Only analgesics are also one of the top 10 most common exposures. Antidepressants are the 14th and alcohols the 15th most common exposure.

4. What exposure routes are most common?

Ingestion is the most common route of exposure (74%), followed by dermal, inhalation, or ocular exposures; bites and stings; and parenteral (intravenous) or aspiration exposures. In an ingestion, the toxin must be absorbed across the gastrointestinal mucosa before toxic symptoms occur. The stomach can serve as a reservoir of toxin for the small intestine, where most absorption occurs. Inhalation injuries from noxious fumes may be immediate or delayed. Hypoxia is the greatest threat to life and occurs owing to airway obstruction caused by edema, laryngospasm, or bronchospasm or to displacement of oxygen by the inhaled gases themselves. Absorption from skin contact is usually slow, unless the skin barrier is disrupted from abrasions, lacerations, or burns. Dermal exposure to corrosives can be very painful and disfiguring, but with few exceptions, it is not a life threat. Despite a rapid blink reflex, the eye is relatively unprotected from exposures. Ocular damage can be immediate and irreversible. Intravenous routes are obviously the fastest routes of exposure. These may occur in IV drug abusers or inadvertently in the setting of home IV therapy.

5. What are the scene priorities for an unknown exposure?

The first priority, as always, is scene safety for the rescuers. Environmental dangers or hazardous material may require special equipment or protective gear. Since most exposures occur in a public or residential setting, however, extraordinary measures will be unnecessary. Obtain as much information as possible from family and bystanders. The time, amount, and route of ingestion are crucial pieces of information. Long-acting or extended release medications are concerns for delayed or prolonged poisonings. Make sure to ask about the patient's illegal and prescription drug use as well as any available drugs or medications on the scene. Try to determine if the ingestion was intentional or accidental. Gather any empty bottles and transport them with the patient. If there is more than one patient, ask about exposures common to all, such as food, work or industrial chemicals, smoke, or heat sources (carbon monoxide). Manage the ABCs, as in any illness, but be aware that a precipitous decline may follow ingestion or exposure.

6. What kind of decontamination can be done in the field?

Remove the patient from the source of exposure! Evacuate the area of potentially inhaled poisons and remove contaminated clothing. Irrigate the skin and eyes with normal saline or plain water. Apply high-flow oxygen by mask. Nebulized inhaled water may help dilute nasopharyngeal irritants. Never try to "neutralize" a base with an acid or an acid with a base. This will only further contaminate the patient, and the reaction is likely to release large amounts of heat and add thermal burns to the initial chemical injury.

7. What are the dangers of drinking the different kinds of alcohol?

Anyone who works in the prehospital setting soon appreciates the damage that alcohol abuse can wreak. Ethanol is the alcohol found in beer, wine, and liquor. Other easily available alcohols are methanol ("canned heat"), isopropyl (rubbing alcohol), and ethylene glycol (antifreeze). All alcohols are CNS depressants and will exhibit the familiar signs of drunkenness: ataxia, nystagmus, slurred speech, emotional lability, and decreased sensorium. Eventually, severe toxic ingestions progress to respiratory depression, pulmonary aspiration, seizures, and coma. Methanol is metabolized to formic acid, which causes visual changes and even blindness beginning 6 to 12 hours after ingestion. Isopropyl alcohol leaves an odor of acetone on the breath. It can cause coma at blood levels that would be only mildly intoxicating with ethanol. Ethylene glycol is sweet tasting and often visually attractive. This makes it appealing to children and animals. It is very intoxicating and can rapidly cause seizures or coma. It binds calcium, which then crystallizes in the kidneys, heart, and central nervous system. The resulting low levels of calcium can result in severe seizures and muscle spasms (rarely including laryngospasm).

8. Many people are taking medication for depression. Are there serious dangers with an overdose of these medicines? How is an overdose treated?

Absolutely. Between 10% and 20% of the general population will become depressed at some point during their lives. It is the most common psychological disturbance. There are several families of medication aimed at relieving the symptoms of depression. The tricyclic antidepressants (TCAs) cause the most concern, while the newer serotonin reuptake inhibitors have a wider safety margin. TCAs include imipramine, amitriptyline, desipramine, and doxepin, among others, and have a confusing array of brand names. Symptoms of overdose include tachycardia, agitation and altered mental status, dilated pupils, and a dry mouth. Cardiovascular complications are life threatening and evidenced by a prolonged QRS over 100 ms, prolonged QT interval, and variable degrees of atrioventricular block. Ventricular tachycardias, torsades de pointes, and marked hypotension can occur. Myoclonic jerking and twitching may be seen. Seizures can be difficult to treat. Careful attention must be paid to the ABCs. Aggressively treat seizures with diazepam, and treat cardiac arrhythmias following ACLS protocols. Hypotension requires volume resuscitation. On long transport times or for refractory symptoms, sodium bicarbonate may be indicated to treat conduction disturbances or hypotension. Phenytoin is used in the setting of resistant seizures and ventricular arrhythmias, although its long loading time makes its use in the prehospital setting unlikely. Sinus tachycardias do not necessarily portend decline and as such do not need particular treatment.

9. Acetaminophen is found in many over-the-counter drugs, so it must be safe, right?

When taken as directed, it is safe and effective. In larger quantities, however, it can be fatal. One of the difficulties with an acetaminophen (APAP) overdose is recognition of the ingestion itself. There are numerous over-the-counter and prescription drugs that are combined with APAP. Most cold or sinus medicines and analgesic prescriptions contain APAP. Consequently, every ingestion is routinely screened for APAP. Twenty extra-strength tablets or 30 regular-strength pills are toxic in an average-sized adult. Since the primary site of damage is the liver, alcoholics or patients with liver damage are at an increased risk for injury. Initially, there may be little evidence of toxic effects; nevertheless, the optimal time for antidote therapy with acetylcysteine is within 8 hours of ingestion.

10. Aspirin is also found in many prescription and over-the-counter remedies. Are there any characteristic findings in an overdose?

The chemical name for aspirin is acetylsalicylic acid. Salicylates are the family of compounds that include aspirin and its cousin preparations of bismuth subsalicylate (Pepto-Bismol), magnesium salicylate (Doan's Pills), methyl salicylate (oil of wintergreen), and other prescription medicines for inflammatory bowel disease and pain control. In an overdose, these medications may form concretions called *bezoars* in the stomach, which may delay and prolong absorption. Thirty tablets of aspirin in an adult is the minimum acute toxic dose; twice that can result in severe intoxication. Initially, patients present with nausea, vomiting, abdominal pain, hyperventilation, and tinnitus, which is a ringing or buzzing in the ears. This can develop over 10 to 15 hours into evidence of worsening mental status, dehydration, and deafness. Symptoms of severe or late salicylism include seizures, respiratory depression, hyperthermia, hypotension, and coma. Treatment is generally supportive and may include advanced management of the airway, IV fluids, and diazepam for seizures. Severe salicylate ingestions require dialysis.

11. How do patients who take too much of their heart medicine present?

Calcium channel blockers are used for hypertension, angina, and heart failure. Several are currently available. The more common ones are diltiazem, verapamil, nifedipine, and amlodipine. These drugs act to slow atrioventricular (AV) node conduction, slow sinus node activity, and cause vasodilatation in both the coronary and peripheral circulations. Consequently, an overdose will present as hypotension and bradycardia. The bradycardia can be the result of varying degrees of AV block or sinus bradycardia.

Beta blockers are another widely prescribed medication used not only for hypertension and heart disease but also for hyperthyroidism and occasionally for migraines. Again, hypotension and bradycardia are cardinal features of an overdose. Hypoglycemia may accompany a beta blocker overdose. Seizures are more common with beta blockers than calcium channel blockers.

Digoxin is used in the treatment of congestive heart failure and atrial fibrillation. Some degree of toxic symptoms is believed to occur in 5–20% of patients on digoxin. Toxicity initially presents with gastrointestinal disturbances. Nausea, vomiting, diarrhea, and abdominal distention are common complaints. In addition, the patient may complain of blurred or yellow-colored vision, lethargy, and confusion. Finally, cardiac conduction disturbances are the most life threatening. Paroxysmal atrial tachycardia with AV block is classic, but any combination of tachycardia and heart block is suspicious for digoxin overdose.

Treatment is similar for all three ingestions. Initial treatment includes cardiac monitoring, IV fluids for hypotension, and atropine for bradycardia. Cardiac pacing may be required. Calcium channel blockers may benefit from IV calcium. Glucose may be helpful in beta blocker overdose. Cardioversion of ventricular tachycardia caused by digoxin toxicity may result in ventricular fibrillation. Magnesium may improve conduction disturbances caused by digoxin.

12. Are there any toxic exposures common to the rural setting?

Pesticides and crop sprays are related to nerve gases and chemical warfare agents. These compounds are called organophosphates and inhibit acetylcholinesterase, which leaves the autonomic nervous system unregulated and effectively "locked on." The result is best remembered by the "SLUDGE" acronym (salivation, lacrimation, urination, diarrhea, gastrointestinal cramping, and emesis). In severe cases, muscle fasciculations and seizures may follow. The initial management is airway protection and patient decontamination followed by IV atropine. Large doses of atropine are often required. Pralidoxime blocks the action of some organophosphates and will typically be given in the emergency department.

Rat poisons contain warfarin or other anticoagulants. In general, a single ingestion in an otherwise healthy person does not cause significant bleeding. There are many potent and long-acting anticoagulants in use, however, and all ingestion victims require transport and evaluation.

13. *Alice in Wonderland* wasn't on the reading list for my paramedic training. Am I too late for tea?

The opposite of an organophosphate poisoning is an anticholinergic overdose. This results in the autonomic nervous system being "locked off." Anticholinergic medications are commonly found in over-the-counter cold and sleep preparations, antihistamines, medication for depression and psychosis, and Jimson weed ("loco weed"). An "anti-SLUDGE" syndrome develops. Characteristics of the classic anticholinergic syndrome are initial CNS excitation followed by depression, fragmented speech, bizarre behavior, visual and possibly auditory hallucinations, hyperthermia from increased activity and decreased sweat production, widely dilated pupils, dry mucous membranes, and tachycardia. These symptoms are commonly remembered by the phrase "hot as a hare, blind as a bat, dry as a bone, red as a beet, and mad as a hatter."

The phrase "mad as a hatter" is a reference to mercury poisoning. Mercury was used in the hat-making process. Because of its effects (memory loss and emotional instability), hatmaking became linked with madness. The mad hatter in *Alice in Wonderland* apparently had an advanced case of this illness.

14. What did Walt Disney know about plant ingestions?

In the classic movie *Fantasia*, the dance of the mushrooms offers a message on the dangers of plant ingestion. These mushrooms are *Amanita muscaria*. Although plant ingestions rank fourth overall, they are not in the top 15 causes of death from ingestion. In fact, plant ingestions are generally benign, with few exceptions. Plant preparations of steeped teas or powdered seeds can be dangerous. Treat the symptoms of the ingestion rather than the ingestion itself. Bring a sample of the plant or preparation to the emergency department if it is available. Mushrooms grow almost everywhere, and poisonous varieties tend to be gastrointestinal irritants. The nondescript white *Amanita phalloides* are dangerous and can result in fatal hepatic necrosis. These are different from the colorful *Amanita muscaria* dancing in *Fantasia*. These mushrooms cause an anticholinergic syndrome.

15. What about street drugs?

Cocaine, amphetamines, and related stimulants are commonly available illicitly, in over-the-counter diet medicines, and by prescription. Patients with significant ingestion show euphoria, mydriasis, agitation and restlessness, tachycardia, and hypertension. They are at risk for seizures, hyperthermia, and ventricular arrhythmias. In some cases, psychosis will develop that is indistinguishable from schizophrenia or the manic phase of bipolar disorder. Myocardial infarction and stroke have occurred owing to cocaine use. Diazepam is the treatment of choice to control vital signs and agitation.

Opiate overdose has a triad of classic symptoms. Narcotics act in the CNS to cause sedation ranging from drowsiness and lethargy to frank coma. Miosis, or pinpoint pupils, is perhaps the best known sign. Respiratory depression poses the greatest life threat. In addition, hypotension, hypothermia, and bradycardia may complicate the overdose. Naloxone is a specific narcotic antagonist used to reverse an opiate overdose. The initial dose, 2 mg IV, may be repeated in cases of suspected severe overdose. There is a risk of precipitating withdrawal symptoms in some patients and in patients on methadone maintenance treatment.

16. Speaking of withdrawal, how dangerous is it?

That depends on what the patient has been taking. Onset of symptoms can vary from a few hours in the case of cocaine and alcohol overdose to one or two days for some opiates. Ethanol is associated with the most common withdrawal syndrome, which may be life threatening. It manifests as intense sympathetic nervous system stimulation. A blood level of zero is not required for withdrawal to occur. In chronic alcoholics, serum alcohol levels over the legal limit of 100 mg/dL may produce symptoms. Ethanol withdrawal has four stages beginning with tremulousness, tachycardia, hyperthermia, and hypertension. This is followed by a progression through seizures, hallucinations, and finally frank delirium. Diazepam or lorazepam is the treatment of choice for sedation and control of autonomic dysfunction.

Opiate withdrawal is much more benign, albeit very uncomfortable. The constellation of symptoms includes rhinorrhea, lacrimation, vomiting, diarrhea, agitation, and mild elevations in heart rate and blood pressure. Piloerection (hair standing on end) is common, while seizures, mental status changes, and hyperthermia are rare. Withdrawal may be precipitated by naloxone use. Naloxone has a short half-life, however, and symptoms should resolve in two or three hours. Severe symptoms may respond to clonidine.

Cocaine or amphetamine withdrawal typically ends with depression and lethargy. No specific treatment is indicated.

17. What are the important inhaled toxins?

Carbon monoxide is produced in a fire and also by gas heaters, engine exhaust, and coal burners. It binds to hemoglobin 200 times more often than oxygen. Hemoglobin bound by carbon monoxide cannot transport oxygen. The earliest symptom is headache followed by dyspnea, irritability and fatigue, tachycardia, confusion, coma, and seizures (with increasing toxicity). Treatment is high-flow oxygen and possibly hyperbaric oxygen.

Cyanide gases from burning plastics or industrial settings is easily absorbed. Patients rapidly decline and complain of headache, nausea, and anxiety. They appear confused, and initial hypertension and bradycardia can progress to hypotension and tachycardia and quickly to apnea. High-flow oxygen and inhaled amyl nitrite are the initial measures. Then sodium nitrite IV and thiosulfate are given. These are all contained in a prepackaged cyanide antidote kit.

18. What should be done for the unknown ingestion?

Careful attention to the airway is paramount to prevent hypoxia and complications from aspiration. Oxygen by mask or nasal cannula, cardiac monitoring, and establishing IV access are routine measures. Naloxone, 2 mg IV, should be given regardless of suspicion for opiate ingestion. Glucose, 25 g IV, is given in case of hypoglycemia due to diabetes or medication. Seizures are treated with diazepam or lorazepam.

BIBLIOGRAPHY

1. Abbott J: Prehospital Emergency Care. New York, Parthenon Publishing Group, 1996.
2. Cox RD: Decontamination and management of hazardous materials exposure victims in the emergency department. Ann Emerg Med 23:761–770, 1994.
3. Erickson TB: Dealing with the unknown exposure. Emerg Med 28(6):74–88, 1996.
4. Jones SA: Advanced Emergency Care for Paramedic Practice. Philadelphia, J.B. Lippincott, 1992.
5. Litovitz TL: 1996 Annual report of the American Association of Poison Control Centers Toxic Exposure Surveillance System. Am J Emerg Med 15:447, 1997.
6. Pimentel L: Cyclic antidepressant overdoses. Emerg Med Clin North Am 12:533–544, 1994.

42. HYPOTHERMIA

Richard Buchanan, B.A., EMT-P, and John Tarr, Jr., M.D.

1. Why do I need to know about hypothermia?

There are very few places in the United States that don't ever get at least a little bit cold, or wet, or both, so hypothermia can occur anywhere. Additionally, the injured, the sick, the young, and the old are particularly susceptible to cold. Therefore, EMS providers must be familiar with causes, prevention, and care of hypothermia.

2. What is hypothermia?

Hypothermia occurs when the core temperature of the body drops below 35°C (95°F). Hypothermia is categorized as mild (32.2–35°C, 90–95°F) moderate (27–32.2°C, 80–90°F), or severe (< 27°C, < 80°F).

3. What causes hypothermia?

Hypothermia occurs whenever the body loses heat into its environment faster than it can produce it. Hypothermia may also result from impaired thermoregulation.

4. What are the mechanisms of heat loss?

Heat is lost by four mechanisms: conduction, convection, radiation, and evaporation, so certain environmental factors can increase loss.

1. Conductive loss is enhanced by direct contact with cold objects (such as lying on snow or a metal surface) and moisture, since water conducts and removes heat much faster than air. For example, conductive heat loss increases 25fold with immersion in cold water.

2. Convective loss is increased by air movement, so windy conditions remove much more heat than calm; thus the concept of wind chill.

3. Loss through radiation increases with removal of clothing and other insulating layers. Radiation may account for more than 50% of heat loss.

4. Evaporative heat loss increases with windy conditions and low humidity.

5. Who is prone to hypothermia?

Patient characteristics that increase heat loss or decrease heat production include increased surface area compared to volume (infants and children), decreased metabolism (elderly, shocky, intoxicated), increased fluid loss (sweating, diarrhea, burns), and being disrobed for evaluation and treatment of illness or injury.

6. How do you prevent it?

Understanding and minimizing the four sources of heat loss is the best prevention. Getting a patient out of the environment causing heat loss is the first step. Removing wet clothing, insulating from cold surfaces, avoiding unnecessary exposure, and providing adequate coverage with warm blankets are simple and effective ways to minimize further heat loss. Effectively treating contributing conditions such as shock and dehydration enhances the body's ability to generate heat. Maintaining a high level of surveillance for sources of continuing heat loss is essential.

7. How do you diagnose it?

Reliable core temperatures are difficult to obtain in the field. Unless tympanic thermometers become easier to use, more reliable, or more accepted, following a simplified clinical assessment is recommended, being cautious to exclude other conditions that might cause a similar clinical picture.

Mild	Poor judgment
	Strong shivering
	Normal blood pressure
Moderate	Little or no shivering
	Arrhythmias
	Pupils dilate
	Stupor/poor perfusion
Severe	No reflex or response
	Significant hypotension
	Maximum risk of ventricular fibrillation
	No pupil response

8. How is hypothermia treated?

Hypothermia is a physiologic derangement much like shock and should be corrected as aggressively.

1. **Localized hypothermia (or frostbite)** is best treated by immersion in water at 100°–108°F. Unless your ambulance is equipped with a hot tub, it may be difficult to accomplish this in the prehospital setting. **Carefully monitored** application of chemical heat packs over dressings can be helpful but is risky and can cause burns. Thawing tissue should not be further traumatized by massage or unnecessary manipulation. Tissue should never be warmed or thawed if there is a danger of refreezing. Rapid transport to a hospital is imperative.

2. **Mild hypothermia** can be effectively treated merely by preventing further heat loss and allowing the patient to generate his own heat through shivering. Hypothermia bags, blankets, or even just a warm ambulance can be used. It is important to expose and examine a patient, but do so under temperature-controlled circumstances.

3. **Moderate and severe hypothermia** must be actively treated, and the treatment may be passive or active rewarming.

Severe hypothermia (< 27°C, < 80°F) is best treated by core rewarming. The best method is cardiopulmonary bypass, as is used in open heart surgery, but obviously not practical or available in the field. Irrigation or lavage of body cavities and hollow viscera (such as peritoneum, stomach, colon, or bladder) is also theoretically possible but is difficult or impossible to accomplish in a prehospital setting.

Administration of warmed IV fluids is reasonable, but the laws of thermodynamics prevent adding much heat by this method. As an example, mixing a liter of water at 90°F with a liter of water at 105°F will give two liters of water at 97.5°F. Since the average human is approximately 60% water, the average total body water of a 70-kg human will amount to about 42 liters. Consequently, a severely hypothermic patient with a core temperature of 90°F will have 42 liters of body water at 90°F. It would take an equal amount (42 liters) of 105°F IV fluids to warm the cold body fluid to 97.5°F, which would incidentally increase body water to 84 liters. It's doubtful that most patients would tolerate this much IV fluid acutely.

In contrast, the average *resting* human ventilates the lungs with approximately 10 liters of air each minute, and the *entire* cardiac output (which averages 5 liters/min) passes through the lungs. Exposing 5 L/min of centrally circulating blood to 10 L/min of warm air is much more doable than giving 42 liters of IV fluids. There are a number of products on the market that can heat and humidify oxygen (104°–113°F), including some that are battery operated. Any EMS agency working in areas that have cold environments should investigate this type of equipment.

9. Should CPR be initiated on the severely hypothermic patient?

This is an age-old question that continues to be debated. Generally, CPR should be initiated for patients in cardiac and respiratory arrest. CPR is insufficient under these circumstances, and transport to definitive care should not be delayed. Also, performing CPR on the severely hypothermic patient will often induce ventricular fibrillation, which will be difficult to treat, since defibrillation is usually unsuccessful. Resuscitation should be continued during transport while attempting to rewarm the patient.

10. Can I mistake hypothermia for death?

You bet you can, and it has occurred. Profoundly hypothermic patients may appear to be dead owing to the dramatically decreased metabolic rate (i.e., slow shallow respirations and bradycardia). Therefore, for all such patients, you should obtain a 60-second rhythm strip documenting asystole before death is pronounced.

11. When should resuscitation of the severely hypothermic patient be terminated?

The statement "a patient is not dead until he or she is warm and dead" is still a good concept. Except in circumstances where the safety of the EMT is in jeopardy or in a triage situation, a patient should be resuscitated until a physician can make a final determination, usually after adequate core rewarming, or as specified by local policies and protocols. Of course, if the patient's torso is frozen solid, resuscitation will probably be unwarranted.

12. At what temperature should ACLS guidelines be followed?

Cardiac medications and electrical therapy generally don't work in patients with core temperatures below 86°F (severe hypothermia). Bretylium has been shown to be the exception, being much more effective than lidocaine for both prophylactic and hypothermic arrest situations. Since perfusion is significantly decreased, the dosages of other medications should be decreased to prevent accumulation and toxicity.

13. Should the severely hypothermic patient be intubated?

Airway is still and always the first priority and should be secured in the hypothermic patient. The concern that endotracheal intubation can cause ventricular fibrillation is overemphasized. In addition, preoxygenation with high-flow oxygen and bag mask ventilation will help prevent this dysrhythmia from occurring. Most research shows that ventilation sufficient to prevent or correct respiratory acidosis minimizes that risk. Endotracheal intubation will facilitate the use of humidified, heated oxygen systems as well as protecting the patient's airway.

14. What prophylactic medications should be given to the hypothermic patient in the pre-hospital setting?

There are a number of medications that have been shown to be appropriate for the moderate or severely hypothermic patient. When establishing peripheral intravenous access, use normal saline instead of lactated Ringer's solution. A hypothermic liver may not metabolize the lactate, resulting in lactic acidosis. Administration of dextrose 50 and naloxone is also indicated. Thiamine (100 mg IV) may also be considered for patients with altered mental status.

15. What special considerations should be given to the hypothermic trauma patient?

The hypothermic trauma patient is a unique challenge. Research shows that because of the physiologic changes associated with hypothermia (impaired coagulation, altered platelet function, and disseminated intravascular coagulation), considerably increased blood loss can occur. The patient most at risk will have blunt or penetrating abdominal trauma as well as hypothermia. Aggressive efforts should be made to rewarm these patients or to minimize their heat loss. Avoid use of cold intravenous fluids, ventilation with cold oxygen, and exposing the patient for long periods of time.

16. Can I cause hypothermia?

Yes. Exposure of the very young and the very old by removal of clothing for relatively brief periods of time will cause hypothermia. Also, the application of wet dressings to a body burn of greater than 10% of body surface area will cause hypothermia.

BIBLIOGRAPHY

1. American Heart Association: Accidental Hypothermia: Textbook of Advanced Cardiac Life Support, 2nd ed. Dallas, TX, AHA, 1990, pp 231–233.
2. Bernabei MD, Alvise F: The effects of hypothermia and injury severity on blood loss during trauma laparotomy. J Trauma 33:835–839, 1992.
3. Danzl D: Hypothermia and Frostbite. In Markovchick VJ, Pons PT, Wolfe RE (eds): Emergency Medicine Secrets. Philadelphia, Hanley & Belfus, 1993.
4. Evanovich K: Hypothermia and trauma. Orthop Nurs 12:33–37, 1993.
5. Hector MD, Melvin G: Treatment of accidental hypothermia. Am Fam Phys 45(2):785–791, 1992.
6. Lawson MN, Lari L: Hypothermia and trauma injury: Temperature monitoring and rewarming strategies. Crit Care Nurs Q 15(1):21–31, 1992.

43. HEAT ILLNESS

Thomas G. Burke, M.D.

1. Name the mechanisms of heat transfer and an example of each one.
There are four ways heat is transferred:

Conduction: Direct transfer of heat energy from warmer to cooler objects (touching an ice cube).

Convection: Heat loss to air and water vapor circulating around object (a cool sea breeze).

Radiation: Heat transfer by electromagnetic waves (the warmth of the sun).

Evaporation: Conversion of liquid to gas and resultant heat loss (sweating). This is the major source of heat transfer (cooling) in humans.

2. Why do humans become hyperthermic?
Humans are a biologic furnace. Food is the fuel, and heat is produced as this energy source is metabolized. Our baseline metabolic function of 50–60 kcal/hr would equal a rise in temperature of 1.1°C (2°F) *every hour* if we had no cooling mechanisms. High environmental temperatures add even more heat energy.

3. Where are the thermostats in the human body?
Thermosensors are in the skin and central nervous system (hypothalamus). Skin has a wide variation in temperature tolerance, but the central regulatory system is much less forgiving and much more important in regulation.

4. What are the main thermoregulatory mechanisms in humans?
Sweating combined with an increased cardiac output and peripheral vasodilation are the most important and quickly regulated mechanisms. The hyperdynamic cardiovascular system delivers heat from the body's core to the skin. Peripheral vasodilation increases the surface area for heat transfer and also provides heat for evaporation of sweat. There is a compensatory splanchnic vasoconstriction, and cardiac output must increase dramatically to maintain a reasonable blood pressure. Because of this, jacuzzis and saunas may be dangerous to persons with cardiac disease.

Sweating provides a water source for evaporation. About 1–2 liters of sweat are typically lost by a person exercising in a hot environment. The amount of sweat that is actually evaporated is decreased in a humid environment because the surrounding air can only absorb a limited amount of moisture. This is why it feels hotter on a humid 80° day in Washington, DC, than it does on a dry 80° day in Denver.

Of note, respiratory countercurrent (heat exchange by increasing the respiratory depth and rate) is a method of heat transfer in all animals. Although pronounced in dogs (who don't sweat), it is fairly ineffective in humans compared to the above mechanisms.

5. What are the predisposing factors for heat illness?
Environmental heat stress is caused by high outdoor temperatures or being in enclosed environments such as cars, tanks, tents, engine rooms, hot tubs, saunas, or factories. **Dehydration** is a result of decreased intake, vomiting, diarrhea, or diuretics. **Inhibited sweating** occurs with occlusive clothing, skin disease, or anticholinergic drugs. **Decreased peripheral blood flow** results from diabetes or atherosclerosis. **Cardiac disease** may inhibit the ability to increase peripheral circulation to provide adequate heat transfer. Several medical conditions also cause increased heat production: hyperthyroidism, malignant hyperthermia, and neuroleptic malignant syndrome. **Alcohol, amphetamines, and obesity** are additional risk factors.

6. What is the difference between fever and hyperthermia?

They have different mechanisms, and it is important to differentiate between the two. Fever changes our body's "set point," and we seek warmer environments (i.e., blankets). Attempts at cooling will cause shivering, rigors, and discomfort. Hyperthermia is caused by an inability to cool the body, and we seek cooler environments (shade).

7. What is heat illness?

Heat-related illness represents a spectrum or continuum of signs and symptoms that may range from quite mild to severe and life-threatening. The disease is called heat cramps in its least severe form, heat stroke in its most severe type, and heat exhaustion in between.

8. Describe heat cramps.

Heat cramps occur in muscles that are fatigued by heavy work and are brought on by prolonged strenuous exercise, as in steel workers, sugar cane cutters, and miners. The onset occurs *after finishing* heavy work and during relaxation. They differ from the cramps of athletes, which occur *during* exercise and relieve with massage and resolve spontaneously. Heat cramps are caused by salt deficiency as a result of copious sweating during exertion and large volumes of hypotonic fluid replacement. Treatment is electrolyte fluid replacement, which can usually be accomplished orally. This is one of the reasons British and German laborers traditionally salt their beer.

9. What are the symptoms and signs of heat exhaustion?

Volume depletion and electrolyte loss. The patient complains of any combination of weakness, fatigue, frontal headache, vertigo, nausea and vomiting, thirst, decreased urine output, and cramps. Temperature is often normal and, if elevated, is usually < 40°C (104°F). Mental function remains intact. Tachycardia, orthostatic hypotension, and clinical dehydration may occur, and the skin is pale, cool and clammy, and may be flushed. Sweating persists and may be profuse.

10. What is the treatment for heat exhaustion?

Rest in a cool, shady spot. Fluid and electrolyte replacement is essential. Rehydration with solutions such as Gatorade, Powerade, or dilute sugar drinks with a half teaspoon of salt per liter can be very effective. If significant hypotension is present, intravenous fluids should be started. The patient should be monitored for further signs of progressive illness because heat exhaustion may progress to heat stroke.

11. What are the two types of heat stroke?

Classic heat stroke is typically seen with high environmental temperatures and often associated with high humidity. Its victims are elderly, debilitated patients and those who live in poorly ventilated houses with limited access to water. Chronic illness such as cardiovascular disease, diabetes, and alcoholism also will inhibit the thermoregulatory systems of the body. Patients have been exposed to heat for a prolonged period, are likely to have been sweating excessively, are dehydrated, and most have stopped sweating by the time heat stroke is manifested.

Exertional heat stroke presents in young otherwise healthy and physically fit individuals who are overtaken by endogenous heat production. Sweating is still present in half of these patients, and they may not be dehydrated despite their loss of thermoregulation.

12. What are the symptoms and signs of heat stroke?

This entity is different from heat exhaustion in that the thermoregulatory mechanisms have failed. Heat stroke is a catastrophic life-threatening emergency that is manifested by hyperthermia, mental status changes, and cardiovascular collapse. Temperature is typically above 40°C, with tachycardia and tachypnea. Blood pressure may be low. Central nervous system dysfunction is evident with bizarre behavior, ataxia, hallucinations, delirium, seizures, and coma. The skin is generally red and hot. High-output congestive heart failure, pulmonary edema, and eventually hypotension will ensue. Hepatic damage is common, but the signs of coagulopathy and jaundice are late findings (> 24 hrs).

13. What is the treatment for heat stroke?

Attention to the ABCs is first and foremost, as usual. The patient then must be removed from the hot environment, disrobed, and cooling measures initiated immediately. The longer the duration of hyperthermia, the greater the tissue damage. Cooling is best accomplished by lightly spraying the exposed patient with water while fanning—with a hand or electric fan—air over their body to facilitate evaporative heat loss. Ice water baths or rubbing the skin with ice is contraindicated because it will cause peripheral vasoconstriction and impaired heat transfer. Establish an IV and infuse ambient temperature normal saline. Transport or evacuate all patients who have an altered level of consciousness or who are unstable.

14. What are means to prevent heat illness?

• Keeping well hydrated is essential to preventing heat illnesses. Rarely will people replace the amount of fluids they lose during exercise or in a hot environment.
• Avoid prolonged exposure to hot environments and rest frequently during strenuous exercise.
• Wear well-ventilated, loosely woven, breathable clothing to keep cool, and wear a hat for protection from direct sun exposure.
• Avoid drugs that predispose to poor thermoregulation, such as amphetamines, diuretics, antihistamines, cocaine, and alcohol.
• Remember that heat illness is completely preventable.

BIBLIOGRAPHY

1. Fogerty WW (ed): Wilderness Medical Society Practice Guidelines for Wilderness and Environmental Emergencies. Merrillville, IN, ICS Books, 1995.
2. Hubbard RW, Gaffin SL, Squire DL: Heat related illnesses. In Auerbach PS (ed): Wilderness Medicine: Management of Wilderness and Environmental Emergencies, 3rd ed. St. Louis, Mosby, 1995, pp 413–445.
3. Tilton B (ed): Wilderness Medicine Handbook, 2nd ed. Pitkin, CO, Wilderness Medical Institute, 1997.
4. Yarbrough B: Heat illness. In Rosen P, et al (eds): Principles and Practice of Emergency Medicine: Concepts and Clinical Practice, 3rd ed. St. Louis, Mosby, 1992.

44. ALTITUDE ILLNESS

Thomas G. Burke, M.D.

1. How is altitude measured, and why are people affected by increases in elevation?

Altitude is measured in feet or meters above sea level. The partial pressure of oxygen (how much oxygen is available in the air we take for each breath) decreases with an increase in altitude. Therefore, the symptoms and signs associated with high altitude are directly and indirectly a result of hypoxia. Each individual has a different response to this hypoxia and, therefore, different susceptibilities to altitude illness. Within a few hours at altitude, a decrease in blood oxygen saturation is detected and ventilation is increased. This result is called the hypoxic ventilatory response (HVR). Altered fluid homeostasis also occurs, and a redistribution of fluid from the intravascular to intracellular and extracellular spaces results in peripheral and, occasionally, pulmonary and cerebral edema.

2. What are the most common syndromes caused by altitude illness?

Altitude illness is a continuum of symptoms and signs that can range from a mild loss of appetite and headache to cerebral and pulmonary edema, coma, and death. For the purposes of classification, these syndromes have been described as mild, moderate, and severe acute mountain sickness (AMS), with severe AMS involving high altitude pulmonary edema (HAPE) and/or high altitude cerebral edema (HACE).

3. Describe the symptoms, signs, and treatments for mild AMS.

Symptoms and signs: Headache relieved by rest and medication, nausea, lassitude, anorexia and insomnia. There are no characteristic physical exam findings.

Treatment: One should never continue to ascend until the symptoms have diminished. It is best to try to acclimatize at the same altitude. It is important to keep well hydrated and continue adequate nutrition even in light of anorexia. Although lassitude may be present, light exercise is often helpful. Headaches can be severe, and ibuprofen, aspirin, or acetaminophen can be beneficial. Sedatives should be avoided because they may mask a further progression of illness. Acetazolamide (Diamox) will help with quicker acclimatization.

4. Describe the symptoms, signs, and treatments for moderate AMS.

Symptoms and signs: Headache not relieved by rest or medication, nausea with vomiting, shortness of breath, fatigue and weakness at rest, anorexia, and insomnia.

Treatment: Descent of at least 1000 feet and sometimes 2000 feet or greater is necessary. Hydration and nutrition are essential. Since hypoxia is the underlying cause of AMS, oxygen will significantly improve symptoms. However, one should never delay descent to wait for supplemental oxygen, because the descent itself is the equivalent of providing additional oxygen. Pain medications for headache and, if persistent vomiting is present, an antiemetic such as prochlorperazine 50 mg by suppository are recommended. Acetazolamide also will be helpful. It is important to closely monitor the patient for deterioration.

5. Describe the symptoms, signs, and treatment for severe AMS, including HAPE and HACE.

Symptoms and signs: All of the above findings plus the following physical findings, which develop as AMS worsens. Ataxia is the most important sign to recognize that AMS is progressing from moderate to severe. Fatigue and personal neglect may progress to the point that the patient is not eating, drinking, or dressing himself. There is dyspnea at rest and tachycardia. HAPE develops insidiously with fluid accumulation in the lungs. A persistent dry cough begins, and scattered rales may be heard on lung ascultation. Late in the illness, a productive cough of blood-tinged frothy sputum may develop. Hypoxia worsens and tachypnea progresses. HACE is manifested by a change in mental status that may include disorientation, somnolence, confusion, combativeness, stupor, and coma. HAPE and HACE can be seen independently, but both are usually present to some degree.

Treatment: Successful treatment depends on early recognition of the progression of AMS. Immediate descent is the treatment of choice. Oxygen is helpful. Pharmacologic intervention includes dexamethazone (Decadron) for HACE. Nifedipine and acetazolamide can be used for HAPE. Medication will not work on its own—descent is necessary.

6. If descent is not an immediate alternative, is there a way to simulate descent?

The Gamov bag is a portable, inflatable, neoprene bag that can be inflated to 2 psi to simulate a descent of 4000–6000 feet. This barometric change usually will improve the patient's symptoms. One or two people may fit in this device, and it provides a temporizing measure until descent can be made.

7. What is acetazolamide, how does it work, and what are its indications for use?

Acetazolamide, or Diamox, is a diuretic that indirectly causes enhanced ventilatory acclimatization and decreases cerebral spinal fluid production. It is the drug of choice for prophylaxis of AMS. It is also indicated for use during rapid ascent (i.e., for those partaking in a rescue effort), for persons with a past history of moderate AMS or HAPE, and for treatment for AMS that has already developed. The dose is 125–250 mg orally twice a day.

8. Does Diamox have any side effects?

Yes. It is a sulfa-based drug and allergies may exist. Since Diamox is a diuretic, it causes polyuria and can lead to dehydration if adequate intake is not maintained. Peripheral paresthesias, myopia, and impotence can also occur. A side effect is that it allows carbon dioxide to be tasted in carbonated beverages and ruins their taste.

9. What is dexamethasone, how does it work, and what are its indications for use?

Dexamethasone is a steroid that has antiinflammatory effects. It is effective in treating AMS and HACE. However, symptoms can rebound once the medication is stopped. Therefore, its use is limited as a prophylactic medication for AMS to those with intolerable side effects from Diamox.

10. What are prevention measures for AMS?

If traveling to 8000 feet and above, ascend slowly. Spend the first 2–3 days at altitude doing moderate exercise. If traveling above 10,000 feet, only ascend 1000–2000 feet per day and have frequent rest days. Climbing to a higher altitude and then descending to sleep helps with acclimatization (climb high, sleep low). Keeping well hydrated is a must. A high-carbohydrate diet (70%) helps reduce AMS symptoms. Avoid sedatives and alcohol while at altitude. Prophylactic use of acetazolamide can be helpful.

11. What is HAFE?

High altitude flatus expulsion. It has brought to ruin many a nights' sleep in a tent while at altitude. Although not extensively studied, HAFE has been described in great detail by mountaineers the world over. It is proposed that intralumenal bowel gas expands with a decreased barometric pressure, causing flatus. Simethicone may assist in decreasing the symptoms.

BIBLIOGRAPHY

1. Fogerty WW (ed): Wilderness Medical Society Practice Guidelines for Wilderness and Environmental Emergencies. Merillville, IN, ICS Books, 1995.
2. Hackett PH, Roach RC: High altitude medicine. In Auerbach PS (ed): Wilderness Medicine: Management of Wilderness and Environmental Emergencies, 3rd ed. St. Louis, Mosby, 1995, pp 1–37.

3. Hackett PH, Rennie D: The incidence, importance and prophylaxis of acute mountain sickness. Lancet 2(7996):1149–1155, 1976.
4. Johnson TS, Rock PB: Acute mountain sickness. N Engl J Med 319:841–845, 1988.
5. Larson EB, Roach RC, Schoene RB, Hornbein TF: Acute mountain sickness and acetazolamide. JAMA 248:328–332, 1982.
6. Tilton B (ed): Wilderness Medicine Handbook, 2nd ed. Pitkin, CO, Wilderness Medical Institute, 1997.

45. OBSTETRIC AND GYNECOLOGIC EMERGENCIES

Jean Abbott, M.D.

1. When should you consider that a woman with medical complaints may be pregnant?

Generally speaking, any woman 14–50 years old may be pregnant unless she's had a hysterectomy. The possibility of pregnancy must be considered in the differential diagnosis, particularly when a woman presents with acute abdominal pain or vaginal bleeding.

2. What is an ectopic pregnancy and how is it diagnosed?

An ectopic pregnancy is a pregnancy that implants and grows outside of the uterus. It causes symptoms in the first 12 weeks of pregnancy, sometimes even before the patient misses a menstrual period. It is a problem because bleeding can be significant, hidden in the peritoneal cavity, and life-threatening. Ectopic pregnancy should be considered in the prehospital assessment in any woman of childbearing age who presents with unilateral or bilateral lower abdominal pain.

3. What causes a miscarriage and how does it present?

Miscarriage, or spontaneous abortion, is relatively common, occurring in about 20% of women who are pregnant as confirmed by chemical tests. Of women who have vaginal bleeding in pregnancy, almost half have normal pregnancies and the other half miscarry. About 80% of miscarriages occur in the first 3 months, and most are caused by abnormal growth of the fetus, due either to chromosomal abnormalities or to abnormalities within the uterus. In the second trimester, after 14 weeks, miscarriage may be more complicated and associated with heavier bleeding. Before the uterus expels tissue, the miscarriage is considered *threatened*. When the cervix opens, miscarriage is considered *inevitable* or *incomplete*. A *completed* miscarriage occurs after all tissue has been expelled. To assess the patient in the emergency department, it is mandatory to bring all the clots and tissue that the patient shows you. Pathologic analysis of this tissue can help to determine if miscarriage has occurred.

4. What prehospital considerations are important in the patient who is a victim of alleged sexual assault?

The paramedic is responsible for treating traumatic injuries and for preserving evidence. All clothes should be brought in with the patient, the police should be notified, and the emergency department should be alerted that a possible sexual assault victim is being transported. The patient needs to be as active a participant in her care as possible, since the trauma has involved powerlessness. Only the history that is necessary to perform a competent medical examination and treatment should be obtained by prehospital personnel.

5. How do vital signs change in pregnancy?

In pregnancy, blood pressure is normally not higher than the patient's baseline before pregnancy. The systolic pressure may be lower by 5 to 15 mm Hg in the second trimester. The pulse usually rises to 80–95 beats per minute in late pregnancy. The respiratory rate and tidal volume increase. The diaphragm rises about 4 cm in late pregnancy, impairing respiratory reserve.

6. How should a pregnant patient be transported?

After 20 weeks, supine positioning can cause hypotension, which occurs when the gravid uterus presses on the inferior vena cava, obstructing venous return. In 20% of pregnant women, this can result in decreased cardiac output, known as the *supine hypotensive syndrome*. For this reason, after 20 weeks, the patient should be transported on her left side or, if immobilized on a backboard, with the backboard wedged and tilted 15° to the left.

7. What are the main causes of bleeding in a woman who is more than 20 weeks pregnant?

The two primary causes of vaginal bleeding in the second half of pregnancy are placenta previa and abruptio placentae. *Placenta previa* is due to low implantation of the placenta near the cervix. As the uterus grows, small bridging vessels overlying the cervix can tear and cause a small amount of bleeding, which is usually painless and bright red. A digital exam of the cervix can cause uncontrolled bleeding and therefore should never be performed in the prehospital arena. *Abruptio placentae* is premature separation of the placenta, which is usually painful and associated with uterine tenderness and contractions. Risk factors for abruptio placentae include trauma to the abdomen, cocaine use, hypertension, and eclampsia. Other causes of vaginal bleeding after 20 weeks include early labor and other local lesions of the cervix.

8. What is preeclampsia and how are preeclampsia and eclampsia differentiated?

Preeclampsia, or pregnancy-induced hypertension (PIH), is a vasospastic condition unique to pregnancy in which the patient develops edema, protein in the urine, and hypertension. The level of hypertension is usually just over the usual "normal" blood pressure of 140/90.

Eclampsia itself is the occurrence of seizures in a pregnant patient with preeclampsia. Eclampsia can occur up to a week postpartum. Vasospasm associated with eclampsia causes injury to multiple organs, including the liver, kidney, and brain. Warning signs for eclampsia include hyperreflexia, visual disturbances, right upper quadrant pain, and severe headache.

9. How should eclamptic seizures be treated?

With diazepam 5–10 mg IV, as with seizures in nonpregnancy. The specific treatment of choice is magnesium sulfate, 4 g of 10% solution IV over 20 minutes in 250 ml of D_5W. During the infusion, reflexes should be monitored and respiratory depression should be treated with ventilation.

10. What else can cause seizures in pregnancy?

Patients can have increased frequency of epileptic seizures; thrombotic strokes or intracranial bleeds; and seizures due to toxins or overdoses. Never forget the possibility of hypoglycemia in the pregnant patient with seizures.

11. How should paroxysmal superventricular tachycardia (PSVT) be treated in pregnancy?

Much the same that it is in nonpregnant women. The first priority should be to ascertain that the tachycardia is indeed primary and is not secondarily caused by hypovolemia, sepsis, fever, or another illness. Adenosine can be used safely in pregnancy, and cardioversion also is safe to the fetus.

12. When do you consider the fetus separately when the mother is critically ill?

After 24–26 weeks, at which point the fetus is potentially viable outside the uterus. Rapid transport for consideration of perimortem cesarean section should be done whenever the dome of the uterus is at or above a position halfway between the umbilicus and the xiphoid.

13. What may cause cardiac arrest in pregnancy?

Causes specific to the pregnancy need to be considered: hypovolemia due to uterine rupture of abruptio placenta, hepatic or splenic rupture, or ruptured ectopic pregnancy lead the list. In addition, pulmonary emboli, amniotic fluid embolus, and other diseases can occur. Cardiopulmonary resuscitation is difficult in pregnancy due to the large mass of the uterus. Up to 26 weeks, the goal should be maximal resuscitation of the mother. After 26 weeks, two patients exist: the fetus and the mother. Fluids should be administered; supplemental oxygen and early intubation are mandatory; the patient should be tilted at least 15° to the left side; and the usual advanced cardiac life support (ACLS) drugs and defibrillation should be employed. Because cardiopulmonary resuscitation has such a dismal outcome, expeditious transport for possible cesarean section or thoracotomy is indicated.

14. In a motor vehicle accident, what are the special risks in pregnancy?

One is abruptio placentae. Also, physical exam signs are diminished in blunt abdominal trauma, and the patient must be considered to have significant injury until proven otherwise. Therefore, when the visibly pregnant patient is in a motor vehicle accident, it is necessary to be aggressive in fluid resuscitation, avoid the supine position, and ventilate with high-flow oxygen. The hospital should be advised if the patient appears to be more than 26 weeks pregnant, since a two-patient resuscitation should be instituted in the emergency department.

15. When do you stop the ambulance with a woman in labor and prepare to deliver?

Imminent delivery should be considered if the patient is bearing down, if there is crowning of the head, or if the patient is a multiparous woman who knows that she is about to deliver.

16. What are the priorities for prehospital delivery of a pregnant woman?

The first priority is to control the speed of delivery and thus the trauma to the maternal perineum. This is done by having the patient pant and putting some gentle counter-pressure against the baby's head to maintain flexion and slow delivery. After the head has delivered, you must check around the baby's neck for the umbilical cord and disengage it or double-clamp and cut the cord if you are unable to remove the cord from around the neck. After the head is delivered, suction the infant's airway and wait for the rest of the delivery. External rotation will occur so that the head will realign with the anterior and posterior shoulders. The anterior shoulder should be delivered first with gentle downward traction on the next contraction, and then upward traction is followed rapidly by delivery of the posterior shoulder and the rest of the baby. Do *not* pull on the baby's neck—gentle guidance is all that is required.

17. Should you wait for the placenta to deliver?

The patient can be transported after delivery of the baby and cross-clamping of the cord. Manual traction on the placenta can cause tearing and incomplete separation of the placenta and uncontrolled bleeding. Therefore, it is best to leave delivery of the placenta to hospital personnel.

18. Name some physiologic changes that occur during pregnancy.

Increased heart rate
Increased respiratory rate
Normal or low blood pressure
Decreased respiratory reserve
Increase venous pressure in legs
Supine hypotension
Loss of abdominal findings such as guarding

19. Summarize the treatment of critical illness in pregnancy.

Early intubation
Aggressive fluid resuscitation
Position on left side/backboard 15° to left
ACLS—normal protocols
Rapid transport after 24 weeks of gestation for consideration of fetal rescue

BIBLIOGRAPHY

1. Abbott J: Complications related to pregnancy. In Rosen P, Barking RM (eds): Emergency Medicine: Concepts and Clinical Practice, 4th ed. St. Louis, Mosby, 1997.

2. Abbott JT, Emmans L, Lowenstein SR: Ectopic pregnancy: The common pitfalls in diagnosis. Am J Emerg Med 8:515, 1990.
3. Cunningham FG, MacDonald PC, Gant NF, et al: Williams' Obstetrics, 19th ed. Norwalk, CT, Appleton & Lange, 1993.
4. Goodwin TM, Breen MT: Pregnancy outcome and fetomaternal hemorrhage after noncatastrophic trauma. Am J Obstet Gynecol 162:665, 1990.
5. Mishell DR: Abortion. In Droegemueller W, et al (eds): Comprehensive Gynecology. St. Louis, Mosby, 1992.
6. Pearlman MD, Tintialli JE, Lorenz RP: Blunt trauma during pregnancy. N Engl J Med 323:1609–1613, 1990.

46. ALLERGY AND ANAPHYLAXIS

Lance W. Jobe, M.D.

1. What is anaphylaxis, and why does it occur?

Anaphylaxis is a rapidly developing immunologic reaction resulting from a few chemical factors that are released systemically by mast cells. It is a continuum of disease that may occur as a mild local reaction or a critical life-threatening systemic disorder. People often refer to a local reaction as an allergy; however, allergy is really a broad term referring to several types of immunologic reactions.

2. Sounds easy enough, but what are mast cells?

Mast cells are individual cells located in connective tissue and concentrated near mucosal surfaces and blood vessels. These cells contain preformed chemicals ready to be released into the surrounding tissue. Since these chemicals initiate a strong immunologic reaction in response to "foreign invaders," the mast cell has been referred to as a sentinel cell. When the antibodies, called IgE, located on the surface of the mast cell contact an antigen, the cell releases its store of chemicals or mediators. This is called Type 1 hypersensitivity (allergic reaction) and generally occurs within 20 minutes of exposure.

3. What is an antigen?

Antigen is simply a name given to the bad guy, the foreign invader, that sets off the whole reaction. For example, penicillin could be an antigen, as can the venom injected as a result of a bee sting.

4. How do these chemical factors affect the body?

Some of the chemicals cause blood vessels to dilate and leak fluid into the surrounding tissues. This may result in swelling (edema) of the face or upper airway. The skin may become erythematous secondary to increased blood flow. Therefore, if the reaction remains local, simple urticaria (hives) may be the only symptom. If the reaction becomes systemic (a chain reaction throughout the body), significant upper airway swelling may occur, or blood pressure may drop precipitously owing to profound vasodilation, resulting in anaphylactic shock or severe bronchospasm, all of which may constitute an immediately life-threatening situation. Thus, airway, breathing, and circulation can all be profoundly affected.

5. If I am giving a drug that a patient has never had before, could he have an anaphylactic reaction?

No. In order for a Type 1 (anaphylactic) reaction to occur, the immune system must have had a previous exposure to the antigen so that it can mass produce a unique antibody that will recognize the antigen on a subsequent exposure.

6. What else besides antibiotics can cause anaphylaxis?

Penicillins are the most common cause, though theoretically any drug may cause an allergic reaction. Worse reactions are associated with the parenteral route of administration. Other common causes include venom (bees, snakes, ants), foods (peanuts, eggs), vaccines (measles, mumps, rubella; tetanus; influenza), latex, and antisera. Some unfortunate souls even experience anaphylaxis with exercise or cold exposure.

7. Can it be difficult to recognize anaphylaxis?

Generally not. Most patients will tell you that they think they're having an allergic reaction, and they are usually right. Furthermore, most patients will have urticaria. It may be important to recognize that rarely patients present with hypotension but no urticaria or mucosal edema. Angioedema, a delayed allergy that is infrequent and most commonly associated with the drugs known as ACE inhibitors, may present without urticaria or facial edema. Other potential airway emergencies, such as foreign body obstruction, epiglottitis, or retropharyngeal abscess, will generally show obvious clues from the history or secondary survey.

8. How should I approach the patient with possible anaphylaxis?

As always, start with the ABCs and remember to review them periodically, since things can change quickly. A definitive airway, endotracheal intubation, may be needed in severe cases. Oxygen should be immediately provided. If the patient is talking, he has a patent airway and he will be helpful in telling you if he is having more difficulty breathing. Also, listen for stridor, hoarseness, and wheezing, and watch for an inability to handle secretions. Diphenhydramine (Benadryl), 50 mg IV or IM, will often provide rapid relief and counteract the effects of some of the chemicals released by the mast cells.

9. What should I do if the airway is compromised?

Immediate action is indicated. Besides preparing to intubate the patient, you should administer epinephrine 1:1000, 0.3 to 0.5 mg subcutaneously, which can be a life-saving action. If the airway is in question, do not wait to establish an IV line before giving the epinephrine. The dose can be repeated every 5 to 15 minutes if symptoms do not improve or if they recur. Racemic epinephrine, 0.5 ml nebulized in 3-ml normal saline, can also be used. If severe airway compromise is present, 1 ml of 1:10,000 epinephrine diluted in 10 ml of normal saline can be given via slow IV push over 3 to 5 minutes. This may precipitate cardiac arrhythmias, however, especially in older patients and those with cardiac problems. A safer approach would be an epinephrine drip of 1–10 mcg/minute.

10. If the patient is wheezing, would albuterol be beneficial?

Yes. In patients with bronchospasm (wheezing), nebulized albuterol should be given, but epinephrine, 0.3–0.5 mg 1:1000 subcutaneously, is the primary or first-line drug.

11. What about pediatric patients?

The only major difference is the dose of medication. The dose of diphenhydramine is 2 mg/kg (max 50 mg). The dose of epinephrine SC is 0.01 ml/kg of the 1:1000 solution (max 0.5 ml). Start an epinephrine drip at 0.1 mcg/kg/minute and titrate to 0.5 mcg/kg/minute.

12. What are the indications for intubation in the field?

Since the airway is lost in anaphylaxis owing to massive tissue edema, intubation can be extremely difficult, and failed attempts may convert a tenuous but usable airway into a completely obstructed airway. For the unresponsive patient in whom attempts with mechanical mask ventilation are unsuccessful, intubation may be necessary. If at all possible, however, patients in distress should be transported immediately to the closest facility. They should be alerted ahead of time so as to prepare for possible cricothyrotomy.

13. We have covered the airway and breathing, but what about circulation?

A blood pressure reading and IV access should be obtained in all patients with allergic reactions. Hypotensive patients will need a bolus of normal saline. In young patients, a liter of fluid and then re-evaluation are adequate. In older patients with possible cardiac problems, not more than 500 ml should be given before reassessing the patient. Any unstable patient should be placed on a cardiac monitor. An epinephrine drip should be administered to those patients who remain hypotensive despite adequate volume resuscitation.

14. If there is a Type 1 reaction, there must be other types as well. Are these important?

Yes and no. There are three other types of allergic reactions; however, they are not important in the emergency setting.

15. Should every patient with an allergic reaction be transported to a hospital for further evaluation?

If any treatment is implemented at the scene, the patient should be evaluated in the emergency department (ED). The reason is that all the medications given in the field are relatively short acting, but the precipitating antigen is not. These patients are usually observed for a period of time in the ED and if they can be discharged home are often placed on a short course of steroids to prevent recurrence.

16. Should I administer epinephrine to a patient who has only hives?

In general, diphenhydramine (Benadryl), 25–50 mg PO or IV, is all that is necessary for this non–life-threatening but uncomfortable condition.

17. What are the relative contraindications to epinephrine?

Hypertension, tachycardia, ischemic chest pain, and a history of angina. If the patient has life-threatening anaphylaxis, however, epinephrine should be administered carefully, beginning with lower dosages.

BIBLIOGRAPHY

1. Cotran R, Kumar V, Robbins S: Diseases of immunity. In Robbins S (ed): Pathologic Basis of Disease. Philadelphia, W.B. Saunders, 1989, pp 163–237.
2. Kinser D: Drug allergy and other drug reactions. In Harwood-Nuss A (ed): The Clinical Practice of Emergency Medicine. Philadelphia, J.B. Lippincott, 1996, pp 934–937.
3. Markovchick VJ: Anaphylaxis. In Markovchick VJ, Pons PT, Wolfe RE (eds): Emergency Medical Secrets. Philadelphia, Hanley & Belfus, 1993.
4. Zull D: Anaphylaxis. In Harwood-Nuss A (ed): The Clinical Practice of Emergency Medicine. Philadelphia, J.B. Lippincott, 1996, pp 929–932.

47. DIABETIC EMERGENCIES

Jedd Roe, M.D.

1. What is diabetes mellitus?

Diabetes mellitus (DM) is the most common endocrine disorder. Because of abnormalities in glucose metabolism, many organs are affected, which leads to multiple complications. Diabetes mellitus occurs in an estimated 2–4% of individuals in the United States. The EMS system is used frequently by patients with diabetes. It is important for prehospital providers to be aware of not only the problems directly associated with diabetes mellitus but also complications related to the disease.

2. What hormones regulate glucose metabolism?

Insulin is produced in the pancreas and is released into the blood stream in response to elevations in blood sugar level. Insulin assists in glucose uptake by the cells, allows excess glucose to be stored in the liver and muscle, and is used in fat synthesis.

Other cells in the pancreas make different hormones that are also important in glucose metabolism. One of these is glucagon. When glucose is not getting into cells, because of either lack of food intake or lack of insulin, the body perceives a fasting state and releases glucagon to attempt to increase the level of blood sugar. Glucagon causes the breakdown of stored sugars in the liver and then of stored body fat, which results in production of ketones as a breakdown product. Ketones are acidic and lead to a lower blood pH (acidosis). It is this process of ketone and acid formation (ketoacidosis) that may lead to one of the acute complications seen in the diabetic.

3. How does diabetes mellitus affect glucose metabolism?

Diabetes mellitus is caused by inadequate amounts of insulin. Since insulin is required for glucose to be transported into cells, the hallmark of the disease is an elevated blood sugar level (hyperglycemia). Owing to a perceived lack of intracellular glucose, compensatory mechanisms (involving the breakdown of stored sugar, protein, and fat) release glucose (and ketone bodies) into the blood stream. As cellular uptake of glucose is inhibited, the blood sugar level rises.

4. What types of diabetes mellitus are there?

Diabetes can be separated into two disease presentations. Type I, also known as insulin-dependent diabetes mellitus (IDDM) or juvenile-onset DM, usually develops prior to early adulthood. The peak age of onset of IDDM is 10 to 14 years. Patients with type I DM produce almost no insulin and consequently may develop markedly elevated glucose levels. Metabolic acids may accumulate in the blood secondary to the breakdown of stored body fat, and ketoacidosis may occur. Patients with IDDM are dependent on insulin therapy for survival.

Type II, or non–insulin-dependent diabetes mellitus (NIDDM), usually occurs in patients older than age 40. Patients with NIDDM are able to produce insulin but do so in decreased amounts. These persons require diet control, oral medication, or additional insulin to control blood sugar levels. Ketoacidosis rarely occurs in patients with type II diabetes because some insulin is produced. Differences between the two types of diabetes are listed in the table.

Comparison of Type I and Type II Diabetes

	TYPE I (IDDM)	TYPE II (NIDDM)
Name	Insulin-dependent diabetes mellitus	Non–insulin-dependent diabetes mellitus
Pathology	No insulin production	Decreased insulin production
Age of Onset	Childhood (Peak age 10–14)	Adulthood (> age 40)
Required Treatment	Insulin	Diet control, oral agents, insulin
Tendency for Ketoacidosis	Strong	Weak

5. Why do diabetic patients access the 911 system?

Either too little or too much sugar in the blood. Abnormally low blood sugar, referred to as hypoglycemia, may result from a decrease in food intake with regular insulin administration, an error in insulin administration, or a combination of both. Patients who are not on insulin but who take certain oral hypoglycemic agents are also at risk for hypoglycemia up to 36 hours after taking these medications.

Unrecognized hypoglycemia can lead to death. The cells of the body, especially the brain, are dependent on glucose to function. Without glucose, the cells may find other sources of energy, but their breakdown products will be toxic to the cells and will cause cell death. Permanent brain damage may occur in patients who survive hypoglycemic events because the cells of the brain do not have the ability to store or use other sources of energy like the rest of the body.

6. What about problems related to too much sugar?

Diabetic ketoacidosis (DKA) is caused by an insufficient amount of insulin. In the liver, stored glucose is released into the blood, causing hyperglycemia. Once these stores have been depleted, body fats containing fatty acids are broken down to form glucose. The resulting by-products of fatty acid breakdown are ketone bodies, which cause the blood pH to become acidic. As glucose levels rise, the kidney's ability to retain glucose becomes overwhelmed, and glucose is lost into the urine. Glucose in the urine causes the kidney cells to draw water and electrolytes out of the blood and into the urine. This causes increased urination secondary to the larger amount of glucose and electrolytes in the urine, resulting in volume loss and dehydration. Volume loss in adult patients with DKA ranges from 4–10 liters.

Diabetic ketoacidosis is a dangerous complication of diabetes mellitus and occurs with greatest frequency in patients up to 19 years of age. The overall mortality is 5–15% per episode. It generally occurs in patients who are insulin dependent but has been reported to be the first manifestation of undiagnosed diabetes mellitus in 20–30% of all cases of DKA. Precipitating causes are found in 70–80% of patients, with infection and medication noncompliance being the most common factors.

7. Does an elevated blood sugar level always lead to DKA?

No. Elevated blood sugar levels (hyperglycemia) can occur in some patients without the development of DKA. Many diabetic patients routinely have an elevated blood sugar level with essentially normal acid-base status. Insulin deficiency, other hormones that regulate glucose, and dehydration can all contribute to hyperglycemia. It is not known why some patients develop ketosis and acidosis and others do not.

Nonketotic hyperosmolar coma (NKHC) is more common in persons older than 60 years of age and is characterized by central nervous system dysfunction associated with severe hyperglycemia and dehydration. Mortality may be as high as 50%. The predominant presentation is abnormal metal status, which may vary from lethargy to coma. Unlike DKA, focal neurologic deficits such as seizures or hemiplegia may occur. These resolve with treatment of the hyperosmolar state.

8. What factors may cause problems in controlling diabetes mellitus?

Many diabetic patients administer insulin to themselves in the morning. If food intake is delayed, hypoglycemia ensues. The blood sugar level may also fall precipitously during exercise because metabolic requirements increase. Common precipitating factors in the development of hyperglycemic states include infection, systemic illness, stroke, and medication noncompliance.

9. What is the major goal of patient assessment?

In assessing a diabetic patient who enters the EMS system, the prehospital provider is generally trying to differentiate hypoglycemia from hyperglycemia. These conditions, which must be recognized promptly and treated appropriately, are frequently identified by history, physical findings, and rapid blood glucose determination (or administration of glucose) in the prehospital setting. The signs and symptoms of hypoglycemia are rapidly reversible; therefore, recognition is the primary goal of patient assessment. Owing to the easily reversible nature of this disease, management may precede a complete patient assessment.

10. Can physical signs be helpful in distinguishing between hypoglycemia and hyperglycemia?

First, remember that many diabetic patients wear medic alert tags, which may provide important clues to the diagnosis in those who are unresponsive. Typically, those patients with hypoglycemia demonstrate pale, cool, clammy skin because of sympathetic nervous system activation. Hypothermia is a common presentation, and the respiratory rate is usually slowed or normal. Mental status changes occur rapidly (minutes to hours); initially, patients may exhibit bizarre behavior, irritability, and combativeness prior to unresponsiveness. Seizures may occur secondary to hypoglycemia and usually resolve with administration of glucose. This presentation may easily be confused with that of an alcohol-intoxicated patient. Because alcoholism may be a factor predisposing to hypoglycemia, a prudent strategy is to assume that hypoglycemia is present whether or not alcohol is involved.

Some of the signs of dehydration seen in DKA have already been described. Other important findings include dry, warm skin and gastrointestinal complaints such as nausea, vomiting, and abdominal pain. A fruity odor on the patient's breath means that ketones are present. Mental status changes are gradual in onset (over several days) and progress from restlessness and lethargy (an apathetic appearance) to unresponsiveness.

11. What other symptoms may be present?

Polydipsia (excessive thirst), polyuria (frequent urination), and polyphagia (desire to eat frequently) are common presenting symptoms of new-onset or worsening diabetes and are also characteristics of the hyperosmolar state and dehydration seen with elevated blood sugar levels. Other associated symptoms include abdominal complaints (nausea, vomiting, and abdominal pain), fatigue, and visual disturbances.

12. Are abnormalities in vital signs common?

Yes, in both hypoglycemia and hyperglycemia. Evaluate the patient for respiratory distress, and assess the rate and rhythm of respirations. A slight increase in respiratory rate is seen early in DKA. Kussmaul's respirations (deep, rapid, and intense respirations) may develop later. Hypoglycemic patients may have slowed or normal respiratory rates. Tachycardia is commonly seen in both hypoglycemic patients and patients with DKA. Irregular or bradycardic rates may represent underlying cardiac disease. Blood pressure may be decreased secondary to dehydration or underlying cardiac disease.

13. What other physical signs are important?

As we have seen, a patient may experience 4–10 liters of volume loss during DKA. The skin should also be assessed for tenting or loss of elasticity, suggesting dehydration. Important facial features may include sunken eyes, a furrowed tongue, and dry mucous membranes. Hypoglycemic patients are usually well hydrated and will have normal skin turgor as well as moist skin and mucous membranes. Abdominal examination in DKA may show nonspecific pain, tenderness, or distention. Focal findings such as right lower quadrant tenderness may also be present. Neurologic deficits may be seen in patients with high or low blood sugar levels.

14. What management strategies are appropriate for diabetic patients?

Any patient with respiratory distress requires airway stabilization and administration of high-flow oxygen by mask. Cardiac monitoring and pulse oximetry (if available) should be utilized.

A rapid blood sugar determination is ideal for all known diabetic patients and all patients with altered mental status, preferably prior to glucose administration. Any adult who is not awake and aware and any patient with a blood glucose reading of 70 or less should receive 50 ml (one amp) of 50% dextrose (D$_{50}$) intravenously. Children should receive 2–4 ml/kg of 25% dextrose (D$_{25}$). Awake patients with glucose levels of less than 70 may be given juice or other oral forms of glucose by mouth, so long as they are competent to administer the liquid themselves without assistance.

Hypotensive patients and other patients with signs of dehydration or hypoperfusion should be given IV fluids such as normal saline (NS) or lactated Ringer's solution to replenish the fluid volume. Children should be given 20 ml/kg of NS as an initial fluid bolus. This should be repeated once if vital signs do not respond. Adults should be given fluid boluses of 500 ml of NS, which can be repeated to a total volume of 2 liters. Fluid replacement is the mainstay of therapy for DKA and NKHC and should be undertaken aggressively owing to the huge amount of fluid volume already lost.

15. What if I can't determine the blood sugar level in the field?

For unresponsive patients with an unknown blood glucose level, IV glucose should be administered.

16. Isn't that dangerous if the blood sugar is already too high?

No. One dose of 50% dextrose has not been shown to have a deleterious clinical effect. The only concern has been the administration of glucose to a patient who is having a stroke. Glucose can exacerbate the amount of damage ultimately produced. Therefore, if hypoglycemia is a real concern in a patient with a potential stroke, glucose determination is preferred prior to administration of sugar. If transport time is short and glucose measurement is not available in the prehospital setting, glucose infusion can be delayed until arrival at the hospital. Otherwise, glucose should be administered.

17. Are there specific considerations for alcoholic patients?

Yes. If there is a possibility that the patient is alcoholic, D$_{50}$ administration should be preceded by 100 mg of thiamine intravenously if this medication is available. Thiamine is utilized as a cofactor in the metabolism of glucose, and alcoholic patients generally have depleted most of their stored thiamine. While controversy exists, some evidence suggests that Wernicke's encephalopathy may be precipitated by a large load of glucose, which then rapidly depletes the small amount of stored thiamine.

BIBLIOGRAPHY

1. Bergenstal RM: Diabetic ketoacidosis: How to treat and, when possible, prevent. Postgrad Med 77:151, 1985.
2. Blanda M, Clancy P: Diabetic emergencies. In Pons P, Cason D (eds): Paramedic Field Care: A Complaint Based Approach. St. Louis, Mosby, 1997, pp 431–438.
3. Feingold KR, Gavin LA, Schambelan M, et al: Diabetes mellitus. In Andreoli TE, Carpenter C, Plum F, et al (eds): Cecil Essentials of Medicine. Philadelphia, W.B. Saunders, 1990, pp 496–505.
4. Hoffman RS, Goldfrank LR: The poisoned patient with altered consciousness in one use of a "coma cocktail." JAMA 274:562–569, 1995.
5. Israel RS: Diabetic disorders. In Markovchick VJ, Pons PT, Wolfe RE (eds): Emergency Medicine Secrets. Philadelphia, Hanley & Belfus, 1993, pp 175–178.
6. Ragland G: Diabetic ketoacidosis. In Tintinalli JE, Krome RL, Ruiz E (eds): Emergency Medicine—A Comprehensive Study Guide, 2nd ed. New York, McGraw-Hill, 1988, p 490.
7. Update in Diabetic Ketoacidosis: Strategies for effective management. Emerg Med Rep 12(10):89–96, 1991.

48. PSYCHIATRIC EMERGENCIES

Lance W. Jobe, M.D.

1. What is a psychiatric emergency?
It is a situation in which the patient's presenting problem stems from disordered thought processes, causing the patient to be a potential danger to himself or others.

2. What are the categories of psychiatric emergencies?
The first is organic. In these patients, disturbed behavior is the result of a well-defined physiologic illness or toxin such as hypoglycemia or alcohol. The second is functional, which has no definable physiologic cause and is thought to result from abnormal intrinsic brain function. Thus, this is a true psychiatric illness.

3. Is it important to distinguish between these two broad categories in the prehospital setting?
It is extremely important to have an understanding of this concept because the treatment will ultimately be very different. It would be considered poor form to bring an out-of-control, delusional patient to the emergency department only to find out later that the patient had a blood glucose of 30 (and all that time was rapidly losing brain cells), which could have been easily treated in the field. Therefore, even if a distinction can't be made in the field, gathering the data that may help make that distinction is very important.

4. Why don't we just give them all dextrose and let the physicians figure it out?
Simply because the information available from or obtained in the field may be the only solid clue to a diagnosis.

5. What are examples of organic causes of psychiatric disorders?
Meningitis, head trauma, hypoglycemia, hypothermia, hypoxia, and arrhythmias. The most common cause of disturbed behavior is alcohol or other drugs.

6. What clues would help differentiate organic causes from a primary mental disturbance?
Obviously, obtaining the history of the current illness as well as the past medical history will often provide initial clues. Searching the scene for drugs, alcohol, and medications can also help. Patients with organic disease often have an altered level of consciousness, whereas patients with a primary mental disorder (PMD) generally do not have an alteration of consciousness. They are usually oriented and have no problems with memory but instead have a disordered thought process. Visual hallucinations, lethargy, and abnormal vital signs (including pulse oximetry) indicate an organic cause. Auditory hallucinations suggest a psychiatric cause. Diagnosing a patient with a PMD who has no previous psychiatric history should be done carefully. Try to ascertain if the changes are acute, since a sudden change over hours or a couple of days is less likely to be attributable to a PMD. Encourage family members to come to the emergency department. If no family is available, try to obtain a phone number of a person who knows the patient.

7. What should I do if an organic cause is suspected?
Checking blood glucose level and pulse oximetry are two simple tests. If results are abnormally low, you can intervene immediately.

8. What is a normal dextrose stick?
Between 70 and 110 mg/dL.

9. Since these patients may be violent or easily prone to violent behavior, how should they be approached?

Clearly identify yourself and explain your purpose. Speak in as calm a voice as possible. Respect the patient's personal space. If the patient backs away, don't immediately try to approach him again; he is telling you to back off. Furthermore, try to ensure that your position and posture do not make the patient feel that he is cornered. Exclude disruptive persons from the scene.

10. Are there any clues to which patients may become violent?

In general, if alcohol or drugs are involved, there is a greater potential for violence. Obviously, situations in which violence has already occurred may be dangerous. Possible warning signals are tense, clenched fists; pacing; avoiding eye contact; loud threatening speech; or startling easily. Most important, if you don't think of violence as a possibility, you won't be able to diffuse it before it starts.

11. Can I physically restrain a patient?

When a patient is a danger to himself or others, physical restraints may be necessary. Obviously, this is not a black-and-white situation, and judicious use of restraints is needed. If restraints are necessary, wait for assistance. (A minimum of five people is desirable, one for each extremity and one for the head.)

12. When are chemical restraints indicated?

If the patient is still thrashing violently despite restraints, he may still be in a position to hurt himself or others. In addition, further medical evaluation and care may be impossible. In these situations, chemical restraints are needed. The drug most often used is droperidol.

13. What do I need to know about depression?

Prehospital personnel are often called to situations in which depression is the underlying reason for the call. Diagnostic criteria are explicitly laid out by the American Psychiatric Association. They quantify symptoms such as feelings of hopelessness, depression, loss of interest in pleasurable activities, sleep disturbance, and decreased concentration and productivity, as well as recurrent thoughts of death. Displays of depression may be as overt as the person standing on a bridge threatening to jump or as subtle as the elderly woman, living alone, who calls because she is "not feeling well." Suicide, of course, is the main life threat that must be addressed and is the eighth leading cause of death in the United States. If there is any concern about depression, the patient should be asked about thoughts of suicide.

14. If I question a person about suicide, isn't there a risk that I'll be giving them the idea?

No. People who are depressed will be thinking about suicide, to some degree, long before you question them.

15. What is bipolar disorder?

Bipolar disorder, or manic-depression, is a mood disorder, just as depression is a mood disorder. People afflicted with bipolar disorder will have episodes of severe depression; however, the depressive episodes are separated by cycles of mania, or elevated mood. In the manic phase, people tend to lose all self-control and to have a hyperinflated self-esteem. They may be out in the street directing traffic or out spending money irrationally (e.g., they may spend all they own, including house and car, in a matter of days).

16. What do I need to know about schizophrenia?

Schizophrenia is a disorder of thought processes. It is characterized by delusions, hallucinations, and disorganized speech and behavior. Delusions are ideas or beliefs that have no factual basis and in general are obviously false. These individuals may also have bizarre, paranoid ideas, which can make them dangerous. The greatest concern, however, is for their own safety. Schizophrenic patients are at high risk for suicide.

17. I've heard about mental health holds (MHHs). Who would qualify for an MHH?

Although there is some variation from state to state (and you should know what the law says in your state), a mental health hold can be placed on a patient who is a risk to himself (suicidal), a risk to others (homicidal), or gravely disabled as a result of psychiatric illness. The MHH allows the patient to be held against his will for a specified amount of time (usually a maximum of 72 hours) in order to evaluate him psychiatrically.

18. Who can place a patient on a mental health hold?

This also varies from state to state but generally includes physicians, police officers, psychiatric nurses or social workers, and psychiatric therapists. Interestingly, EMTs and paramedics are usually not included, even though they often contact patients who need to be placed on holds. Thus, they are required to involve the police in placing a hold in the field.

BIBLIOGRAPHY

1. American Psychiatric Association: Diagnostic and Statistical Manual of Mental Disorders, 4th ed. Washington, DC, American Psychiatric Press, 1994.
2. Harwood-Nuss AL: The Clinical Practice of Emergency Medicine. Philadelphia, Lippincott-Raven, 1996, pp 976–986.
3. Markovchick VJ, Pons PT, Wolfe RE: Emergency Medicine Secrets. Philadelphia, Hanley & Belfus, 1993, pp 419–428.

49. MANAGEMENT OF THE VIOLENT PATIENT

Julie Seaman, M.D.

1. What is the rate of injury sustained by prehospital providers as a result of violent patients and violent scenes?

Approximately 10% of paramedics become victims of violence every year. Over a 10-year career, essentially all medics have at one time been a victim of violence.

2. What are some causes of violent behavior?

- Hypoxia
- Metabolic disorders (hypoglycemia, hypercalcemia)
- Drug ingestion (anticholinergics, cocaine, amphetamines, PCP, ethanol)
- Postictal state
- Acute psychosis
- Withdrawal from opiates or ethanol
- Central nervous system disorders (intracranial hemorrhage, mass or infection, stroke)
- Fear

3. How does one approach the violent patient?

- Assess the scene before beginning patient care. Often, it is necessary to await police assistance and control of the scene before attending to injured or ill persons. Patient care and transport can often be expedited if one waits the few extra minutes for police to arrive and attend to non–patient care issues, freeing the medic from worry about non-medical issues.
- Approach the patient in a professional and respectful manner. Position yourself near an exit and stay more than an arm's length from the patient. Be aware of potential weapons. Use confident calming words in an effort to diffuse anger, lessen fear, and control violence.
- Do not let yourself by affected by verbal insults, threats, and aggression. Becoming angry will worsen the situation by leading to poor decisions and poor patient care. It unnecessarily causes excess stress and will eventually lead to job dissatisfaction and burnout.

4. How does one use physical restraint without harming the patient or oneself?

- Use overwhelming force by enlisting the help of others. Utilize police officers, firefighters, and medics simultaneously to help restrain the patient.
- Grasp clothing and large joints. Avoid pressure to the neck and chest.
- Restrain the person in a supine position or on his side, never prone.
- Once restraints are in place, obtain IV access, administer oxygen, and perform a Dextrostix test or administer glucose.

5. What injuries can the actual restraints cause?

- Asphyxiation: Hobble or hogtie restraints have been associated with asphyxiation. With this type of restraint, the patient is placed in a prone position and has the wrists handcuffed behind the back; the ankles are bound; and then the bound wrists and ankles are attached together. Transporting the patient in this position limits diaphragmatic and chest wall motion. The energy expended in struggling against the restraints and positional work of breathing leads to metabolic acidosis, respiratory muscle fatigue, and subsequent death. Most reported deaths result from rapid asystolic arrest. Therefore, hobble restraints should not be used by EMTs. Instead, a patient should be restrained on his side or in a supine position in cases of trauma with need for spinal immobilization.

• Aspiration: All patients who need field restraints should be assumed to be at high risk for vomiting and aspiration. All patients should be restrained left side down unless there is a contraindication, such as a need for spinal immobilization.

• Ischemia: One must routinely reevaluate the restraints to assess limb ischemia, especially during long transports.

6. **What if the patient continues to struggle violently, requiring multiple people for restraint?**
   After IV access, oxygen administration, and a glucose test or dextrose administration, chemical restraint should be considered.

7. **What medications can be used for chemical restraint?**

	Initial Dose	Onset	Peak Effect	Duration
Haloperidol (Haldol)	2–5 mg IM	10–30 min	30–45 min	12–38 hr
Droperidol (Inapsine)	2.5–5 mg IV/IM	3–10 min	30 min	2–4 hr
Diazepam (Valium)	2–5 mg IV	< 2 min	3–4 min	15–60 min (1st dose)
Lorazepam (Ativan)	1–3 mg IV/IM	1–5 min IV 15–30 min IM	15–20 min IV 30–60 min IM	6–24 hr 6–24 hr
Midazolam (Versed)	1–3 mg IV/IM	1–5 min IV 15–20 min IM	5–30 min IV 15–30 min IM	2–6 hr 2–6 hr

8. **What is the best medication for chemical restraint?**
   Droperidol (Inapsine) is currently the preferred medication for chemical restraint. It is unlikely to cause respiratory depression, is an excellent antiemetic, has minimal extrapyramidal effects, is approved for IV use, and has a rapid onset of action. The dose for chemical restraint is 2.5–5 mg IV or IM. This is 2 to 8 times the antiemetic dose for droperidol.

9. **What are the side effects and contraindications of haloperidol and droperidol?**
   • Extrapyramidal symptoms may consist of dystonic reactions, motor restlessness, and parkinsonian signs and symptoms. Dystonic reactions are most common in children, whereas parkinsonian symptoms predominate in the elderly. Treatment is with diphenhydramine (Benadryl, 25–50 mg IV/IM/PO) or benztropine (Cogentin, 1–2 mg IM/PO).
   • Hypotension may develop in an overdose.
   • Premature ventricular contractions, ventricular arrhythmias, torsades de pointes, and bradycardia have been reported with overdose.
   • Seizure threshold is believed to be lowered with haloperidol and probably with droperidol.
   • Neuroleptic malignant syndrome (NMS), a rare side effect, consists of hyperthermia, autonomic instability, rigidity, and mental status changes. Prehospital treatment should focus on airway control and efforts to cool the patient.
   • Haloperidol and droperidol are contraindicated in those patients with severe parkinsonism, pregnancy, and a history of NMS or anaphylaxis. These medications cross the placenta and have been shown to be teratogenic and fetotoxic in animals. Relative contraindications are seizures or ingestion of medications that lower the seizure threshold (cocaine, amphetamines, tricyclic antidepressants, Ultram, and so forth).

10. **What medication is most useful in cocaine or amphetamine intoxication?**
    Benzodiazepines are the treatment of choice in this situation. They raise the seizure threshold, calm the agitated patient, and may help decrease catecholamine release from the brain. Benzodiazepines can cause respiratory depression and hypotension; therefore, incremental dosing, continuous airway monitoring, supplemental oxygen, and frequent vital sign reevaluation are needed. Beta-blockers such as propranolol should be avoided because they may lead to unopposed alpha blockade. This can cause worsened vasoconstriction and ischemia.

BIBLIOGRAPHY

1. Olsen K: Poisoning and Drug Overdose, 2nd ed. Norwalk, CT, Appleton & Lange, 1994.
2. Omoigui S: The Anesthesia Drug Handbook. St. Louis, Mosby, 1992.
3. Paramedic Pages: Dangers in EMS. http://www.netally.com/matic/ems/danger.htm.
4. Stratton SJ, Rogers C, Green K: Sudden death in individuals in hobble restraints during paramedic transport. Ann Emerg Med 25:710–712, 1995.

50. OVERVIEW OF SHOCK

Robert F. McCormack, M.D.

1. What is shock?

Shock is inadequate perfusion of bodily tissue. The cells are deprived of oxygen, which results in anaerobic metabolism. Because of the inadequate circulation, lactic acid and other toxic metabolites are produced and accumulate. Cellular dysfunction ensues, followed by cellular death and organ failure.

Shock may be clinically diagnosed by "end organ" dysfunction, such as confusion or oliguria, or, more commonly, by vital sign abnormalities, such as hypotension and tachycardia.

2. What causes shock?

Perfusion of organs demands an intact circulatory system, a normally functioning heart, sufficient red blood cells and volume, and adequate air exchange through the lungs. Breakdown of any one of these four components can lead to shock.

3. What are the different types of shock?

There are many different classifications of shock. In this section, we will be dealing primarily with *hypovolemic* shock, which refers to loss of volume due to hemorrhage, but it may also result from cellular fluid shifts or dehydration. *Cardiogenic* shock refers to pump failure due to infarction, contusion, or valvular dysfunction. *Neurogenic* or capacitance shock results from loss of vascular tone because of sympathetic denervation. *Septic* and *anaphylactic* shock are a combination of hypovolemia from third spacing of fluid and loss of vascular tone. *Obstructive* shock refers to cardiac tamponade, tension pneumothorax, or pulmonary embolus, situations in which blood return to the heart is impaired.

4. Why does loss of vascular tone cause shock?

Blood vessels are in a state of dynamic control between the sympathetic and parasympathetic nervous systems. The usual capacity of the intravascular space is approximately 5 liters for the average 70-kg adult male (70 ml/kg). Loss of sympathetic tone due to an injury to the spinal cord causes vasodilation, which can greatly increase the intravascular space. The same amount of volume in a larger space causes the blood pressure to drop with resultant inadequate tissue perfusion.

5. How do you differentiate the types of shock clinically?

Take the blood pressure and pulse, and touch the patient. Hypotension, tachycardia, and cool moist skin are the result of hypovolemic or cardiogenic shock. Hypotension, tachycardia, and warm dry skin are caused by neurogenic or septic shock.

6. How do you manage hypovolemic shock?

The initial treatment of hypovolemic shock is administration of up to 40 ml/kg of crystalloid. If hemorrhage is the cause, the bleeding must be controlled as part of the therapy. External bleeding should be controlled by compression or use of tourniquets if the patient is exsanguinating. Internal bleeding will need AGGRESSIVE surgical management.

7. Is oxygen helpful in the treatment of shock?

Absolutely! Oxygen should be administered via a nonrebreather bag-mask reservoir to maximize the inspired oxygen concentration. Since the oxygen-carrying capacity of the remaining hemoglobin may be compromised by hemorrhage or low-flow states, it is of critical importance to maximize the oxygen in the remaining blood and the oxygen delivery to the cells.

8. Why is fluid therapy helpful?

It can transiently maintain perfusion in severe shock, but it is only a TEMPORIZING measure. Time is of critical importance. Continued loss of intravascular volume with normal saline volume replacement will produce an oxygen-carrying deficit as the patient becomes more anemic. When bleeding continues, transfusion with red blood cells and surgical management is the only way to improve the situation.

9. Are there better things to give than normal saline?

Not initially, but whole blood is much better than normal saline for the treatment of hemorrhagic shock. It stays in the intravascular space and increases oxygen-carrying capacity. It should be given for hemorrhagic shock if the vital signs do not normalize after 40 ml/kg of crystalloid are administered.

10. Can I get my hands on blood products?

Not at this time. Blood products need to be refrigerated and carefully maintained. It is not practical to provide blood in the prehospital setting. Research is currently underway into a number of artificial hemoglobin products that may prove very useful in the prehospital setting. The only time blood or blood products may be administered in the prehospital setting is when patients are being transferred to a higher-level trauma care facility.

11. Why does my "know-it-all" partner say he doesn't want an IV if he gets shot in the chest?

Recent research has questioned the use of aggressive fluid resuscitation in penetrating chest trauma. The concept is that as blood pressure increases, the rate of bleeding in the noncompressible chest vessels increases or the higher pressure dislodges tenuous clots. The study has some methodologic problems and needs to be confirmed. The downside of "overresuscitation" is noteworthy, however, and fluid resuscitation should probably be tempered to the minimal amount necessary to maintain adequate perfusion.

12. In a trauma patient, why do I care about the other causes of shock?

Hypovolemia is the most common cause of shock in the trauma patient, but other causes need to be considered as well. A tension pneumothorax can cause profound shock that can be immediately reversed if diagnosed and treated. As the pressure in the hemithorax increases with tension pneumothorax, the vena cava collapses, decreasing venous return to the right heart. The drop in venous return causes a drop in cardiac output, and the result is signs of shock. Needle decompression of the hemithorax equalizes pressures and allows "normal" venous return. Successful needle decompression produces rapid dramatic changes in the vital signs and clearly can be life saving in the prehospital setting.

Neurogenic shock may be present in a patient with a spinal injury. Administration of a fluid bolus may normalize vital signs. Be aware that hypovolemic shock may coexist with spinal shock, however.

Cardiogenic shock may result from a massive cardiac contusion. You want to be certain that you are treating the right type of shock with the right intervention.

13. How do I relieve a tension pneumothorax?

See the thoracic trauma chapter for more details.

14. Why doesn't anyone like MAST pants anymore?

Military anti-shock trousers (MAST) are controversial. Recent studies show no clear benefit in the trauma patient, and in some cases they may even be harmful. Theoretical arguments similar to the IV fluid resuscitation controversy (about increasing bleeding in the chest or abdomen) have been proposed. In addition, compartment syndrome and other complications have been described.

15. What is the definitive management of hypovolemic shock?

The definitive management of hypovolemic shock is hemorrhage control and replenishing of lost blood components. In the case of a self-limited hemorrhage, hemostasis is obtained by the body and an increase in production of blood cells and clotting factors replenishes the deficit. In the case of ongoing bleeding, surgery is usually required to control the bleeding physically, and loss of blood components often requires replacement. It needs to be emphasized that continued bleeding can quickly deplete the body's supply of red cells and clotting factors and that supplementation alone cannot adequately correct for continued hemorrhage. Therefore, surgery must be available in a timely manner when required.

BIBLIOGRAPHY

1. Bickell WH, Wall WJ, Pepe PE, et al: Immediate versus delayed fluid resuscitation for hypotensive patients with penetrating torso injuries. N Engl J Med 331:1105–1109, 1994.
2. Kline JA: Shock. In Rosen P et al (eds): Emergency Medicine. Concepts and Clinical Practice, 4th ed. St. Louis, Mosby, 1998, pp 86–106.
3. Mattox KL, Bickell W, Pepe PE, et al: Prospective MAST study in 911 patients. J Trauma 29:1104–1112, 1989.
4. PHTLS: Basic and Advanced Pre-hospital Trauma Life Support. Shock and Fluid Resuscitation. St. Louis, Mosby, 1994, pp 152–187.
5. Schmidt RD: Shock. In Markovchick VJ, Pons PT, Wolfe RE (eds): Emergency Medicine Secrets. Philadelphia, Hanley & Belfus, 1993, pp 13–17.

51. GENERAL TRAUMA PRINCIPLES

John Lawrence Mottley, M.D.

1. What is a traumatic injury?

Trauma may occur when any external energy source is applied to the body. The energy sources may be mechanical, thermal, or radioactive. The vast majority of traumatic injuries result from mechanical energy transfer. In everyday discussion, the meanings of the terms "trauma" and "mechanical injury" are identical. Thermal and radioactive injuries are discussed elsewhere.

2. What is mechanical injury?

Mechanical injury, or "trauma," results when an object strikes a human body or vice versa. Energy transfer from this collision results in deformation of some or all of the body. (It may also result in deformation of the object, as in a windshield shattered by the head of an occupant.) If the energy imparted to the body is sufficient, damage to tissue will occur.

3. What are the common types of traumatic tissue injuries?

Trauma to the tissue ranges from contusions (bruises), which are the result of capillary blood vessel breakage, to actual disruption of the surface and deeper layers of the soft tissue (lacerations). Skeletal tissue (bone and teeth) will fracture if sufficient force is applied. Hollow organs (e.g., gastrointestinal tract, bladder, heart) may rupture, and solid organs (e.g., liver, spleen) may fracture is sufficient force is applied to the body.

4. How is the mechanism of trauma classified?

Trauma is commonly divided into blunt and penetrating trauma.

5. What is penetrating trauma?

Penetrating trauma, a.k.a. the Knife & Gun Club, is caused by external objects penetrating the exterior surface of the body and causing damage to deeper structures. In the case of bullets or other projectiles, the offending object may remain within the body.

Penetrating trauma is comparatively easy to treat—you just follow the hole(s) and pathways to determine which organs may have been injured.

6. What are the most common sites of overlooked entry wounds?

Both stab and gunshot wounds can be overlooked on cursory physical exam, especially if small-caliber bullets or narrow instruments (such as an icepick) were used. The axilla, groin and buttocks, oropharynx, and scalp are the most common sites of missed entry wounds. There is no substitute for palpating the scalp with gloved hands to find such wounds. The back and buttocks must be examined on every patient suspected or known to have sustained a penetrating injury; the optimal time for examination of the back is when logrolling the patient onto the backboard.

7. What is blunt trauma?

Blunt trauma occurs when only energy is transferred to the body, and there is no penetration of the deeper tissues, although surface lacerations are not uncommon. Blunt trauma is the more challenging type to treat: With no holes to guide you, the physical exam, the mechanism of injury, your experience, and this book are your guides to successful treatment.

8. How does treatment of the trauma patient differ from that of the medical patient?

The trauma patient who requires an operation to repair a life-threatening injury is a patient for whom a few precepts are essential. First, time is of the essence, and the time that counts is the time it takes to get to the operating room. While it is fair to say that no one wants a surgeon, it is nevertheless true that some patients need a surgeon. For those critical patients, the role of EMS is to minimize the time spent in the field. Such patients should have a primary survey performed (correcting any abnormal findings therein), be immobilized on a longboard and placed into the ambulance, and be expeditiously transported to the nearest *appropriate* receiving emergency department. All other evaluations and treatments (if any) should take place en route.

9. What is an appropriate Emergency Department (ED) for trauma patients?

There is no simple answer to this question, but there are guidelines. In a system with designated trauma centers, defined trauma patients should be brought to the nearest trauma center. The total prehospital time from injury to trauma center arrival should be less than 60 minutes. In systems without designated trauma centers, the patient is generally taken to the nearest hospital. Since time to the operating room is the important measure, however, it may be appropriate for either online or offline medical control to direct such patients to specific hospitals based on OR availability. Such decisions should be made based on predefined criteria.

10. What do I do if a trauma patient demands to go to a nontrauma center?

This is a very difficult question and often puts the prehospital provider in a difficult situation. The following position has been taken by the New York State Department of Health:

As always, the Department's first concern is to ensure the best care for each patient while protecting the right of the patient to choose the provider of that care or, indeed, to choose not to accept care at all.

It is essential that such a decision by a patient be an informed decision. Informed consent is a guiding ethical and legal principle of medical care that the Department vigorously supports.

It is axiomatic that a patient cannot make an informed judgment unless he/she fully understands the risks and benefits of the course of treatment suggested by the provider. In the major trauma patient, this is often not possible. A number of factors interfere with the normal process of informed consent. First, the patient's injuries may result in an alteration of the patient's mental status. Such an alteration may result either directly from an injury to the head or indirectly due to injury to other areas of the body resulting, for example, in shock or extreme pain. Obviously, a patient with an altered mental status is unable to make an informed judgment, nor is the pre-hospital provider trained to determine the patient's capacity to do so.

Secondly, the time constraints required to effectively treat trauma patients are extreme. Effective trauma care is measured in minutes. The nationally recognized principle of the "golden hour" of trauma care requires that optimum patient care can be achieved if the patient reaches definitive trauma center care as expeditiously as possible. The time required to list and explain the risks and benefits of the various transport alternatives in a meaningful manner would prevent the patient from receiving this optimal care.

Third, and perhaps most important, informed consent requires that the patient be informed of the suggested and alternative courses of action, and the risks and benefits of each. Yet, in the pre-hospital setting, the provider is a certified Emergency Medical Technician, not a licensed physician. The scope of training of an EMT does not include knowledge of the complications, alternatives, or even the likely outcome of a particular course of action, much less the range and likelihood of reasonably known complications. Thus, since the information needed to make an informed judgment in the pre-hospital setting is unavailable, an informed judgment—by definition—cannot be made.

In the absence of informed consent, the provider should follow the course of action of a reasonable and prudent EMT. Such course of action is clearly laid out in the State Emergency Medical Service Basic Life Support protocols. All EMTs are required to follow these protocols.

Lastly, it is important to remember that the decision made by the EMT is the hospital destination. Once at the appropriate hospital, the patient will be cared for by a licensed physician, who can accurately determine the capacity of the patient to make an informed judgment, and provide the information necessary for that informed judgment to be made.

For the reasons outlined above, it is the position of the Department that trauma patients, as defined in the State Emergency Medical Service Basic Life Support protocols, be transported in accordance with those protocols, even if the patient objects.

This nicely summarizes the issues faced by the EMT. Each EMS system should have a policy in place describing how this situation should be handled by the EMT.

11. Can trauma center patients be accurately identified in the field?

Usually, but not always. While EMS providers can accurately identify patients whose abnormal vital signs identify them as trauma center candidates, some trauma patients have vital signs that are initially normal. Traditionally, the mechanism of injury has been used as an indirect indicator of severe trauma. Recent data have cast doubt on at least some of these mechanism-of-injury criteria in blunt trauma.

12. If the paramedic's judgment is as good as any other method of identification, why do we have written trauma triage guidelines?

So your medical director gets sued and not you. If paramedic discretion is the basis for trauma triage, every mistriage can be questioned and the individual paramedic held to account.

13. What other factors enter into the trauma triage equation?

Patients at higher risk of complications or patients who are more difficult to assess should more often be brought to a trauma center. Examples include the elderly and the very young and patients with comorbid factors such as diabetes or pregnancy.

14. How long is too long to remain on the scene?

In a situation that does not involve entrapment or other difficult extrications, ten minutes or less is the ideal time frame. We often may not know scene arrival time to the minute, however. A useful operational parameter points out that at the time you ask yourself, "How long have I been on scene?" you've been on-scene too long.

15. What interventions should be performed on scene?

The airway should be assessed and opened if not patent, while maintaining cervical spine precautions. High-flow oxygen should be administered. An oral or nasopharyngeal airway or endotracheal tube should be placed if the airway is unstable and there are no contraindications. Breathing should be assessed and assisted if less than 10 breaths per minute. Circulation should be assessed by palpating the pulse at the carotid and radial pulses. CPR should be started if the patient is apneic and pulseless. Some advocate placing the defibrillator for blunt traumatic arrest in hopes of finding unsuspected ventricular fibrillation. Given the low survival rate of blunt traumatic arrest, it will likely do no harm to do so. Lastly, the patient should be placed on a backboard (or other spinal immobilization device), loaded into the ambulance, and started en route to the hospital. *ALL* other interventions—including IV placement, cardiac monitoring, and secondary assessment—should be performed while en route to the appropriate hospital.

16. How useful is the oxygen saturation monitor in the trauma patient?

Oxygen saturation monitors make the EMT feel better, but not the patient. The sicker the trauma patient, the less useful the O_2 sat becomes. Oxygen saturation monitors are notoriously unreliable in shock states, which are marked by peripheral vasoconstriction. Bad data are worse than no data at all because they may prevent you from using alternative means of patient assessment. Remember: The treatment for hypoxia is oxygen, not (necessarily) intubation. All trauma patients should be given 100% O_2 by nonrebreather mask or via ET tube when indicated.

17. How long should an on-scene basic life support unit wait for a responding paramedic unit?

Generally speaking, not long at all. Given that definitive treatment is surgery, the basic life support (BLS) unit should not wait once the patient has been packaged for transport. In the rare patient with an unstable airway (obstruction, tension pneumothorax, or apnea), the BLS should wait for advanced life support (ALS) to arrive only if the ALS unit's estimated time of arrival is *clearly shorter* than the travel time to the hospital.

18. If fluid replacement for the hypovolemic patient still the standard of care?

Yes, but recent research has begun to question the effectiveness of fluid resuscitation prior to surgical control of bleeding. The argument is that fluids dilute the clotting factors and increase blood loss by raising the blood pressure. This research is not yet definitive, and treatment protocols generally continue to call for IV fluid.

In any case, there is no controversy in external bleeding. In such cases, when the bleeding site is known and controlled, aggressive IV resuscitation is clearly indicated.

BIBLIOGRAPHY

1. Baxt WG, Berry CC, Epperson MD, et al: The failure of prehospital trauma prediction rules to classify trauma patients accurately. Ann Emerg Med 18:1–8, 1989.
2. Bickell WH, Wall WJ, Pepe PE, et al: Immediate versus delayed fluid resuscitation for hypotensive patients with penetrating torso injuries. N Engl J Med 331:1105–1109, 1994.
3. Blackwell TH: Prehospital care. Emerg Med Clin North Am 11:1–14, 1993.
4. Kingsland R, Rosen P: Multiple trauma. In Markovchick VJ, Pons PT, Wolfe RE (eds): Emergency Medicine Secrets. Philadelphia, Hanley & Belfus, 1993, pp 355–358.
5. New York State Department of Health EMS Rules.
6. Mattox KL, Bickell W, Pepe PE, et al: Prospective MAST study in 911 patients. J Trauma 29:1104–1112, 1989.
7. Schmidt J, Moore GP: Management of multiple trauma. Emerg Med Clin North Am 11:29–52, 1993.
8. Walls RM: Airway management. Emerg Med Clin North Am 11:29–52, 1993.

52. HEAD INJURIES

Peter T. Pons, M.D.

1. What is the single most important observation to make when evaluating a patient who has sustained head trauma?

The patient's level of consciousness and what it has done over time. Specifically, you want to determine what the level of consciousness was at the time of the trauma, what it was immediately after the trauma, and what has it done since your arrival. A decreasing level of consciousness is the earliest and most important sign of increasing intracranial pressure. A patient who was knocked out as a result of the head trauma and is now awake is much less worrisome than a patient who was awake initially and is now becoming unresponsive. The level of consciousness provides one of the best and earliest clues to the potential severity of the injury.

2. The books all teach about checking the pupils. Where does that fit in?

Checking the pupils is an important part of the physical examination. A dilated pupil is an ominous finding suggesting increased intracranial pressure and brain stem herniation. Unfortunately, pupillary dilatation is a late sign of increased intracranial pressure. Therefore, the ideal is to recognize the subtle change in level of consciousness that indicates increased intracranial pressure before the pupil dilates and the diagnosis becomes apparent to all.

3. What are the common causes of increased intracranial pressure after head trauma?

The brain is enclosed within the confines of the rigid skull. Therefore, anything that occupies space inside the skull will cause an increase in intracranial pressure. Space can be taken up by hematomas in the subdural, epidural, or intracerebral locations or by diffuse swelling of the brain tissue.

4. You mentioned herniation of the brain as a complication of increased intracranial pressure. Can you give a little more detail?

As the pressure inside the cranium increases, the brain is compressed by the hematoma or swelling. Eventually, the pressure will become so great that either the intracranial pressure will exceed the ability of the vascular system to perfuse the brain or the brain will be pushed through some of the small openings in the skull. Both these complications lead to permanent damage or death.

5. How can I tell the difference between subdural, epidural, and intracerebral hematomas clinically?

It is almost impossible to tell the difference between these various hematomas without performing computed tomography. The textbooks teach that in a patient with a subdural hematoma, after trauma occurs, the patient sustains a loss of consciousness and remains unconscious. The classic history for a patient with an epidural hematoma is that the patient loses consciousness at the time of the trauma, then wakes up and has a "lucid" period. Some time later, he loses consciousness again. Intracerebral hematomas can present with loss of consciousness or neurologic abnormalities related to the area of the brain that is injured. Unfortunately, there is significant overlap in the presentation of all these entities, and clinical differentiation is virtually impossible.

6. How can I tell the difference between a patient who has sustained a serious head injury and one whose altered mental status is from alcohol ingestion?

This can be extremely difficult. The intoxicated patient frequently is a victim of head trauma for a variety of reasons, including falling, driving while intoxicated and getting into an accident, or being assaulted. Unfortunately, many of these patients will present with altered mentation, which could be from the alcohol or could be from the trauma. The guiding principle should be to assume the worst possible injury consistent with the mechanism and treat the patient accordingly. This means that many patients whose only problem ultimately turns out to be alcohol intoxication will undergo cervical spine immobilization and, in some cases, endotracheal intubation in the field and computed tomography of the brain in the emergency department (ED).

7. How should I describe the patient who has a head injury?

There are many terms that are commonly used to describe the patient who has an altered level of consciousness. These terms include comatose, lethargic, stuporous, semicomatose, unresponsive, and so forth. The best way to describe the patient is to relate how the patient responded to a stimulus, since these terms mean different things to different people. For example, "The patient followed my verbal commands correctly," or "The patient did not follow any verbal commands but pushed my hand away in response to a sternal rub," or "The patient had no response to any stimulus."

8. What about the Glasgow Coma Scale (GCS)?

This is a scoring system that attempts to quantify the patient's level of consciousness in an objective fashion by assigning point scores to various observations. This has the advantage of yielding reproducible results rather than depending on a variety of terms that may mean different things to different observers. The GCS is scored as follows.

Eye opening	4—spontaneously
	3—to command
	2—to pain
	1—does not open eyes
Verbal response	5—oriented and conversant
	4—confused conversation
	3—inappropriate words
	2—incomprehensible
	1—none
Motor	6—follows commands
	5—localizes pain
	4—withdrawal from pain
	3—decorticate (flexion) posturing
	2—decerebrate (extension) posturing
	1—no motor activity

9. So how does the GCS relate to my patient clinically?

Rescoring the GCS over time and obtaining a series of results can help determine if the patient is improving or deteriorating. In addition, a severe head injury is defined as a score equal to or less than 8, a moderate head injury as a score between 9 and 12, and a minor head injury as a score greater than 12. It should be noted, however, that a patient who is dead still has a score of 3!

10. If I think someone has a serious head injury, what should the management be in the field?

First, assess the mechanism of injury for the potential presence of a spine injury. If there is concern about spine trauma, the spine should be immobilized. Supplemental high-flow oxygen should be provided and the patient's blood pressure maintained to assure cerebral perfusion. If the mental status is decreased or there is concern about increased intracranial pressure, endotracheal intubation should be performed to protect the airway, help assure oxygen delivery, and potentially permit hyperventilation.

11. Can you tell me about the use of lidocaine before intubation of head-injured patients?

Intubation has been shown to produce a sudden, although short, increase in intracranial pressure. There have been a number of studies in animals demonstrating that lidocaine administered intravenously can decrease this reflex response. There are no studies showing that this same effect occurs in humans, but based on the animal studies, lidocaine is administered prior to intubation in the hope that it does help.

12. I've heard that head-injured patients should no longer be hyperventilated. Is that true?

Yes, to a certain extent. Routine hyperventilation of a patient with a head injury is not recommended because it causes vasoconstriction and can actually decrease cerebral perfusion. On the other hand, if a patient is showing signs of increased intracranial pressure and herniation, mild to moderate hyperventilation can still be used to buy some time during transport. Mild to moderate hyperventilation can be accomplished by bagging the intubated patient at a rate of approximately 20–24 breaths per minute.

13. Is there anything else that can be done in the field to decrease intracranial pressure?

When spinal immobilization does not prevent it, the head of the patient can be elevated approximately 30°. In addition, diuretics such as mannitol and furosemide can be administered according to local protocol to help decrease the intracranial pressure.

14. What are some minor head injuries?

One of the most common injuries confronted in the prehospital setting is the scalp laceration. Although not usually serious, it can be a source of major blood loss. The scalp is extremely vascular, and failure to control hemorrhage from a "simple" scalp laceration can lead to hypovolemic shock. Bleeding from the scalp can usually be controlled by digital pressure. The one problem that arises is when there is concern about a potential skull fracture in association with the laceration. In this situation, pressure can be applied to the intact scalp and skull around the injured area and in this fashion control the hemorrhage.

15. Does a dilated pupil always mean that there is herniation of the brain?

No. The dilatation of a pupil must be evaluated within the context of the trauma sustained and the other findings of the physical examination. A dilated pupil with a normal mental status does not indicate increased intracranial pressure. The pupil can be dilated as a result of a direct blow to the globe causing traumatic mydriasis, which on close observation is seen as an irregular rather than a perfectly round pupil.

BIBLIOGRAPHY

1. Buloock R, Chesnut R, Clifton G, et al: Guidelines for the Management of Severe Head Injury. New York, Brain Trauma Foundation, 1996.
2. Chesnut RM: The management of severe traumatic brain injury. Emerg Med Clin North Am 15:581–604, 1977.
3. Eisenberg HM, Aldrich EF (eds): Management of head injury. Neurosurg Clin North Am 2:1–501, 1991.
4. Feldman Z, Kanter MJ, Robertson CS, et al: Effect of head elevation on intracranial pressure, and cerebral blood flow in head-injured patients. J Neurosurg 76:207–211, 1992.
5. Newton E. Head trauma. In Markovchick VJ, Pons PT, Wolfe RW (eds): Emergency Medicine Secrets. Philadelphia, Hanley & Belfus, 1993, pp 365–369.
6. Teasdale G, Jennett B: Assessment of coma and impaired consciousness: A practical scale. Lancet 2:81–84, 1974.

53. SPINAL CORD INJURIES

Scott Bolleter, EMT-P, I/C

1. A whole chapter on spinal cord injury?

Yes, that's right! A whole chapter devoted to selected spinal cord injury (SCI) issues and the initial prehospital management of a potentially devastating injury. This chapter will change the way you currently think about providing care to those who present with SCI.

2. What do I need to know about immobilization?

How often do you actually see a patient "immobilized"? With absolutely no patient movement? I suggest that you have rarely seen such a thing, yet you use that term in documentation. I recommend caution on this point from an informed legal perspective. What *is* actually occurring is *spinal motion restriction (SMR)*. The patient's movement has been restricted in such a manner that the possibility of further injury is lessened. This motion restriction is accomplished by the use of various pieces of equipment, teamwork, and patient education. SMR, as always, is dependent on local protocol and routine.

From a procedural standpoint, little or nothing changes. Picture yourself, however, as a defendant in a case involving a spinal cord injury. The patient involved in the litigation is the once-intoxicated noncompliant individual you really did try to help. Now visualize the attorney demonstrating how the patient was "moving" while immobilized. By use of patient and receiving-staff testimony, several eyewitnesses, an on-scene amateur video, and a simple demonstration using your equipment and a model, the plaintiff's attorney will show you in fact *lied* on your documentation. The patient *was* moving.

Now imagine a completely different scenario. Your defense attorney begins the cross-examination. She points out your numerous attempts to comfort and console the patient. Your counsel directs the jury toward your efforts to educate the patient about the risk of movement. She additionally demonstrates how you *restricted the patient's motion* following local protocol and the standard of care. Though you were unable to control this violent patient completely (through no fault of your own), you clearly restricted the patient's motion in an effort to limit and/or prevent injury. The change in terminology may appear insignificant, but the adjustment might well make a substantial difference in the outcome of the lawsuit.

3. Is this much ado about nothing?

Spinal motion restriction has been a very hot topic for some time now. There has been a great deal of discussion and some research about whether there is a need to restrict the vast numbers of patients who currently find themselves on backboards in the United States. Some protocols in select EMS systems currently allow prehospital personnel to determine whether SMR is indicated. The following is a compilation from several of the more common protocol approaches to this dilemma.

SMR may not be indicated when all the following criteria are met.

1. The patient is an adult.
2. The patient is able to communicate in such a manner that there is no possibility of misunderstanding or misinterpretation.
3. The patient is pain free, meaning no subjective complaint of neck pain and no objective finding of tenderness on palpation.
4. The patient has not ingested any substance that might interfere with his or her interpretation of pain.
5. The mechanism of injury does not suggest SCI.

It is not difficult to see that utilization of this protocol is still significantly limiting and thus results in the continued use of SMR for most patients.

4. How about the patient with penetrating neck trauma? Do I have to apply spinal motion restriction devices in these cases?

As a general rule, no. With victims of shootings and stabbings, if no spinal cord injury is found initially, they are usually not going to develop one. This is because of the difference in mechanism of injury between blunt and penetrating injury and the forces and energy involved. With blunt injury, significant force and energy are applied to the vertebral column and spine, resulting in disruption of the integrity of the supporting structure of the vertebral column. Thus, even if a cord injury did not occur at the time of the trauma, the lack of structural integrity of the spinal column could permit movement of damaged vertebrae and subsequent spinal cord injury if spinal motion restriction is not employed. With penetrating neck trauma, on the other hand, damage is usually limited to the path of the penetrating object and usually does not cause structural support disruption. Thus, subsequent neurologic injury is very rare.

5. What is the current thinking on the use of the rigid spine board?

There are studies that suggest that our current approach to SMR utilizing the rigid spine board might actually be detrimental to a segment of our patient care population. The size of the study clearly suggests that more research is indicated. There is consensus among most providers that the long spine board is extremely uncomfortable and that there is a correlation between excessive time spent on the board and additional complications.

Is there an alternative to the rigid spine board? At present, there are several alternatives to the "board," and more are currently under development. Without doubt, the trend is to achieve SMR with the recognition that it can be accomplished with a measure of comfort and no further harm. Full-body vacuum splints are certainly not an end-all but do point to one approach that meets a direct need. Obviously, protocol adjustments will meet selected concerns, as will additional education and training for the provider. As for the majority of potentially complex extrications, the various devices available on the market today are still, for the most part, subservient to the rigid spine board for at least the initial phase of activity. With further research and development, the rigid spine board dilemma may one day give rise to discussions on the most comfortable way to achieve SMR.

6. What clinical signs and symptoms should I look for that suggest spinal cord injury?

First, evaluate the mechanism of injury to see if it has the potential to produce a spinal column or cord injury. Next, determine what complaints the patient voices. Any complaint of numbness, tingling, pins and needles, weakness, or paralysis should be presumed to be due to a spinal injury until proven otherwise. The physical examination will, of course, provide important information as well. Evaluate the patient for sensory abnormalities and motor function. As before, any abnormal findings should be presumed to be resulting from a spinal cord injury. The presence of priapism (persistent erection) is thought to be pathognomonic of spinal cord injury. Patients with very high cervical cord injuries may develop respiratory compromise.

7. I've heard about spinal shock. What should I do about it?

Spinal shock (also referred to as neurogenic shock) may develop as a result of spinal cord injury when sympathetic tone to the vascular system is lost. This results in vasodilatation and hypotension, often with a normal heart rate. Since most of these patients could, and often do, have other associated injuries, however, hypotension must be presumed to be secondary to blood loss, and the patient should be treated for hemorrhagic shock. Spinal shock is therefore a diagnosis of exclusion, once hemorrhagic causes of shock have been eliminated.

8. When there is airway compromise, what is the best method of intubation?

When confronted with an SCI patient in need of a patent airway, there is little question that time is of the essence. SCI patients with high cervical injury or progressive secondary cord injuries are at a great risk for the development of respiratory compromise. The prudent provider should always maintain a watchful eye for progressive changes in neurologic findings that may suggest pending respiratory embarrassment. Research suggests that the method of airway management most familiar to the provider will be that which is employed. Further discussion points out that oral intubation (with appropriate personnel, in-line stabilization, and rapid-sequence medications) when necessary does not appear to create additional neurologic complications or deficits. In fact, given the experience base of today's provider, it may be the preferred method. The following is an outline of one approach that may be used to secure the airway of an SCI patient with respiratory compromise.

1. Manual stabilization and motion restriction to maintain neutral positioning (throughout procedure).

2. Preoxygenation with a bag-valve mask, oral airway, and cricoid pressure.

3. Sedation and paralysis (as indicated by patient presentation).

4. Removal of the anterior portion of the cervical collar (posterior portion left in place).

5. Oral intubation with direct visual observation of the vocal cords (cricoid pressure as needed).

6. Confirmation of tube placement.

It should be noted that additional methods of airway management that do not cause extension, flexion, or lateral motion are quite acceptable. Other management techniques that do not require direct visualization include blind nasotracheal intubation, digital intubation, and the lighted stylet (i.e., the TrachLight). In the patient in whom respiratory arrest has not occurred but a patent airway must be provided, nasotracheal intubation may be appropriate. Care must be taken to insure that patient movement and any *relative* contraindications have been taken into consideration. The key factors that are the underlying framework for successful airway management are teamwork and flexibility on the part of the providers.

9. What is a neutral position, and does it change from patient to patient?

A neutral position is when the eyes are at a 90° angle to the spine. The head is neither flexed nor extended, and the spinal column's natural "in line" position is maintained. In adult and pediatric populations, the ability to achieve a neutral position changes depending on the relationship between the occipital region of the skull and the patient's shoulders. Ask several associates to lay supine on the floor. Carefully examine the relationship between their shoulders, their occiput, and the floor. Note that some will rest their heads in a neutral position, without aid. Some, however, will need padding behind the occiput (I have seen as much as 5 inches) to maintain the head in the correct position (eyes at a 90° angle to the spine). The pediatric patient (depending on age and size) is most often the direct opposite of the adult. This is quite easy to understand because infants and children have disproportionately larger heads when compared to the body. Thus, padding the pediatric patient's body brings the head into a neutral position.

10. Is there such a thing as secondary cord injury?

Yes. When discussing insult to the spinal cord, the conversation is often limited to the initial trauma. Recent research points to secondary cord injury resulting from ischemia and post-traumatic membrane changes as a significant concern. When the neutral position is achieved in any patient, there is a maximal amount of space available for the cord within the spinal canal. This space is reduced as the patient extends or flexes. If we consider normal anatomy, it is quite simple to see that any disruption or displacement could and does create a compromise in blood flow. This compromise in blood flow, in combination with edema and a failure to achieve neutral positioning, may be the cause for significant *additional* progression of the injury.

11. Is there anything else that can be done to minimize this secondary injury?

Clinical experience and research indicate that spinal cord injuries benefit from appropriate oxygenation (the treatment of hypoxia), and for situations involving prolonged prehospital times (hours), the administration of methylprednisolone may help reduce edema and decrease secondary injury. Certainly, the argument can be made that aggressive management is favored over the "wait-and-see approach." Prehospital intervention with SMR to limit or prevent injury, drug therapies directed at cessation of the spinal cord destruction, and follow-through at tertiary care facilities are proven factors in the reduction of morbidity and mortality.

12. If I am going to give methylprednisolone, how do I administer it?

The dose of steroid is extremely high. The drug must be administered within 8 hours of the time of injury. A loading dose is given first in the amount of 30 mg/kg of body weight administered intravenously over 15 minutes. There is a 45-minute waiting period, then 5.4 mg/kg per hour are given for each of the next 23 hours.

13. Are there any additional concerns that should be addressed?

Yes, age-related index of suspicion. There is research that concludes that in the pediatric population, an insult known as SCIWORA (spinal cord injury without radiologic abnormality) exists, and, if the provider is not versed in the kinetics of the mechanism of injury, the insult can go untreated until the deficit is noted. It is absolutely imperative for us to inspect each individual thoroughly for the signs of occult injury. It makes little difference if the injury is apparent initially or if the insult progresses insidiously. Deficit is, after all, deficit. A fair amount of supportive literature exists that maintains that even though the preponderance of SCI occurs to the 16 to 33-year-old active male, we must continue to insist on a high index of suspicion for all other patient care populations.

BIBLIOGRAPHY

1. Anderson D, Hall E: Pathophysiology of spinal cord trauma. Ann Emerg Med 22:987–992, 1993.
2. Bracken MB, Shepard MJ, Collins WF, et al: A randomized, controlled trial of methylprednisolone or naloxone in the treatment of acute spinal-cord injury. Results of the Second National Acute Spinal Cord Injury Study. N Engl J Med 322:1405–1411, 1990.
3. Committee on Trauma, American College of Surgeons: Advanced Trauma Life Support. Chicago, American College of Surgeons, 1993, pp 47–59, 191–203.
4. Criswell J, Nolan J: Emergency airway management in patients with cervical spine injuries. Anaesthesia 49:900–903, 1994.
5. Davis J, Phreaner D, Hoyt D, Mackersie R: The etiology of missed cervical injuries. Trauma J 34(3): 342–346, 1993.
6. Diliberti T, Ronald W: Evaluation of the cervical spine in the emergency setting: Who does not need an x-ray. Orthop 15(2):179–183, 1992.
7. Hadley M, Zabramski J, Browner C, Rekate H, Sonntag V: Pediatric spinal trauma: Review of 122 cases of spinal cord and vertebral column injuries. Neurosurg J 68:18–64, 1988.
8. Spivac JM, Weiss M, Cotler J, Call M: Cervical spine injuries in patients 65 and older. Spine 19(20):2302–2306, 1994.
9. Tator H, Fehlings M: Review of the secondary injury theory of acute spinal cord trauma with emphasis on vascular mechanism. Neurosurg J 75:15–26, 1991.
10. VanBuren RL, Franklin C: Respiratory complications after cervical spinal cord injury. Spine 19 (20):2215–2219, 1994.

54. THORACIC, ABDOMINAL, AND PELVIC TRAUMA

Robert F. McCormack, M.D.

1. What do you mean by thoracic trauma?

The thorax is enclosed within the rib cage and contains many essential organs including the heart, lungs, trachea, esophagus, and great vessels. In addition, the upper abdominal organs, particularly the spleen and liver, lie in the lower thoracic cage. Therefore, any injury below the nipple line anteriorly or below the inferior border of the scapula posteriorly can injure both chest and abdominal organs.

2. What are the deadly dozen?

The deadly dozen refers to the twelve possible major injuries to the thoracic organs. The immediate threats to life are airway obstruction, open pneumothorax, tension pneumothorax, massive hemothorax, and cardiac tamponade. Potential threats to life include traumatic aortic rupture, flail chest, bronchial disruption, myocardial contusion, diaphragmatic tear, esophageal injury, and pulmonary contusion.

3. What should I look for when I examine the chest?

First, observe the patient for signs of respiratory distress. Then look at the chest to evaluate the rate, depth, and symmetry of chest wall expansion. Note if there are any segments of the chest wall that have paradoxic motion, indicating a flail segment. Also look for any penetrating wounds and entry and exit wounds. Next, place your hands on the patient and palpate the ribs and chest wall to check for subcutaneous emphysema and bony crepitus. Finally, if the noise level in the area permits, auscultate the chest for the presence or absence of breath sounds as well as any abnormal sounds such as stridor or wheezing. Don't forget that any chest wall findings such as penetrating wounds or possible rib fractures located below the level of the nipples anteriorly or the tip of the scapulae posteriorly should be considered to be potential abdominal wounds as well.

4. How about when I examine the abdomen and pelvis?

Observe the abdomen, flank, and back for obvious penetrating wounds. Then palpate the abdomen, looking for tenderness, especially over organs such as the liver and spleen. Palpate the pelvis and gently compress the pubic rami in the midline and laterally over the iliac crests to determine tenderness or instability. Remember that early in the course of many injuries, the abdominal examination can be unremarkable in the face of significant trauma. The presence of alcohol and other distracting painful injuries such as fractures can be misleading and mask findings of tenderness.

5. How do I treat thoracic trauma?

The mainstay of prehospital treatment of thoracic trauma is really the basics: A patent airway, high-flow oxygen via a nonrebreather bag reservoir mask, adequate circulation, a brief secondary survey, immobilization if necessary, placement of an IV line (or two) en route, and early notification of the receiving hospital. Airway obstruction should be treated as it is discovered. Intubation may be necessary. It is important to consider other potential injuries. You may suspect a pneumothorax or tamponade clinically and be able to prepare the hospital team for the patient's arrival. Prehospital management of thoracic trauma is usually the same regardless of the specific injury, with the exception of tension pneumothorax.

6. How do I diagnose tension pneumothorax and treat it?

Tension pneumothorax is a true life-threatening emergency! It should be treated as soon as it is diagnosed. Tension pneumothorax develops when air enters the pleural space through a laceration of the lung, a bronchial tear, or the chest wall and cannot escape. As more air enters the space, the pressure builds and eventually shifts the mediastinum, collapsing the vena cava and decreasing blood return to the right heart. Loss of blood return causes a drop in cardiac output, resulting in hypotension and tachycardia.

Tension pneumothorax is diagnosed by the absence of breath sounds over the hemithorax, hypotension, and tachycardia. Subcutaneous emphysema is often palpated and may be massive. Tracheal shift away from the affected side may or may not be apparent. Needle decompression is achieved with a 14-gauge 2-inch Angiocath on a 3-ml syringe with 2 ml of normal saline in the syringe with the plunger removed. The needle is introduced into the second intercostal space at the midclavicular line. Passage of air through the water medium represents adequate decompression. Vital signs should normalize quickly. Remain alert for recurrence of the tension and decompress again if symptoms return. Failure of the vital signs to normalize may occur with concomitant hypovolemic shock. If the patient is intubated, another sign of tension pneumothorax is greater backpressure or decreased compliance to bagging. In such patients, decompression may be accomplished by inserting a large Angiocath into the fourth intercostal space (midaxillary line), without the need for a one-way valve.

7. What do I do for the other injuries?

Rapid transportation is the most important therapy. Administer high-flow oxygen to all patients with suspected chest or abdominal injuries. Massive hemothorax will require large-volume resuscitation and surgery. Cardiac contusion and tamponade may improve with administration of a relatively small fluid bolus. Flail chest and pulmonary contusions may require endotracheal intubation.

8. Is giving fluid really bad?

Yes and no! Recent research has questioned the use of aggressive fluid resuscitation in penetrating chest trauma. The concept is that as blood pressure increases, the rate of bleeding in the noncompressible chest vessels increases or the higher pressure dislodges tenuous clots. The study has some methodologic problems and needs to be confirmed. The downside of "overresuscitation" is noteworthy, however, and fluid resuscitation should probably be tempered to the minimal amount necessary to maintain adequate perfusion. Fluid therapy should be titrated to a blood pressure of 90 mm Hg systolic. Continuous aggressive administration of crystalloid after reaching a blood pressure of at least 90 mm Hg systolic may also be harmful to patients with large pulmonary or myocardial contusions.

9. What are the indications for a "slash" thoracotomy?

There is no indication for this procedure in the field. Also known as an emergent thoracotomy, this heroic surgical procedure is rarely successful. The indications are penetrating trauma to the chest with witnessed loss of vital signs. Treatable findings are cardiac tamponade or isolated cardiac puncture wounds. Success rates are low and related to the time between loss of vital signs and thoracotomy. In the setting of blunt trauma, thoracotomies are rarely helpful and usually not indicated. A patient found in the field in traumatic arrest due to blunt trauma will stay that way. If vital signs are lost during transport, a "slash" thoracotomy on arrival to the ED may be indicated in cases of penetrating trauma to the chest or abdomen. Isolated head-injured patients will not benefit from thoracotomy.

10. How does a stab wound to the left chest injure the spleen?

Remember that the spleen and liver lie in the lower chest. During exhalation, the diaphragm can rise as high as the nipple line. Any of these structures can be injured with a stab wound or gunshot wound.

11. What is the difference between blunt and penetrating abdominal trauma?

The first thing to remember about abdominal trauma is that symptoms may develop late. Early symptoms of pain, distention, guarding, and rigidity suggest massive internal bleeding.

Blunt abdominal trauma usually injures the solid organs, with spleen injury being most common. Abdominal tenderness can indicate serious intra-abdominal injury.

Penetrating wounds often injure the bowel and can present with a normal abdominal exam. Peritonitis is a late complication of bowel injury that can have catastrophic results. All penetrating wounds to the abdomen require ED evaluation. Remember, serious stab wounds may have very benign outward appearances.

12. Who goes to the operating room?

Anyone who continues to bleed, such as a patient with chest injuries in which the output from the chest tube remains high. Patients with cardiac tamponade need a cardiac window to be created to relieve the pressure and surgery to identify and correct the bleeding site. Most gunshot wounds to the abdomen need exploration. The management of abdominal stab wounds is more complicated, but they often need exploration. Any penetration or rupture of the gastrointestinal tract or the urogenital tract needs surgical repair.

13. Who needs a trauma center?

Any person who has sustained a substantial mechanism of injury, such as high-speed motor vehicle accidents, falls from great heights, substantial burns, or stab or gunshot wounds to the head, neck, or torso. Other indications are any trauma patient who has abnormal vital signs or evidence of a chest or abdominal injury; patients with amputations (replant center) or neurovascular compromise of an extremity due to trauma; and patients with significant head injuries with loss of consciousness, altered level of consciousness, or focal neurologic findings.

In accordance with the golden hour, direct transport to a trauma center is the best choice. If the ABCs can be maintained, bypassing a local hospital to go directly to a trauma center is probably the best decision. These decisions need to be made in the context of local protocols, other available methods of transport, and level of training of the ambulance crew.

14. How do I diagnose and treat a pelvic fracture?

A pelvic fracture should be suspected in anyone with pelvic pain on movement or with compression of the pelvic girdle. Motor vehicle accidents (particularly lateral collisions), being struck by automobiles, falls, and bicycle/motorcycle accidents are common mechanisms of pelvic injury. It is important to suspect pelvic injuries because they can result in massive blood loss. Unstable pelvic bones can cause continued arterial and venous bleeding that can go unnoticed. If transport times are prolonged, military antishock trousers (MAST) can act as an excellent splint for an unstable pelvis and help to control bleeding.

15. What is the definitive management of pelvic fractures?

Pelvic fractures may require external fixation in the emergency department or operative fixation. Bleeding from the fractures may require large blood transfusions as well as angiography to embolize the bleeding sites.

16. How is trauma care different when the patient is pregnant?

Simple: Be more careful! You are now dealing with two patients. Even minor trauma to the gravid abdomen can result in dire consequences. All pregnant women with trauma to their abdomen need evaluation in the ED and often need fetal monitoring. The signs of shock may be delayed because of the increased maternal blood volume. Remember, fetal viability is determined by maternal viability. Save the mother first. In the third trimester, position the mother in a modified left lateral decubitus position to facilitate venous return to the heart. Fetal heart tones of less than 120 or more than 160 beats per minute usually indicate significant fetal distress.

BIBLIOGRAPHY

1. Jackimcyzk K: Blunt chest trauma. Emerg Med Clin North Am 11:81–96, 1993.
2. Jorden RC: Chest trauma. In Markovchick VJ, Pons PT, Wolfe RE (eds): Emergency Medicine Secrets. Philadelphia, Hanley & Belfus, 1993, pp 376–380.
3. Marx JA: Penetrating abdominal trauma. Emerg Med Clin North Am 11:125–135, 1993.
4. Mattox KL, Bickell W, Pepe PE, et al: Prospective MAST study in 911 patients. J Trauma 29:1104–1112, 1989.
5. Read RA, Moore EE: Abdominal trauma. In Markovchick VJ, Pons PT, Wolfe RE (eds): Emergency Medicine Secrets. Philadelphia, Hanley & Belfus, 1993, pp 380–386.
6. Read RA, Moore EE: Hemorrhage in pelvic fractures. In Markovchick VJ, Pons PT, Wolfe RE (eds): Emergency Medicine Secrets. Philadelphia, Hanley & Belfus, 1993, pp 386–390.

55. PEDIATRIC TRAUMA

John P. Marshall, M.D.

1. What is the most common cause of death in children?

Trauma is the most common cause of death in children between the ages of 1 and 14 years. Beyond infancy, encounters with motor vehicles—as an occupant, cyclist, or pedestrian—are the most common cause of death, followed closely by penetrating injuries (primarily gunshot wounds), which have been increasing in frequency. During infancy, homicide accounts for the most pediatric deaths. Traumatic injury is more common in summer and occurs more frequently to boys than girls. Children from low socioeconomic settings also appear to be at higher risk. Falls, burns, and drowning occur more frequently in children than in adults.

2. Aren't cervical spine injuries uncommon in children?

Actually, no. Studies have demonstrated that children account for 1–10% of all cervical spine injuries. Therefore, any child with a history of significant trauma should be immobilized in the field prior to transport simultaneously with resuscitative efforts.

3. What are the common causes of cervical spine injury in children?

Spine injury may result from moderate to major motor vehicle collisions, falls from greater than 8 to 10 feet, trauma above the clavicles, trauma associated with neurologic findings including loss of consciousness and altered mental status, diving injuries, and multiple trauma. In addition, any child who complains of neck pain in association with minor trauma should be immobilized.

4. How do I immobilize a child?

In larger children, immobilization can be achieved using pediatric-sized rigid cervical collars such as the Stiff-Neck or Philadelphia collar. Smaller children should be immobilized with a KED (Kendrick extrication device)-type board if available. Blankets and sandbags are also an option. Because of a proportionally larger occiput, small children are difficult to immobilize in an anatomically correct position. Therefore, efforts should be made to align the external auditory meatus with the shoulders using padding under the back and shoulders. Infants can also be successfully immobilized in a pediatric car seat if available.

5. What are the signs of airway obstruction in children?

Airway obstruction is usually manifest by hoarseness, stridor, high-pitched voice, chest and abdominal retractions, grunting, nasal flaring, and drooling. Children who are speaking normally or crying vigorously are unlikely to have an obstructed airway.

6. When should I insert an airway in a child?

Airways should be used only in comatose or semicomatose children or in children requiring bag-valve-mask ventilation, since the risk of vomiting and aspiration is somewhat higher in children. Nasal airways are better tolerated in the patient with an intact gag reflex. Appropriate airway size can be estimated by measuring the airway against the side of the child's face. An oral airway should extend from the corner of the mouth to the angle of the jaw. A nasal airway should extend from the corner of the mouth to the tragus of the ear. In children, oral airways should not be inserted backwards and rotated owing to the risk of trauma to the teeth and mouth. Rather, the tongue should be pulled forward and the airway inserted in the physiologic position.

7. How does intubation differ in children of different ages?

Field intubation has a lower success rate when attempted on children. Nasotracheal intubation is frequently very difficult in children owing to the acute angle of the nasopharynx and the anterior and superior position of the larynx, and it should probably not be attempted. Therefore, oral intubation should probably be the procedure of choice for comatose children in whom bag-valve-mask ventilation has failed or who are at substantial risk for aspiration.

Laryngoscope blade size can be estimated based on the child's age: newborn to 18 months, #1 blade; 18 months to 10–12 years, #2 blade; 12 years and up, #3 blade. A straight blade is generally recommended for children younger than 2 to 3 years old because their larynx is typically anterior and high.

Endotracheal (ET) tube size can be estimated by using a tube the size of the child's little finger or by the equation: (age/4) + 4. Children younger than 8 years old should be intubated only with uncuffed tubes owing to the normal physiologic narrowing at the cricoid cartilage, which should adequately prevent aspiration. Children who are 8 years and older require a cuffed tube. As a final note, confirmation of tube placement always requires auscultation over the stomach in addition to both axillae, since esophageal intubation can mimic tracheal intubation by transmitting false breath sounds to the lungs. If available, end-tidal CO_2 detectors should be used to confirm proper tube placement.

8. What if intubation is unsuccessful?

If bag-valve-mask ventilation and endotracheal intubation are unsuccessful, needle cricothyroidostomy can be performed with the approval of medical control. The space between the cricoid cartilage (Adam's apple) and thyroid cartilage is palpated. This is the cricothyroid membrane. A 12- or 14-gauge IV catheter can be inserted through this space by entering the skin and angling the needle 45° downward toward the lungs. The needle should be aspirated continuously until air is returned. An adapter from a 3 or 3.5 ET tube can be attached to the end, and the child may be bagged through this. Alternatively, if pressurized oxygen is available (25–50 psi), a "Y" connector can be attached to the IV and oxygen lines. The third unused port is then occluded for 2 seconds to permit inflation of the lungs and released for 4 to 5 seconds to allow for exhalation. This type of ventilation can be used only for 30 to 40 minutes before the buildup of carbon dioxide becomes toxic. Unless absolutely necessary, this procedure should not be attempted in children with significant neck trauma because the procedure becomes exponentially more difficult with any distortion of the anatomy.

9. What are the injuries associated with severe chest trauma? What signs should alert you to them?

As in adults, chest trauma can produce tension pneumothorax, open pneumothorax, and, less commonly, flail chest, in addition to a number of other complications that cannot be diagnosed or treated in the prehospital setting such as pulmonary contusion. General signs of critical chest injury include asymmetry of chest wall movement, retractions, nasal flaring, grunting, asymmetry of breath sounds, crepitance, rib deformity, and chest wall abrasions. All patients with significant chest or head trauma should receive high-flow oxygen by mask.

It is important to remember that external evidence of chest injuries is often lacking in children owing to the compliance of their chest wall. Ribs in children tend to bend rather than break. Thus, internal injury such as pulmonary contusion is a more common injury than rib fractures in flail chest.

An important clue in the detection of respiratory compromise is an increasing respiratory rate. Careful initial and repeated determination of the patient's respiratory rate can help provide early recognition that the patient's respiratory status is compromised or deteriorating.

10. Does shock manifest itself differently in children compared with adults?

Unlike adults, in whom blood pressure can be used as a reliable measure of shock, children frequently will not demonstrate hypotension until they have lost 40% of their blood volume. Tachycardia is a much more sensitive indicator of shock in children, although confounding factors such as fear, pain, fever, and hypoxia can also produce a rapid heart rate. Circulating volume can be quickly assessed by checking capillary refill. The nail bed or thenar eminence (at the base of the thumb) can be compressed for 5 seconds, then released. With adequate circulating blood volume, the color should return within 2 seconds. A table of age-based pediatric vital signs can be very helpful. Roughly, maximum pediatric heart rates are 180 bpm for neonates to infants 1 year old; 150 bpm from 1 to 3 years old; 130 from 3 to 7 years old; and 120 from 7 to 14 years old. Heart rates that exceed these maximums should be considered signs of significant hypovolemic shock. A quick estimation of minimum normal blood pressure in children can be made with this equation: $(2 \times age) + 80$.

11. What about using a pneumatic anti-shock garment (PASG)?

As with adults, the use of a PASG is indicated principally for the stabilization of pelvic or femur fractures, particularly in the setting of hypotension. The PASG may be placed with the patient on the backboard after the cervical spine has been immobilized. If a patient with these fractures is stable and requires prolonged transport, the trousers may be placed prior to transport and inflated if the patient appears to become unstable. The pitfall of PASG in children is that the correct size is frequently unavailable, and an adult-sized PASG should not be used on a small child.

12. What if an IV line is difficult to place?

Placing an IV line can be particularly difficult in children. The easiest sites for placing a percutaneous IV line are the antecubital fossa, the interdigital vein of the dorsum of the hand between the fourth and fifth digits, and the greater saphenous vein at the ankle. Access should be attempted on scene only if the transport time is greater than 15 minutes. An unstable child will probably be better served by rapid transport with IV access attempts made en route only. If no venous access is possible and the child is in desperate need of fluids, an intraosseous line may be placed on the order of medical control. These lines should be used only in children younger than 6 years of age and are extremely painful. Thus, it is generally reserved for the child who clearly needs fluid emergently and has an altered mental status. A 16- or 18-gauge, ½ inch bone marrow needle should be used. The puncture is made one fingerwidth distal to the tibial tuberosity (the insertion of the patellar tendon) on the anterior aspect of the tibia. The leg is placed in a 30° flexed position, and the needle is introduced with the bevel up. The needle should be directed toward the foot at a 45–60° angle to the surface of the tibia. Placement should be confirmed by aspiration of bone marrow. When flushed, the line should flow easily without swelling around the site. If the line appears to be in good position, fluid and medications can be infused through it effectively. Complications from this procedure can be severe; therefore, the line must be discontinued when adequate venous access has been established.

13. How do I give IV fluids to a child?

Any child with evidence of shock should receive prompt fluid resuscitation. The initial recommendation is to administer a bolus 20 ml/kg of isotonic fluid, either lactated Ringer's or normal saline. The appropriate volume of fluid should be run wide open or bolused using a 50-ml or 60-ml syringe. If the child's clinical picture or vital signs fail to respond to this initial bolus, a second bolus, also at 20 ml/kg, can be given. It should be noted that the total blood volume for a child is 80 ml/kg. Therefore, any child who fails to respond to two fluid boluses should be assumed to be in severe hypovolemic shock and may require immediate surgical intervention. A third crystalloid bolus should not be used, since further therapy will probably require colloid solutions or blood products. Heart rate and blood pressure should be followed closely during transport. If the child's weight is not available from individuals on the scene, a Broselow tape may be used to estimate the child's weight using the child's height. For children one year of age or older, you can roughly estimate weight with the following formula: $wt = (age \times 2) + 8$.

14. How is the Glasgow Coma Scale (GCS) modified for children?

In addition to observing pupillary response and movement of extremities, you should perform a brief mental status examination for all pediatric trauma patients. This may be as simple as asking the child his name. An adequate response to questioning is sufficient to establish appropriate mentation. This process may be more difficult in the nonverbal or preverbal child. The AVPU mnemonic (**A**lert, responds to **V**ocal stimuli, responds only to **P**ainful stimuli, **U**nresponsive) can, in the primary survey, be used without alteration; however, the verbal and motor portions of the GCS require modification for these patients. (The eye opening response is unchanged.) The motor response is only slightly modified: A score of 6 is associated with *spontaneous intentional movement*, and a score of 5 is *localized withdrawal to pain*.

The entire verbal response scale is modified as follows:

Appropriate words or social smile, fixes and follows	5
Cries but consolable	4
Persistently irritable or inconsolable	3
Restless, agitated	2
None	1

15. How does the small size of children affect outcome after a traumatic event?

Physiologically, children have less substantial subcutaneous tissue and relatively thin skin when compared with adults. In addition, small body size increases the ratio of surface area to body mass. Because of these differences, children are much more prone to hypothermia than their adult counterparts. Great care should be taken in the field to avoid hypothermia, including the use of ambulance heaters, blankets, and warmed intravenous fluids. Exposure should be minimized, since hypothermia greatly increases oxygen consumption. With falling body temperature, the body tissues become refractory to treatment, the central nervous system becomes depressed, and coagulation becomes impaired. Children who present with extreme hypothermia to the point of coagulopathy have only a 50% survival rate.

16. What are the common signs of child abuse?

Unfortunately, child abuse is not uncommon in our society. It occurs in all socioeconomic classes and almost always presents with a history of accidental trauma. While certain injuries are considered specific for child abuse, the most important piece of information is the history given by the parents. This should be recorded meticulously in any setting where child abuse is suspected because an inconsistent history given at different points of evaluation can be an important clue to child abuse. Physical findings inconsistent with the given history are also an important clue to abuse. Specific physical findings associated with abuse include burns limited to the groin area, second-degree burns in a characteristic shape (e.g., an iron), second-degree burns with a sharp line of demarcation and no splash marks, bruises in characteristic shapes (e.g., a belt), unexplained sudden changes in level of consciousness, multiple bruises of different ages, multiple bruises in a nonambulatory infant, or swelling out of proportion to the severity of the described injury.

A refusal of care in the setting of suspected child abuse can be a particularly difficult situation for EMS personnel. Close contact with medical control is essential, as is knowledge of your local and state laws. The police need to be involved early if child abuse is strongly suspected and a parent is refusing care. If the child is in critical condition, medical control may be able to authorize immediate transport while the police are being dispatched. Technically, however, a child cannot be transported or treated against the will of a parent without a court order. Again, consult your local laws for exact details.

BIBLIOGRAPHY

1. Burg J, Fleisher GR: Prehospital care of the injured child. In Eichelberger M (ed): Pediatric Trauma: Prevention, Acute Care, Rehabilitation. St. Louis, Mosby, 1993, pp 99–112.
2. Graneto JW, Solgin DF: Transport and stabilization of the pediatric trauma patient. Pediatr Clin North Am 40:365–380, 1993.
3. Mayer T: Transportation of the injured child. In Mayer T (ed): Emergency Management of Pediatric Trauma. Philadelphia, W.B. Saunders, 1985, pp 508–522.
4. Meyer P, Carli P: Transport of the severely injured child. Int Anesthesiol Clin 32:149–170, 1994.
5. Polhgeers A, Ruddy R: An update on pediatric trauma. Emerg Med Clin North Am 8:267–290, 1995.
6. Rhule R: Advanced pediatric resuscitation. In Reisdorff EJ, et al (eds): Pediatric Emergency Medicine. Philadelphia, W.B. Saunders, 1993, pp 34–51.
7. Yurt R: Triage initial assessment, and early treatment of the pediatric trauma patient. Pediatr Clin North Am 39:1083–1093, 1992.

56. INTERPERSONAL VIOLENCE

Kim M. Feldhaus, M.D.

1. Child abuse, domestic violence, elder abuse. These are social service and law enforcement issues, not health issues, right?

Wrong. Research reveals that more than 3 million children yearly are reported to social services as possible abuse victims, and child abuse results in 2000 to 3000 deaths each year. More than half of all women will experience abuse from an intimate partner or ex-partner at some point in their lives, and 30% of women have experienced domestic violence within the past year. Elder abuse affects at least 4% of the United States population. For these children, women, and elderly persons, injuries and illnesses due to abuse will affect their lives more frequently than hypertension, cancer, and diabetes. Interpersonal violence has tremendous health implications in the United States today.

2. Define child abuse.

Child abuse is defined by the Child Abuse Prevention and Treatment Act of 1974 as the physical or mental injury, sexual abuse, negligent treatment, or maltreatment of a child younger than the age of 18 by a person who is responsible for the child's welfare. Child abuse includes direct actions to injure the child as well as lack of responsible care resulting in injury or illness.

3. List the categories of child abuse.

Child abuse can be divided into (1) physical abuse (also known as nonaccidental trauma), (2) emotional abuse, (3) sexual abuse, and (4) neglect. Of these, neglect is the most common, although most cases of maltreatment that you will encounter involve physical or sexual abuse.

4. Why does child abuse occur?

Abuse of children is thought to have a multifactorial etiology. The three major factors are "right parent, right child, right day." Parents who abuse their children were often abused themselves and are poorly equipped to deal with day-to-day stress. Isolated parents with no support systems have an increased risk of being abusers. Children who require extra attention are at increased risk for abuse: fussy infants, developmentally delayed or physically disabled children, hyperactive kids, or children with chronic diseases. Other factors associated with abuse include drug or alcohol abuse in the family, socioeconomic disadvantage, and increased stress due to financial problems, unemployment, and so forth.

5. You are called to see a 10-month-old with a probable femur fracture. What historical factors should make you suspect child abuse?

The key to identifying physically abused children correctly is that the history of the injury is inconsistent with your physical examination. In this case, a nonambulatory child has no plausible way of fracturing his or her femur. Knowledge of basic developmental milestones (i.e., the age at which children roll over, sit up, and walk) is useful in matching injury with history.

Other clues to child abuse include a history of minor trauma with extensive physical injury, injuries with no explanations (magical injuries), injuries attributed to other siblings, history of self-injury, a history that changes over time, and delay in seeking treatment for a significant injury.

6. In examining a child in whom I suspect abuse, what should I look for?

First and foremost, examine the entire child if possible. (In older children, modesty and respect for the child's privacy may prevent you from performing a complete exam.) Bruises or injuries to the back and buttocks are commonly seen in abused infants and may be missed if a complete exam is not performed. Look for bruises, burns, bony tenderness or deformities, and facial and mouth injuries.

7. Children get bumps and bruises all the time! I can't suspect child abuse in every kid I see!

You are right. Some bruises should raise your suspicion of child abuse, however. Patterned bruises (from a strap, a loop or cord, or a hand), linear bruises, bruises in different stages of healing, and bruises in a young infant (especially a nonambulatory infant) are possible indications of abuse. In addition, bruises from physical abuse often occur in atypical places: cheeks, ears, inside the mouth, neck or trunk, upper legs, or genitalia. Accidental bruises usually occur over a bony prominence such as the knees, tibias, elbows, chin, or forehead.

8. What about trauma from burns? What are the characteristics of abusive burns?

Burns are frequently seen in abused children. Suspicious burns are those that are symmetric (both hands or feet), have clear lines of demarcation (since the leg or arm was held in hot water), or are patterned (from a cigarette, iron, and so forth).

9. What is "shaken baby syndrome"?

Children who are victims of "shaken baby syndrome" are usually younger than 2 years (most are younger than 6 months). The child is forcibly and repeatedly shaken, resulting in rib fractures, thoracic and lumbar vertebral body fractures, and intracranial injuries such as hemorrhage. Often, EMS is called because of an unresponsive child or a child with seizures or apnea.

10. When should neglect be suspected?

EMS providers are the only health care workers who routinely evaluate patients in their home; this gives them the opportunity to observe their living conditions. Neglect should be suspected when the home is unsanitary (with garbage, animal, or human excrement present), lacks heat or plumbing, has fire hazards, or has sleeping and living arrangements that are cold, dirty, or inadequate. There may be evidence of poor child supervision or supervision by another child. Neglected children are frequently undernourished and dirty, demonstrate poor personal hygiene, and may be inadequately dressed for the weather.

11. What is the appropriate management of an abused child?

First and foremost, attend to the child's medical needs. Police intervention may be required if the parents of a child known or suspected to be abused are refusing care or transport of their child. Carefully document the home conditions, interactions between child and parent, all injuries, and your suspicion of abuse. Communication of your concerns to the hospital staff is critical. In addition, all states require that *suspected* child abuse be reported to a child welfare agency or the District Attorney's office immediately. Check your local protocol regarding how this report should be filed.

12. What is the definition of domestic violence?

Domestic violence in a broad sense refers to all violence occurring within a family unit. By this definition, partner abuse, child abuse, and elder abuse are subsets of domestic violence. More commonly, however, domestic violence refers to the victimization of one partner by his or her intimate partner or partners. Partner violence (PV) is a more specific term. Partner violence includes both physical acts, such as battering and sexual assault, and nonphysical acts of coercion and control, such as emotional abuse, economic abuse, threats to harm children and property, or prevention of access to health care or prenatal care. Most battered women state that the nonphysical abuse was more humiliating and distressing to them than the beatings.

13. What are the risk factors for partner violence?

Partner violence occurs in all socioeconomic classes and in all races. Women who are younger than 30 years old, single, divorced, separated, or pregnant or who abuse drugs or alcohol may be at increased risk. It is unclear, however, if some of these "risk factors" lead to partner abuse or are a result of living in an abusive situation. While these women may be at increased risk for violence, it is important to remember that partner violence affects ALL women. *The only true risk factor is being female.*

14. Wait a minute! Are you saying that men are *never* victims of partner abuse?

Men certainly are injured as a result of domestic violence. In any conflict that has escalated to the point of violence, the persons involved become mutual combatants, and injury may be inflicted on a man by his female partner. The female is 13 times more likely to be injured than the male, however, and 30% more likely to be killed. Ninety-five percent of victims of partner violence are women, and the pattern of recurrent nonphysical and physical abuse (the battering syndrome) occurs almost exclusively in women.

15. I know some of the women I treat have been battered by their partners. Why won't they tell me?

Women may not reveal the abuse for a number of reasons. They may be embarrassed and humiliated that this is happening to them. There may be cultural or religious beliefs that lead the woman to believe that this is normal or to be expected. She may have been told that she deserves the abuse. Perhaps her abuser has threatened to harm her, her children, or other loved ones if she discloses the abuse to others, or she may believe that no one can help her. In addition, it is important to discuss this issue in private; battered women may be afraid to disclose the abuse when their abuser is present. Treating the patient with respect, compassion, and support will encourage disclosure.

16. Are there some clues to partner violence that may be present in a patient's history?

Most important, a history that is inconsistent with the physical exam findings should raise your suspicion for PV. Also consider partner abuse in patients with threatened miscarriages (due to abdominal trauma), suicidal intentions or attempts (frequently occurring after a "fight" with a partner), patients who are depressed or who show evidence of drug and alcohol abuse, patients with frequent calls for chronic pain complaints, and patients who report no prenatal care (their partners may prevent them from accessing care). Half of all rapes in women 30 years of age or older are part of a battering syndrome.

17. Describe the physical exam clues that may be present in a victim of PV.

Common injury patterns include injuries to the face, neck, throat, chest, breasts, abdomen, and genitals. Any injury that does not fit the history obtained is also suspicious for abuse. Other suspicious physical exam findings include evidence of sexual assault or frequent, recurrent sexually transmitted diseases.

18. How can I increase my recognition of partner abuse?

First, ask about partner violence. Any woman with an injury should be specifically asked *who* injured her. Second, raise your level of suspicion in women without injuries. Remember the clues that might be present in the history or physical exam. If you think there may be partner abuse, ask about it.

19. Give some examples of *inappropriate* comments or questions to ask women regarding partner violence.

EMS personnel should be conscious of how they inquire about partner violence. Asking questions in a judgmental, accusatory, or humiliating way only compounds a difficult situation. Common examples of statements or questions to avoid include the following. "What did you do to him?" "What did you do that made him so mad?" "This has happened before, and you are still married to him?" "Why didn't you tell anyone?" "You let him do that to you?" "I wouldn't let anyone do that to me." "Why don't you just leave?"

20. What do I do if my patient has an injury caused by her partner?

First, treat her injuries. Second, document her history and injuries carefully. Third, communicate your findings to the hospital staff. Many hospitals have protocols to help victims access community resources and shelters if needed. In addition, mandatory reporting or partner violence to the police is required in some states.

21. Who has more shelters available to them—animals or battered women?

There are three times as many animal shelters as there are shelters for battered women.

22. I can't believe it. My patient wants to stay with her assailant. Why doesn't she just leave him?

Why a woman stays in an abusive relationship is a question that we can't stop asking. It is the wrong question to ask, however. It implies that the woman is to blame and that if she would just leave, everything would be OK. In fact, battered women are most likely to be killed when they are in the act of leaving or after they have left their abuser. There are many other valid reasons why a woman stays in an abusive situation. She may have no money or job skills, nowhere else to go, or no local support system, or she may feel that she must stay to protect her children. Rarely do we ask the assailant why he batters his partner!

23. Name the types of elder abuse.

Abuse of the elderly includes (1) physical abuse, such as beating, unreasonable physical constraint, or deprivation of food and water; (2) emotional abuse, such as threats of abandonment or institutionalization; and (3) material exploitation, such as theft of social security checks or embezzlement.

24. What historical information should make you concerned about elder abuse?

Similar to child abuse, an injury that is inconsistent with the history in an elderly person should cause concern. Abused elders often delay in seeking medical care, miss medical appointments, or appear fearful of their caregivers.

25. What are the physical indications for elder abuse?

Multiple injuries in various stages of healing, inconsistent injuries, burns or bruises that are patterned or are in unusual locations, or evidence of sexual abuse.

26. What are the signs of neglect in an elderly person?

Elderly persons who are unkempt, dirty, or unshaven; those who have soiled, torn, stained, or bloody clothing; and those with evidence of malnutrition or dehydration may be victims of neglect.

27. You are called to see a debilitated, frail woman who is bedridden and aphasic. What attitudes or actions on the part of the caregiver would make you suspicious of abuse?

Elderly victims of abuse are frequently abused by their caregiver. Abusive caregivers may have an attitude of anger or indifference toward the elder; they may seem overly concerned about the cost of the medical care; or they may try to limit the victim's interaction with medical providers.

28. What is "self-neglect"?

Self-neglect is seen in a competent individual who is capable of caring for himself or herself yet refuses to do so or in an individual who is disabled yet refuses to accept assistance in basic activities of daily living. So long as the person retains decision-making capabilities and competence, he cannot be forced to accept assistance or placement into nursing facilities.

29. Do I have any legal responsibilities when caring for an abused elderly person?

While the legal response varies, every state has legislation that provides for the protection of abused elderly, prosecution of the perpetrators of abuse, and legal protection for those who are mandated to report elderly abuse. In many states, suspected elder abuse must be reported to adult social services.

BIBLIOGRAPHY

1. Abbott J, Johnson R, Koziol-McLain J, et al: Domestic violence against women: Incidence and prevalence in an emergency department population. JAMA 273:1763–1767, 1995.
2. American College of Emergency Medicine Policy Statement: Domestic violence: The role of emergency medical service personnel. Ann Emerg Med 27(6):845, 1996.
3. Giardino AP, Christian CW, Giardino ER: A Practical Guide to the Evaluation of Child Physical Abuse and Neglect. Thousand Oaks, CA, Sage Publications, 1997.
4. Jones J, Dougherty J, Schelble D, et al: Emergency department protocol for diagnosis and evaluation of geriatric abuse. Ann Emerg Med 17(10):1006–1015, 1988.
5. Kercher EE: Issues of personal violence. In Pons P, Cason D (eds): Paramedic Field Care: A Complaint-Based Approach. St. Louis, Mosby, 1997, pp 693–702.
6. Muelleman RL, Lenaghan PA, Pakieser RA: Battered women: Injury locations and types. Ann Emerg Med 28(5):486–492, 1996.
7. Salber PR, Taliaferro E: The Physician's Guide to Domestic Violence. Volcano, CA, Volcano Press, 1995.
8. Sebastian S: Domestic violence. In Harwood-Nuss A (ed): The Clinical Practice of Emergency Medicine, 2nd ed. Philadelphia, Lippincott-Raven, 1996, pp 1557–1559.
9. Whitworth JM: Child abuse. In Harwood-Nuss A (ed): The Clinical Practice of Emergency Medicine, 2nd ed. Philadelphia, Lippincott-Raven, 1996, pp 1138–1140.
10. Wilt S, Olson S: Prevalence of domestic violence in the United States. J Am Med Wom Assoc 51:77–82, 1996.

57. THERMAL BURNS

Marilyn K. Bourn, R.N., M.S.N., EMT-P

1. How do most adults and children get burned?

Nearly three-fourths of all unintentional burn deaths are as a result of house fires. Of this group, children and the elderly are the most likely victims. Alcohol and drug intoxication have been reported as contributing factors in as high as 40% of all house fires. Children are often burned from playing with matches, cigarette lighters, and other ignition devices. Injuries from accidental and intentional scalding are also common forms of burns in children.

2. How are the layers of the skin related to the depth of injury?

The epidermis, or outermost layer of the skin, is damaged when a minor, first-degree injury such as sunburn occurs. This injury will heal quickly due to the regeneration of epithelial cells. The dermis, or second layer of the skin, contains appendages such as nerve endings, hair follicles, sebaceous glands, and sweat glands. Consequently, when damaged, as in a second-degree burn, blisters form, and the tissue is hypersensitive and very painful. If infection is prevented, second-degree wounds usually heal within 3 weeks. Full-thickness, or third-degree burns, affect the epidermis, dermis, and subcutaneous tissue. These burns are often leathery, charred, and firm. Because the epithelial, or regenerative cells, are damaged these wounds do not heal spontaneously. Regeneration from the wound border, which causes severe scarring, or skin grafting is needed.

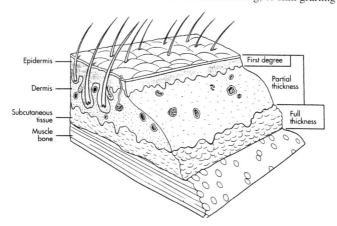

Skin anatomy and burn depth. (From Mann R, Heimbach DM: Emergency care of the burned patient. In Auerbach PS (ed): Wilderness Medicine: Management of Wilderness and Environmental Emergencies. St. Louis, Mosby, 1995, with permission.)

3. Is there such an injury as a fourth-degree burn?

Yes. A fourth-degree injury not only destroys the three layers of the skin but also damages the deep underlying structures such as muscle and bone. This type of deep injury usually happens as a result of electrical injury or prolonged exposure to a heat source (e.g., a lower leg pinned under the exhaust pipe of a motorcycle for an extended time). Repair of this type of injury is sometimes impossible, and amputation may be required.

4. Why does it take several days or even longer to determine how deep a burn injury goes?

It is not unusual for burned tissue to appear charred, blistered, have clothing melted into it, or be covered with dirt. Consequently, it may take several days of wound cleaning and debridement before the wound can be assessed clearly. In addition, it may take several days before the real extent of the injury can be determined.

5. What are epithelial cells and how do they function?

Epithelial cells, which are responsible for regenerating a new surface, will begin to work within a few hours following a burn. Along the margins of a wound new cells develop and begin to migrate toward the center to cover the gaps and heal the wound. Infection must be prevented to allow this spontaneous process to progress.

6. Describe third spacing as it applies to burn injuries.

Numerous local and systemic hemodynamic changes occur as a result of a serious burn. Within the first hour following a burn, due to changes in permeability, pressures, and filtration, an immediate and rapid increase in fluid occurs in the burned tissue. Plasma shifts from the intravascular space to the interstitial space, which causes edema to develop in the burned tissue. In severe burns this fluid shift also will occur in nonburned tissue (i.e., the respiratory tract) causing the complication of pulmonary edema.

7. Why does the seriously burned patient go into shock?

Burns resulting in damage to 35–40% of the total body surface area (TBSA) invariably cause tissue dysfunction known as "burn shock." Burn shock results from the decrease in plasma volume from third spacing, decreased cardiac output, increased systemic vascular resistance, and pulmonary edema. These changes last approximately 24–48 hours, during which time aggressive fluid resuscitation is required to prevent potentially fatal shock.

8. Does burn shock occur rapidly?

No; it is relatively slow. If the patient goes into shock rapidly, look of other mechanisms of injuries such as pelvic fractures or internal hemorrhage from blunt trauma.

9. Is it really necessary to use some type of scale to estimate the amount of burned tissue?

Yes. Because large burns are so "visual" and grossly unpleasant to look at, it is common for the health care provider to overestimate the extent of injury unless an objective scale is used.

10. Does it matter if we estimate the extent of burn in the prehospital setting?

Yes, but not at the expense of delaying transport. Accurate estimation of TBSA is necessary first to determine appropriate prehospital destination and later to guide fluid resuscitation. Several simple methods can be used to determine the TBSA. If, however, one of the simple formulas cannot be immediately recalled, you should simply but completely describe to the base station personnel the location of the burns; they can calculate the TBSA and assist in determining proper destination and initial field care.

11. What is the Rule of Palms?

When burns are scattered and only cover small areas around the body, the Rule of Palms works well. The patient's palm represents approximately 1% of TBSA. Therefore, irregularly dispersed burns can be easily and objectively estimated.

12. What is the Rule of Nines?

The most commonly used and simple formula to determine the TBSA. Each portion of the body is either 9% (anterior chest) or 18% (anterior chest and abdomen) of the TBSA. Because children have a relatively larger head and smaller legs, the Rule of Nines is adjusted accordingly. Add each percentage to determine the TBSA.

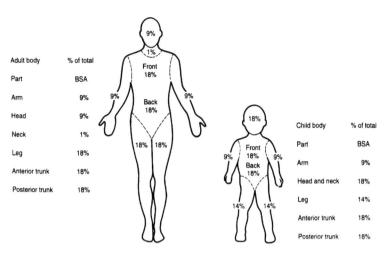

Adult body	% of total
Part	BSA
Arm	9%
Head	9%
Neck	1%
Leg	18%
Anterior trunk	18%
Posterior trunk	18%

Child body	% of total
Part	BSA
Arm	9%
Head and neck	18%
Leg	14%
Anterior trunk	18%
Posterior trunk	18%

Adult and pediatric "Rule of Nines."

13. What is the Lund and Browder Chart?

Probably the most accurate of the charts but the hardest to use. Save this one for the emergency department or the intensive care unit.

14. Do patients commonly get burns of the respiratory tract?

No. The respiratory tract is very efficient at cooling down (or warming up) the air we breathe. Consequently, the trachea, bronchi, and alveolar sacs are protected from heated air. Superheated air saturated with water—steam— is a whole different situation. Because the water can carry as much as 200 times more heat, steam can cause significant damage to air passages and lung parenchyma. The respiratory complications of burns are from inhaling toxic production of combustion, resulting in pneumonia or pulmonary edema.

15. How can you tell if someone has an inhalation injury?

Most often, victims with inhalation injury will have been exposed to smoke in an enclosed space for a prolonged time. A high index of suspicion should include those who have been in an enclosed space with burns to the face, soot in the mouth or upper airway, raspy voice, difficulty breathing, or cough productive of soot or blood tinged mucous.

16. How do you manage inhalation injuries in the field?

Respiratory complications are the major cause of death in thermal injuries. Half of the patient will be dead at the scene. All patients with burns should receive high-flow oxygen (preferably humidified) via non rebreather by reservoir mask or endotracheal tube. Patients with the signs and symptoms of inhalation injury and upper airway obstruction such as stridor should be intubated before edema in the upper airway causes total obstruction.

17. What is the best thing to do for a chemical burn?

Stop the exposure! Chemicals can burn the skin locally as well as cause systemic toxicity from their absorption. Remove the chemical as rapidly as possible from the skin. Be sure to protect yourself from exposure in the process. Brush away any powder before irrigation and then irrigate with *massive* amounts of water. Also, protect yourself against exposure or contamination by wearing proper protective clothing. Gather any information that is available about the chemical source and provide it to the receiving hospital.

18. Is it true that low voltage electricity can't kill a person?

No. Voltage, amperage, current, and resistance are all factors that determine the degree of injury associated with electrical injuries. Injuries from household current, which is low voltage (< 1000 volts and 60 cycles per second) can be serious because of the victim's inability to let go of the electrical source, thus causing prolonged exposure.

19. If you know the location of the entrance and the exit wounds, can you trace the path the electrical current took through the body?

Another myth about electricity. It is true that electricity will often follow pathways of least resistance (i.e., the nerves) through the body. It is not true, however, that you can always predict the pathway of the current based on the location of the entrance and exit wounds. The best assumption to make about the pathway is to assume the worst until proven otherwise.

20. Does the extent of external injury give an indication of the extent of internal damage?

The damage at the level of the skin is only the tip of the iceberg. In situations in which there is significant skin resistance, such as dirty or calloused hands and feet, skin resistance is high, causing a concentration of heat and significant surface level injury (fourth degree). Wet or thin skin such as the lips and tongue, with minimal resistance, may show little surface damage but there may be severe underlying injury.

21. Describe the "classification of burns" and its impact on prehospital care.

The "classification of burns" may seem purely academic, but it is not. These classifications can help the prehospital provider and the receiving emergency department with appropriate triage and destination decisions. According to the American Burn Association (ABA), major burns should be treated at a burn center; moderate burns can be adequately managed in a general hospital; and minor burns are treated on an outpatient basis.

Classification of Burns

MINOR BURN INJURIES	MODERATE UNCOMPLICATED BURN INJURIES	MAJOR BURN INJURIES
Partial-thickness burns over < 15% adult total body surface area (TBSA) or < 10% child or elderly TBSA	Partial-thickness burns over 15–25% adult TBSA or 10–20% child or elderly TBSA	Partial-thickness burns over > 25% adult TBSA or > 20% child or elderly TBSA
Full-thickness burns of ≤ 2%	Full-thickness burns of < 10%	Full-thickness burns involving ≥ 10% TBSA
No functional or cosmetic risk to areas of specialized function, such as the eyes, ears, face, hands, feet, or perineum	No functional or cosmetic risk to areas of specialized function, such as the eyes, ears, face, hands, feet, or perineum	All burns involving eyes, ears, face, hands, feet, or perineum that may result in functional or cosmetic impairment
		All inhalation injuries
		High-voltage electrical burns
		All burns complicated by fractures or other trauma
		All burns in immunocompromised or debilitated individuals

22. What are some of the home remedies used on burns? Are they OK?

Many bad and some good home remedies are used on minor burns. Anything from butter to toothpaste, lard to bacon fat has been put on burns. Regretfully, these home remedies usually just contaminate the wound and make it impossible to assess the depth of injury. Petroleum jelly, burn cream, and antibiotic ointments are also used and, although contamination is not as bad, visual assessment remains difficult. Clean cool water is still the best home and prehospital treatment.

23. Describe the priorities in care for a minor burn.
1. Be sure the mechanism of injury correlates with the visible injury. Don't overlook the potential for something more serious, such as child abuse.
2. Apply a cool, moist (sterile if possible) dressing to stop the burning process, or immerse the burned area in cool clean water.
3. Do not apply any ointments or home remedies.
4. Leave blisters intact.

24. Are wet dressings or dry dressings better for a major burn?
That's probably the most frequently asked and controversial question about prehospital management of burns.
- Generally it is recommended that dry sterile dressings be applied to large burns (> 15%) to prevent further contamination and hypothermia.
- Cool, moist sterile dressings will stop the burning process, help hydrate the tissues, and lessen pain. However, the risk of hypothermia is very high. Therefore moist dressings are usually *not* recommended.
- Since wet dressings are contraindicated in major burns, sterile dry dressings or clean sheets should be used and the pain controlled with adequate doses of morphine sulfate.

25. Describe commercial burn dressings and whether they should be used in the field.
Commercial burn dressings were developed as a possible solution to the wet vs. dry issue. The dressings are usually impregnated with a water-soluble gel, which helps to stop the burning process but does not evaporate, thus decreasing the risk of hypothermia. The cost of the product, which may be as much as $300–600, must be weighed against need and frequency of use. Commercial products may be particularly useful in situations in which rescue or transport is prolonged.

26. How much fluid is needed to begin resuscitation of the burn-injured patient?
Large, even massive, amounts of intravenous fluids are needed to resuscitate the severely burned patient. The Baxter (Parkland) Formula is the most universally accepted formula used to initially guide fluid resuscitation:
   4 ml Ringer's Lactate/kg body weight/% TBSA burned in the first 24 hours
   ½ administered in the first 8 hours
   ½ administered in the next 16 hours
   (many prehospital agencies use normal saline instead of Ringer's)
The above amount calculated is for use over 24 hours; thus, massive volume infusion in the prehospital setting is almost never needed.
   A slightly more simple formula is recommended by the ABA for prehospital use:
   Over 15 years of age: 500 ml per hour
   5–15 years of age: 250 ml per hour
   Under 5 years of age: no IV

27. Should you place an IV through burned tissue?
It is preferable to avoid inserting an IV through burned tissue; however, sometimes in major burns it can't be avoided. Consider an external jugular vein; avoid using lower extremities. In children an intraosseous line may be necessary. Do not delay transport to start an IV.

28. Why shouldn't you give the burn victim fluids by mouth?
As part of the shock compensatory mechanism, blood is shunted away from the gastrointestinal tract and displaced to more vital organs. Thus, digestive processes are slowed dramatically, resulting in a paralytic ileus ("paralyzed gut"). Any fluids, foods, or medications given by mouth will *not* be transported through the gastrointestinal tract normally, and complications such

as vomiting or abdominal distention may occur. All prehospital fluids and medications should be given only through an IV.

29. How should pain be addressed?
The pain associated with burns can be excruciating. Covering the wound and elevating the extremities will begin to help. However, large amounts of narcotics such as morphine are typically needed to manage the pain. Be sure to monitor the blood pressure and respiratory status.

30. Is hyperbaric oxygen useful in burns?
The use of hyperbaric oxygen (HBO) therapy in the management of the burn victim is controversial. HBO therapy is recommended for patients whose carboxyhemoglobin level exceeds 25%. This reduces the half-life of carboxyhemoglobin from 250 minutes (on room air) to 30 minutes (at 3 atmospheres). In patients who have sustained a significant inhalation injury and also have thermal burns, physiologic monitoring and aggressive resuscitation is very difficult to carry out in an HBO chamber. Thus, a significant and potentially fatal delay in burn management may occur.

31. Does dry ice cause a burn or a frostbite?
Good question. Dry ice, which is solid carbon dioxide, causes frostbite on direct contact with skin. The dermal injury resembles a thermal burn but is managed like the frostbite injury that it is.

32. What is the difference between a surgical intensive care unit and a burn ICU? Does it matter where the patient is admitted?
Both surgical ICUs and burn ICUs are staffed by highly qualified specialists. However, burn units are staffed by physicians, nurses, rehabilitation therapists, respiratory therapists, psychiatrists, social workers, nutritionists, and other specialists who are educated on every aspect of burn care. Burn centers also require specialized equipment for the acute care, surgical repair, and rehabilitation of the burn victim. Burn centers are the ideal place to care for severely burned patients.

Injuries Requiring a Referral to a Specialized Burn Facility after Initial Assessment and Treatment at an Emergency Department

---

- Second- and third-degree burns > 10% body surface area (TBSA) in patients under 10 or over 50 years old
- Second- and third-degree burns > 20% TBSA in other age groups
- Second- and third-degree burns with serious threat of functional or cosmetic impairment that involve the face, hands, feet, genitalia, perineum, and major joints
- Third-degree burns > 5% TBSA in any age group
- Electrical burns, including lightning injury
- Chemical burns with serious threat of functional or cosmetic impairment
- Inhalation injury with burn injury
- Circumferential burns of the extremity and chest
- Burn injury in patients with preexisting medical disorders that could complicate management, prolong recovery, or affect mortality
- Hospitals without qualified personnel or equipment for the care of children should transfer burned children to a burn center with these capabilities
- Any burn patient with concomitant trauma (for example, fractures) in which the burn injury poses the greatest risk of morbidity or mortality. However, if the trauma poses the greater immediate risk, the patient may be treated in a trauma center initially until stable, before being transferred to a burn center. Physician judgment will be necessary in such situations and should be in concert with the regional medical control plan and triage protocols.

Adapted from National Burn Institute: Advanced Burn Life Support and Pre-Hospital Burn Life Support Course. Omaha, NE, National Burn Institute, 1991.

BIBLIOGRAPHY

1. Braen GR: Thermal injury. In Rosen P, Barkin RM (eds): Emergency Medicine: Concepts and Clinical Practice, 3rd ed. St. Louis, Mosby, 1992.
2. Boswick JA (ed): The Art and Science of Burn Care. Rockville, MD, Aspen Publishers, 1987.
3. Herndon DN: Total Burn Care. Philadelphia, W.B. Saunders, 1996.
4. International Technical Information Institute: Toxic and Hazardous Industrial Chemicals Safety Manual. Tokyo, ITII, 1985.
5. Mann R, Hemibach DM: Emergency care of the burned patient. In Auerbach PS (ed): Wilderness Medicine: Management of Wilderness and Environmental Emergencies. St. Louis, Mosby, 1995.
6. National Burn Institute: Advanced Burn Life Support and Pre-Hospital Burn Life Support Course. Omaha, NE, National Burn Institute, 1991.
7. Olshaker JS, Tek D (eds): Environmental Emergencies. Emerg Med Clin North Am 10:211–475, 1992.
8. Trofino RB: Nursing Care of the Burn-Injured Patient. Philadelphia, F.A. Davis, 1991.
9. US Department of Transportation: Hazardous Chemical Data. Washington, DC, US Coast Guard, 1985.

XII. Pediatrics

58. FIELD APPROACH TO INFANTS AND CHILDREN

F. Keith Battan, M.D.

1. Can children be cared for as if they were small adults?

No. Children up to about age 14 are different in terms of anatomy, physiology, and immunologic, intellectual, and emotional maturity. The smaller the child, the more this is true.

2. Why can pediatric calls be anxiety-provoking?

- Few hours are devoted to pediatrics in initial emergency medical technician (EMT) and paramedic training.
- Continuing medical education devoted to pediatrics is uncommon.
- Only about 10% of 9-1-1 calls are for pediatric patients and, of those, only about 10% are for critically ill children.
- Tensions can be high simply because the patient is a child. Identifying with the patient, e.g., thinking that he or she looks like your own child or neighbor, may impede good judgment.

3. Where can problems arise in caring for children?

The smaller the child, the more difficulty there may be with airway control and intravenous access. Failure to manage the airway effectively is the greatest cause of preventable morbidity and mortality for children with medical and traumatic emergencies.

4. Describe the approach to a critically ill or injured child in the field.

- Stay calm. If you manage the ABCs well and in turn, nothing will be overlooked and all vital functions of the child will be maintained. You have the ability to effectively resuscitate a critically ill child.
- Managing the airway effectively is paramount. Use noninvasive means first (head positioning, chin lift/jaw thrust, suctioning, an oral airway if unconscious, bag-mask ventilation), followed by oral intubation (if < 12 years old), or rarely, needle cricothyrotomy. Use cervical spine precautions if indicated.
- Ensure adequate oxygenation and ventilation (see chapter 59).
- Check peripheral perfusion (see question 5). If abnormal, obtain vascular access and begin 20 ml/kg normal saline bolus.
- Note mental status and pupillary size and reactivity.
- Keep the patient warm: use blankets, overhead lights, and turn the heat up in the ambulance. Undress only what is necessary to examine the patient.
- Transport the patient to the most appropriate facility with pediatric expertise.

5. How is circulation assessed?

Six signs are available to assess adequate tissue perfusion in children:
1. Level of consciousness (LOC).
2. Capillary fill time (CFT). Unless the child is hypothermic or in shock, the CFT should be < 2 seconds.

3. Warmth of the extremities. If hands or feet are cool, find the most distal point where extremities are warm.

4. Quality of the pulses. Are they normal, bounding, thready, absent?

5. Age-dependent heart rate. Shocky children are tachycardic (or scared, febrile, in pain, or need an operation).

6. Skin color: pale, blue, gray, mottled.

If two or more of these signs are abnormal, the patient is in shock and should be treated accordingly.

6. How helpful is blood pressure in determining shock in a child?

A fall in blood pressure is a *late* finding in children due to their great ability to increase their systemic vascular resistance, which shunts blood to central circulation. Blood pressure is maintained until up to 50% of intravascular volume is lost. During the period when there is compromised tissue perfusion but before the blood pressure has fallen below normal for age, vital organs such as the heart, kidneys, liver, and brain are suffering insults. This is compensated shock. When the blood pressure also falls, decompensated shock is present, and irreversible shock may occur.

Therefore you must diagnose shock by the clinical signs mentioned in question 5.

7. What are the best sites for IV access?

In children, the antecubital vein can almost always be seen and/or palpated and allows the maximal size of catheter to be used. Another good site is the saphenous vein, above the medial malleolus. Hand veins are generally visible but permit only a small catheter to be used. Scalp veins are suboptimal due to their small size. If within protocols, the external jugular and femoral veins are good sites for access.

At a minimum, 22-gauge catheters should be used because they allow quick flash-back into the hub to determine entry into the vein and allow much higher flow rates than a 24-gauge catheter.

Intraosseous (IO) needles provide rapid and effective entry into the venous circulation and should be used in any critically ill child younger than 5 in whom peripheral IV access cannot be rapidly obtained.

8. What type of fluids are best for pediatric patients?

Only two types of fluids are necessary for pediatric patients: isotonic crystalloid (almost always normal saline), and dextrose-water. Normal saline should be used for all patients requiring IV fluids.

For documented or suspected hypoglycemia, $D_{10}W$ can be used in infants, $D_{25}W$ for toddlers (made by diluting $D_{50}W$ 50:50 with saline or sterile water), or D_{50} for older children. All of these dilutions can be dosed in a volume of 4 ml/kg of body weight.

Any child with altered mental status is hypoglycemic until proven otherwise.

9. How is a neurologic assessment carried out in a child who can't talk?

Various pediatric equivalents of the Glasgow Coma Scale exist for preverbal children. The best way to assess mental status in infants and toddlers is to evaluate their general level of consciousness: Is the child alert, responsive, and aware of surroundings? Does the child recognize his or her parents? Is the child appropriately afraid of emergency medical services (EMS) personnel?

10. What is the AVPU system?

A fast, easily-reproducible method of determining LOC:

A   Alert
V   responsive to Verbal command
P   responsive only to Painful stimulus
U   Unresponsive to voice or pain

11. **How can I become more familiar with the care of critically ill children?**
   - Do clinical rotations in a pediatric emergency department, visiting the pediatric intensive care unit or transport service whenever possible.
   - Take advanced life support courses such as PALS (pediatric advanced life support).
   - Take Emergency Medical Services for Children (EMS-C) prehospital care courses; contact your state's EMS division for availability.
   - Use self-paced instructional programs from EMS-C such as video workbooks or interactive videodisk technology; contact your state's EMS division or the National EMS-C Resource Center.

12. **What aids are available to help in the field care of children?**
   - Use of a "cor card" or preprinted sheet with drug doses, equipment sizes, and vital signs based on age or weight has been shown to improve speed and accuracy.
   - A length-based emergency tape provides accurate and rapid dose determination and equipment sizes based on the child's length when placed on the tape.
   - Texts covering educational resources, protocols, equipment lists, and other aspects of pediatric prehospital care are listed in the bibliography.

13. **What are some transport tips?**
   - Assess the scene for hints of abuse, neglect, or ingestions.
   - Never delay transport for history-taking.
   - Weight estimate in kg = (age in years × 2) + 8.
   - Hypotension (minimum systolic BP) = (age in years × 2) + 70. Never wait for hypotension to diagnose and treat shock!
   - Limit your examination to the essentials, using a toe-to-head approach to increase compliance.
   - The airway must be stabilized and initial efforts at optimizing ventilation and oxygenation initiated prior to loading the child for transport; all else may be done in the ambulance.
   - A developmental approach will aid good care, e.g., an unresponsive 2-day-old child is likely to be septic, hypoglycemic, or have congenital heart disease, but an unresponsive 2-year-old is likely to have sustained accidental or nonaccidental trauma or have meningitis.

BIBLIOGRAPHY

1. American Academy of Pediatrics and American College of Emergency Physicians: Advanced Pediatric Life Support: The Pediatric Emergency Medicine Provider Manual. Elk Grove Village, IL, AAP/ACEP, 1993.
2. American Academy of Pediatrics and American Heart Association: Pediatric Advanced Life Support Provider Manual. Elk Grove Village, IL, AAP/AHA, 1997.
3. Baker MD, Avner JR: Prehospital care. In Fleisher GR, Ludwig S (eds): Textbook of Pediatric Emergency Medicine, 2nd ed. Baltimore, Williams & Wilkins, 1993, pp 74–92.
4. Battan FK: Educational resources. In Luten R, Foltin GL (eds): Pediatric Resources for Prehospital Care, 3rd ed. Arlington, VA, National Center for Educational in Maternal and Child Health, 1993.
5. Eichelberger M, Ball J, et al: Pediatric Emergencies: A Manual for Prehospital Care. Englewood Cliffs, NJ, Brady, 1992.
6. Glaeser P: Five-year experience in prehospital intraosseous infusions in children and adults. Ann Emerg Med 22:1119–1124, 1993.
7. Lillis K: Prehospital intravenous access in children. Ann Emerg Med 21:1430–1434, 1992.
8. Losek JD, Bonadio WA, et al: Prehospital pediatric endotracheal intubation performance review. Pediatr Emerg Care 5:1–4, 1989.
9. Seidel JS, Henderson DP, et al: Pediatric prehospital care in urban and rural areas. Pediatr 88:681–690, 1991.

59. RESPIRATORY EMERGENCIES IN INFANTS AND CHILDREN

Joan Bothner, M.D.

1. Why are infants and children more at risk than adults for respiratory distress?

Failure to manage the airway is the greatest cause of preventable morbidity for children with medical emergencies. There are multiple differences between the adult and pediatric airway. The tongue is large, easily displaced, and the most common cause of airway obstruction in the unconscious child. Because infants are obligate nose-breathers, any obstruction of the nasopharynx can lead to significant respiratory distress. The small caliber of the upper airway in children makes it vulnerable to occlusion due to a variety of problems (croup, foreign bodies), and the narrowness of the airway results in greater baseline resistance to flow. Any decrease in size of the airway increases resistance dramatically and leads to increased work of breathing. The tonsils and adenoids of children are large and easily traumatized. The cartilaginous rings of the trachea are incompletely formed, and the trachea is easily compressible. The larynx is funnel-shaped, and the cricoid ring (below the vocal cords) is the narrowest portion of the pediatric airway, making obstruction due to infections such as croup more likely. The epiglottitis is short, narrow, angled away from the trachea, and is located higher in the airway than in adults. The lower airways are also small and are easily occluded. Because infants and small children breathe with their diaphragms and minimally with their chest wall muscles, any abdominal distention will decrease effective respiration.

2. How are these differences clinically relevant?

Children will adopt a position of comfort, and any child in distress who is moving air adequately should be left in the position that they assume. Gentle suctioning of secretions in the nares with a bulb syringe or suction catheter may greatly diminish respiratory distress in an infant with nasal congestion. Infants should be placed in a sitting position, (i.e., in an infant safety seat) and not transported supine. Because the tongue is large and easily obstructs the airway, correct positioning in infants and children with respiratory distress is essential. The head tilt-chin lift should be performed if airway management is indicated. If ventilation does not improve, reposition. Care must be taken not to hyperextend the neck, because the airway is easily collapsible. Straight laryngoscope blades are used in children for several reasons. The high position of the larynx makes the angle between the base of the tongue and the glottic opening more acute. A straight blade creates a direct visual plane from the mouth to the glottis and is useful in picking up the floppy pediatric epiglottis. The high position of the glottis makes it more likely that an endotracheal tube may get caught at the anterior aspect of the cords and makes it difficult to visualize the cords if the neck is hyperextended. Endotracheal tubes in children younger than 8–10 are not cuffed, due to the narrowing below the cords. A simple visual estimate of the appropriate sized endotracheal tube is the diameter of the child's fifth finger. The following formula is also useful:

$$\frac{\text{Endotracheal Tube}}{(\text{mm i.d.})} = \frac{\text{Age (years)} + 16}{4}$$

3. What are the signs of respiratory distress in infants and children?

Tachypnea is the most common sign. It occurs as a response to hypoxia and hypercapnea but also can occur with pain, anxiety, fever, or metabolic acidosis (as in diabetic ketoacidosis). Tachycardia also occurs and is nonspecific. Normal respiratory rates vary by age, and upper limits of normal are 60 in a newborn, 40 in older infants, and 30 in children younger than school age.

234

Intercostal, subcostal, substernal, supraclavicular, and suprasternal retractions are common due to the use of accessory muscles. Suprasternal retractions are indicative of significant obstruction. Grunting is heard in young infants in an attempt to generate "auto-peep" in disease states associated with collapsed alveoli, such as bronchiolitis or pneumonia. The position of comfort that the child assumes is often indicative of the diagnosis; children with upper airway obstruction sit with the airway in a "sniffing" position, while those with lower airway disease lean forward supporting the thorax with the arms ("tripoding") to recruit use of the chest wall muscles.

4. What are some warning signs of impending respiratory failure?

Marked retractions, decreased or absent breath sounds, increasing tachycardia, decreasing respiratory rate or effort, and mental status changes, including irritability, agitation, and lethargy. Worsening signs include hypotonia, pallor, head-bobbing, decreased level of consciousness, and bradycardia. Cyanosis is an extremely late sign of respiratory distress in children.

5. How does one assess a child with a complaint of respiratory distress?

The first step is to obtain an adequate history, which needs to include the speed of onset of the symptoms; the presence of a fever, cough, sore throat, or hoarseness; any history of a potential foreign body aspiration; past medical history; and any current medications.

The most important skill to develop is that of observation. All children with complaints of respiratory distress should be allowed to assume their position of maximal comfort, and "looking before touching" will yield much useful information. The child's level of activity and mental status should be noted. Is the child alert, irritable, lethargic, apathetic, or unresponsive? An alert, engaging toddler is not in much respiratory distress. What is the patient's color—pink, pale, mottled, cyanotic? What is his work of breathing? What is the respiratory rate and the respiratory effort? Is the child retracting or assuming a certain position? Is there flaring of the nostrils? Are there any associated noises such as stridor or wheezing? What is the quality of the respirations? Is there good chest wall excursion with each breath? Does the child have a prolonged phase of respiration? Prolonged inspiratory times are associated with upper airway obstructions, such as croup, and a prolonged expiratory phase is associated with lower airway disease such as bronchiolitis and asthma. Is the child drooling, which also occurs with upper airway disease? All of this information can be obtained by observation alone. Use of a stethoscope often leads to an uncooperative child, and auscultation of the chest should be done last. Sounds are transmitted throughout the chest of a small child, and breath sounds should be assessed very laterally, in the axillae. Auscultation may reveal wheezes, rates, and decreased breath sounds. Bradycardia is due to severe hypoxia, and immediate airway management is necessary.

6. What are the general management principles for children with respiratory distress?

- Supplemental oxygen is always indicated regardless of the pulse oximeter reading.
- Prepare equipment for bag-valve-mask and intubation appropriate for the child's age and size.
- Allow the child to assume a position of comfort. Infants should be upright if possible.
- Intravenous access is not necessary in most children with respiratory distress unless very severe.
- Avoid agitating the child.
- Be prepared to suction.
- Most pediatric patients needing airway management can be bag-valve-mask ventilated.
- Do not attempt intubation if the airway can be managed with positioning and bag-valve-mask ventilation.
- Avoid being at the scene for unnecessarily prolonged times.

7. When does a child with respiratory distress need assisted ventilation?

There is no absolute answer to this question. Clinical assessment is the key. The most important parameter is the child's mental status. If children are apathetic or unresponsive, they need airway management. One also should assess the quality of the respirations, including respiratory rate (a decreasing rate is a bad sign), retractions, chest rise, and air entry. Signs of fatigue, another parameter, include lessening respiratory rate, decreased air entry, decreasing retractions, decreased noise (as with stridor), and lessening responsiveness.

8. What are the keys to proper airway management in children?
- Proper positioning is crucial. The tongue and tissues of the oropharynx easily obstruct the upper airway in children with altered mental status. Avoiding flexion or hyperextension is often all that is necessary in obtunded children.
- The child probably has eaten recently. Be prepared with suction. Remember to use cricoid pressure to avoid aspiration of stomach contents if the child needs to be intubated.
- Most pediatric patients can be bag-valve-mask ventilated. If a child needs assistance, bagging is always the first step. If unable to ventilate, reposition. If still difficult, reposition again and consider suction. Avoid excessive pressure, but remember that adequate ventilation is that which gets good chest wall excursion, usually at a tidal volume of 10–15 ml/kg.
- If significant abdominal distention occurs, consider a nasogastric tube.
- Intubation should always be controlled. Orotracheal intubation is preferred in children, due to the small size and friability of the nasopharynx and the high and anterior position of the vocal cords. Proper positioning is crucial to adequate visualization of the glottis. Choose an appropriate size tube; in children with upper airway disease, have a tube that is a half size smaller available. The child's heart rate should be monitored continuously during intubation attempts since mechanical stimulation of the airway or hypoxemia will cause significant bradycardia. If bradycardia occurs, the patient should be ventilated immediately with 100% oxygen.
- Assessment of proper endotracheal tube placement may be difficult in small infants. Look for symmetric chest excursion, equal breath sounds over both axillae, absent breath sounds over the stomach, adequate heart rate, and adequate saturation by pulse oximeter, if available.
- If the endotracheal tube is properly placed but lung expansion is inadequate, problems may include a too small tube with a large leak, poor lung compliance (as with near-drowning or pulmonary edema), or inadequate tidal volume. Remedies include changing to a larger tube, occluding the pop-off valve on the resuscitation bag, and delivering more volume while assessing chest wall movement. Also consider obstruction of the endotracheal tube and suction.

9. How common is croup and what are the signs of croup?
Croup is the most common cause of infectious upper airway obstruction in children. Only 10% of children with croup require hospital admission, and less than 5% require intubation. Croup classically affects children who are younger than 18 months and occurs most commonly in fall and winter. The typical presentation is worsening respiratory distress occurring at night and characterized by cough and stridor in a child who has cold symptoms. Fever is variable and may be high. Drooling is uncommon, but barking cough and hoarseness are frequent. Differentiation of stridor—a high-pitched inspiratory noise—from wheezing is important to assure optimal therapy.

10. Describe the recommended management of croup.
Beta-agonists used for wheezing and asthma are not indicated in the management of croup. Prehospital treatment includes allowing the child to assume his position of comfort, delivering humidified oxygen or air, and transporting with minimal agitation. Intravenous access is not indicated. Nebulized epinephrine (usually racemic epinephrine) can be given for children with markedly increased work of breathing or significant stridor at rest. Assessment of respiratory status is as described earlier in this chapter. Racemic epinephrine works by decreasing airway edema, has a documented relapse potential, and is not indicated for children with minimal stridor

or barking cough only. The dose of racemic epinephrine, 0.5 ml in 3 ml of sterile water, is standard for all children.

11. Is epiglottitis common? Name some of its symptoms.

The incidence of epiglottitis has decreased markedly since the introduction of the *Hemophilus influenzae* vaccine, and many prehospital care providers will never see a case. Epiglottitis due to other bacteria does occur but is not as rapidly progressive. The classic disease occurs primarily in children age 3–7 and has a rapid onset with a high fever, drooling, sore throat and inability to swallow, preference for the sitting position with the head extended, and no cough. Presence of a cough is reassurance that epiglottitis is *not* present. The frightening thing about epiglottitis is the potential for complete airway obstruction, due to pooled secretions, marked swelling of the upper airway, laryngospasm, and fatigue.

12. What are the keys to prehospital management of epiglottitis?

Minimizing agitation, allowing the child to keep his position of most comfort, and rapid transport. Oxygen should be supplied as tolerated. Intravenous access is not indicated and is probably contraindicated in most patients. If the child obstructs or becomes unresponsive, bag-valve-mask ventilation should be attempted. Most children with epiglottitis can be bagged. Intubation is indicated for inability to ventilate with a face mask and should never be done electively in the field.

13. Are foreign bodies a problem in children?

Foreign body aspiration should be suspected in infants and children who develop the sudden onset of respiratory distress associated with gagging, coughing, stridor, or wheezing. Coins, marbles, balloons, hot dogs, round candies, raisins, nuts, and grapes are frequently aspirated. The symptoms will reflect where the object has lodged—from gagging and drooling if the object is in the esophagus, to complete airway obstruction if the object is in the trachea. If the obstruction is incomplete (the child is crying or coughing), management includes supplemental oxygen, allowing the position of comfort, minimizing agitation, and rapid transport. Relief of airway obstruction should be attempted only if signs of complete obstruction are present, including ineffective cough (loss of sound), increased respiratory difficulty accompanied by stridor, cyanosis, or loss of consciousness. In children younger than 1 year of age, five back blows with the head dependent are followed by five chest thrusts. In children older than 1 year, abdominal thrusts are indicated. If the infant or child loses consciousness and the foreign body is not expelled, attempt bag-valve-mask ventilation. If unsuccessful, attempt to visualize the foreign body with a laryngoscope and remove with Magill forceps. If still unsuccessful, attempt vigorous bag-valve-mask ventilation. Intubation also can be attempted, and if the foreign body cannot be removed, it may be possible to push it into a bronchus. Percutaneous needle cricothyroidostomy may be necessary.

14. What is bronchiolitis?

A viral infection of the lower airways affecting infants and children younger than 2 years of age. It occurs most commonly in winter and is characterized by tachypnea, tachycardia, variable degrees of respiratory distress, nasal congestion, and wheezing. Bronchiolitis is most severe in very young infants and those with a history of prematurity, congenital heart disease, bronchopulmonary dysplasia (a chronic lung disease that occurs in premature infants), other underlying lung diseases, and inadequate immune function, such as occurs with infection with the human immunodeficiency virus. Infants younger than 3 months may present with apnea. Cough, rales, and wheezing may be present. Hypoxemia is common. The classic bronchiolitic is a "happy wheezer"—tachypneic, mildly retracting, smiling and interactive, well hydrated, and wheezing away.

15. What is the prehospital management of a patient with bronchiolits?

Supplemental oxygen is always indicated. Place the infant upright or in a sitting position. Nasal suctioning can make a huge difference in small infants who are still obligate nose-breathers.

Intravenous access is rarely necessary. Because a significant proportion of patients with bronchiolitis will respond to beta-agonists, a trial of albuterol is warranted in patients with significant respiratory distress. Recommended doses of albuterol vary from 0.1 to 0.3 mg/kg by nebulization diluted in 2.5 ml of normal saline. This may be repeated as necessary if the infant remains severely distressed. Continuous positive airway pressure by face-mask may help some infants with significant obstruction but with adequate respiratory effort. Steroids and antibiotics are not indicated.

16. How is pediatric asthma managed?

Asthma is a common pediatric respiratory illness. Optimal prehospital management includes supplemental oxygen, allowing the child to assume a position of comfort, and nebulized albuterol. Magnesium sulfate has not been well studied in children and is not included in the prehospital setting. Subcutaneous epinephrine may be helpful in patients with severe distress, and albuterol can be safely given continuously to pediatric patients.

BIBLIOGRAPHY

1. American Academy of Pediatrics and American College of Emergency Physicians: Advanced Pediatric Life Support Provider Manual. Elk Grove Village, IL, AAP/ACEP, 1993.
2. American Academy of Pediatrics and American Heart Association: Pediatric Advanced Life Support Provider Manual. Elk Grove Village, IL, AAP/AHA, 1997.
3. Belfer RA: Group A beta-hemolytic streptococcal epiglottitis as a complication of varicella infection. Pediatr Emerg Care 12:203–204, 1996.
4. Brownstein D, Shugerman R, Cummings P, et al: Prehospital endotracheal intubation of children by paramedics. Ann Emerg Med 28:34–39, 1996.
5. Eichelberger M, Ball J, et al: Pediatric Emergencies: A Manual for Prehospital Care. Englewood Cliffs, NJ, Brady, 1992.
6. Ledwith CA, Shea LM, Mauro RD: Safety and efficacy of nebulized racemic epinephrine in conjunction with oral dexamethasone and mist in the outpatient treatment of croup. Ann Emerg Med 25:331–337, 1995.
7. Tobias JD: Airway management for pediatric emergencies. Pediatr Ann 25:317–330, 1996.

XIII. Prehospital Skills

60. PREHOSPITAL INTERVENTIONS: WHAT WORKS

Herbert G. Garrison, M.D., M.P.H., and Ronald F. Maio, D.O., M.S.

1. What does "what works" mean?

"What works" refers to interventions currently used in prehospital care that are effective in changing the outcome for a patient with a common emergency medical condition.

2. What does "effective" mean?

An effective intervention improves patient outcome when it is applied in usual and customary settings outside of a laboratory or research setting.

3. Does "effective" mean the same thing as "efficacious"?

No. Efficacious refers to an intervention that improves patient outcome when used in a controlled environment. The best example of an efficacy study is the randomized clinical trial, in which the investigators are aware of and may control the circumstances and events that affect the study's outcome. Interventions that are efficacious in controlled circumstances may not be effective in the real world.

4. Why is there so much interest in efficacy and effectiveness?

While there has always been some interest in efficacy and effectiveness, the outcomes movement has increased interest tremendously. The increased interest is also a reflection of what consumers now deem important. There is a reluctance among employers, insurance carriers, and individuals to pay for a health care service or intervention if they do not know that it improves outcomes.

5. What is the outcomes movement?

The seminal event for the modern outcomes movement was Paul Ellwood's 1988 Shattuck lecture to the Massachusetts Medical Society. In his presentation, Dr. Ellwood, who is famous for his advocacy of managed competition, described the many conflicts in health care that resulted from (1) variations in the use of expensive interventions and (2) limited information on which interventions truly improved the health of patients. To resolve these conflicts, Dr. Ellwood proposed a new "technology of patient experience" that would revolve around the monitoring of outcomes.

6. What are the four components of Dr. Ellwood's outcomes management technology?

1. Development of standards and guidelines.
2. Routine, widespread measurement of disease-specific clinical outcomes and patient functioning and well-being.
3. Collection of clinical and outcomes data on a massive scale.
4. Analysis and dissemination of findings from a continually expanding database.

7. Is outcomes management a way to control the escalating costs of health care?

Yes. Also in 1988, Arnold Relman, MD, former editor of *The New England Journal of Medicine*, pointed out that we are now in an "era of assessment and accountability." He noted that the monitoring of outcomes would provide a way to guide the best use of ever scarcer health care resources.

8. What does all of this have to do with me?

An entire emerging medical intervention system has been created and implemented with little analysis of its overall effectiveness in managing the many conditions for which treatment is offered in the prehospital or out-of-hospital setting.

9. Until now, what types of outcomes have prehospital researchers used in their investigations?

The predominant outcome used in prehospital research has been survival. Most emergency medical services (EMS) investigations have focused on whether a prehospital intervention reduced the number of deaths that occurred in the patients receiving the intervention. The classic examples of conditions studied using survival as an outcome are cardiac arrest and multiple trauma.

10. Is survival the best outcome to study in determining which prehospital interventions work?

Yes and no. A major part of the EMS mission remains the saving of lives when an emergency medical condition has threatened to end the life of a patient. However, although most patients to which EMS responds do not have an acutely life-threatening condition, the care that EMS provides may help to relieve pain and dyspnea, prevent disability, provide reassurance and satisfaction, and be cost-effective. For most prehospital interventions, though, whether these alternative outcomes are affected remains unknown because they have not been measured in any systematic fashion.

11. Are there any prehospital interventions that do work?

As noted by Dr. Dan Spaite: "Despite a plethora of EMS 'research,' only two specific interventions have been proven to impact outcome in any prehospital patient population—early CPR and early defibrillation in the setting of out-of-hospital, nontraumatic cardiac arrest." Others argue that the EMS component of trauma care systems improves survival for the multiple trauma patient.

12. If we don't really know what works, how do medical directors for EMS systems determine what to use?

Most likely, medical directors and others rely on the recommendations of guidelines produced by groups such as the American College of Emergency Physicians, the National Association of EMS Physicians, and the American Heart Association. In North Carolina, for example, medical directors can choose from a long list of optional skills and medications but usually only allow the use of skills and medications that are recommended by published guidelines.

13. Should we stop all the prehospital interventions we are providing now and that we innocently think make a difference?

No. Systems should rely on their medical directors to provide guidance on what prehospital interventions to employ. Many medical directors will decide to maintain the present interventions since they are recommended by current guidelines. Others may drop the interventions for which they personally lack confidence and for which positive effectiveness studies are lacking.

14. Is there a consensus document that medical directors and systems can use to provide guidance on what skills to allow their providers to use?

The National EMS Education and Practice Blueprint, which was released in 1993, is a consensus document that recommends which skills should be used by four levels of prehospital providers: first responders, EMT-basics, EMT-intermediates, and EMT-paramedics. The blueprint indicates provider skills for the following core elements: patient assessment, airway, breathing, circulation, musculoskeletal, children and obstetrics/gynecology, behavioral, medication administration, neurologic, environmental, EMS systems, ethical/legal, communications, documentation, safety and triage and transportation issues.

15. Have there been any formal efforts to improve prehospital effectiveness studies?
In April 1994, the National Highway Traffic Safety Administration sponsored a workshop entitled "EMS Outcomes Evaluation: Key Issues and Future Directions."
The discussants recommended the following activities to improve EMS outcomes evaluation:
1. Identifying specific patient conditions that warrant the focused attention of EMS outcomes evaluation
2. Improving methods of characterizing patient severity and case mix
3. Identifying condition-specific and age-related outcomes for EMS
4. Supporting the use of evaluation methods for determining valid and reliable outcomes
5. Promoting the development of population-based data users
6. Providing EMS outcomes information to end-users and stakeholders
7. Building a constituency for EMS outcomes evaluation
8. Identifying barriers to change in EMS programs and policies

BIBLIOGRAPHY

1. Birnbaum ML: Resurrection isn't everything. Prehosp Disaster Med 6:287–288, 1991.
2. Garrison HG, Benson NH, Whitley TW, Bailey BW: Paramedic skills and medications: Practice options utilized by local advanced life support medical directors. Prehosp Disaster Med 6:29–33, 1991.
3. Garrison HG, Brice JH, Evans AT: Prehospital interventions: Analysis of research design and patient outcomes. Prehosp Disaster Med 7(suppl):16S, 1992.
4. Iezzoni LI (ed): Risk Adjustment for Measuring Health Care Outcomes. Ann Arbor, MI, Health Administration Press, 1994.
5. National Emergency Medical Services Education and Practice Blueprint. Columbus, Ohio, National Registry of Emergency Medical Technicians, 1993.
6. National Highway Traffic Safety Administration: EMS Outcomes Evaluation: Key Issues and Future Directions: Proceedings From the NHTSA Workshop on Methodologies for Measuring Morbidity Outcomes in EMS. NHTSA, 1994.
7. Schoenbaum SC: Toward fewer procedures and better outcomes. JAMA 269:794–796, 1993.
8. Spaite DW: Outcome analysis in EMS systems. Ann Emerg Med 22:1310–1311, 1993.
9. Vibbert S: What Works. Knoxville, TN, Whittle Direct Books, 1993.

61. INTRAVENOUS ACCESS

Anne Clouatre, B.A., EMT-P, and John C. Riccio, M.D.

1. How long has the concept of intravenous therapy existed?
Information that dates back to 1628 describes a blood transfusion performed by Dr. Giovanni Francisco Colle, an Italian physician. Twenty-six years later, Dr. Francisco Folli reportedly performed a blood transfusion also. He used animal blood vessels, a silver tube, and a bone cannula.

2. Does everyone need an intravenous line?
No. Intravenous access is not without complications, cost, and pain.

3. Why should an intravenous line be started?
To gain direct access to a patient's circulatory system, which may allow the following to be accomplished:
• Administration of medications
• Replacement of fluid
• Phlebotomy for blood samples for laboratory determinations

4. What kind of equipment is needed?
Typical materials include the following:
• 70% isopropyl alcohol or povidone-iodine pads
• Gauze sponges
• Tourniquet/blood pressure cuff
• Various sizes and styles of tape
• Various sizes and styles of intravenous catheters
• Gloves and other body substance isolation gear
• Intravenous tubing set
• Intravenous fluid(s)
• Equipment for obtaining blood samples

5. What are some optimal peripheral sites to use?
When starting a peripheral line, the veins in the upper extremities are usually the best choice. There are many options from which to choose, the veins are easily accessible, and the upper extremities are most comfortable for the majority of patients.

Unless the patient is critically ill, it is best to start the line in the most distal vein. In case the initial puncture does not work, other, more proximal sites are available. Furthermore, leakage problems may result if the clinician initially fails at a proximal puncture and then tries a distal site in the same extremity.

6. What steps should be followed to start a peripheral intravenous line?
1. Confirm the need to establish an intravenous line
2. Choose the appropriate fluid, tubing, and catheter
3. Connect intravenous fluid and tubing; flush air out of the line
4. Maintain aseptic technique and observe body substance isolation requirements
5. Choose appropriate site for puncture and tourniquet above site
6. Prepare the site using alcohol or povidone-iodine pads
7. Puncture site and insert catheter
8. Draw blood samples if necessary
9. Briefly occlude the area above the catheter to connect intravenous tubing

10. Open intravenous tubing to confirm that fluid will infuse
11. Look for swelling around the site of insertion to rule out infiltration
12. Tape the intravenous set-up to prevent dislodgment
13. Adjust the intravenous line to an appropriate flow rate

7. What are some of the complications of intravenous therapy?

Infection such as cellulitis   Circulatory overload
Thrombophlebitis   Extravasation resulting in tissue damage and sloughing
Local infiltration   Catheter shear
Hematoma   Arterial puncture
Pyrogenic reactions   Venous thrombosis
Air embolism

8. What kind of findings preclude starting an intravenous line in a given extremity?

If the extremity has burns, trauma, thrombosis, cellulitis, phlebitis, sclerosis, or massive edema, an intravenous line should be started elsewhere. If the patient has had a mastectomy or has an indwelling, surgically placed fistula or shunt, the opposite arm should be used to start the line. The vessel that is used to start a line should not empty into the traumatized area; fluids could be lost out of the trauma site.

9. If the arm veins are inaccessible, is there another peripheral choice?

The external jugular vein may be a good alternative. It is easily visualized and is relatively constant in its anatomic position.

10. Are there any suggestions to keep in mind when starting an external jugular line?

Yes:
1. Know your anatomic landmarks.
2. To promote venous distention, use your finger to tamponade the vessel at the base of the neck.
3. If no cervical spine trauma is suspected, turn the patient's head to the side and try to lower the head (Trendelenburg position).
4. Once you have successfully placed the catheter, be sure to place pressure just past the tip of the catheter while preparing to attach the intravenous tubing. This will help prevent air from being drawn into the vein and consequently will help to avoid introducing an air embolism.

11. I've started the intravenous line but it won't run. I'm sure I saw a flash and that I am in the vein. What could be wrong?

Any number of things, most of which are easily corrected. The following questions help to troubleshoot the problem:
- Is the stopcock open?
- Is the tourniquet/blood pressure cuff off the patient's arm?
- Is the IV solution hanging up high enough?
- Is something pinching off the tubing?
- Is the stretcher wheel sitting on top of the tubing?
- Is the drip chamber completely full?
- Has the patient moved and occluded the catheter tip?

12. What can be done to confirm that the intravenous catheter is in the vein?

1. Lower the bag of fluid *below* the level of the IV site; if the catheter is in, some blood will come back into the intravenous tubing. *Or:*
2. Attach a syringe to the nearest port by the puncture site. Draw back on the syringe and look for blood coming back into the tubing. If blood is visible, the catheter is probably in the vein. *Or:*

3. Attach a syringe to the nearest port to the puncture site and draw back. You should see blood but, in addition, reinject the fluid that you just drew back. Look and palpate carefully around the puncture site. You should *not* see any swelling when you reinject the fluid. If you do, the line is probably not patent.

13. What can be done about swelling around the puncture site?

The fluids have probably infiltrated, which can be confirmed by lowering the IV bag or drawing back with a syringe. If no blood is in the tubing, the line is probably not patent. It should be shut off immediately and the catheter removed. Pressure is applied to the puncture site and the site dressed appropriately. Document what happened and, if possible, start another line.

14. Can't the line be left in, especially if the patient is critically injured and we are low on EMS personnel?

Yes. If you are dealing with a critical patient and do not have time to pull the line, just shut it off. When activities slow down, pull it, apply pressure, and dress the site according to protocol. Document your actions appropriately.

15. As I punctured the vessel, the back end of the catheter flew off. As I attached the intravenous tubing, I noticed that the blood was bright red. It then began to work its way up the tubing toward the intravenous fluid. What is happening?

It sounds like an inadvertent arterial puncture. You should immediately shut off the line and pull the catheter. Apply direct pressure to the puncture site for at least 5 minutes or until the bleeding is stopped. Document and report the events appropriately.

16. What should I do if I accidentally give medications or fluids in the interstitial space instead of into the vein where they belong?

Immediately shut off and pull the line. Some fluids and medications cause no problems when they extravasate. Others, however, can be toxic and cause local necrosis of tissue. Notify the physician about this complication in case additional therapy such as an antidote is indicated.

17. What are the best sites in which to start an intravenous line in children?

Good peripheral intravenous sites include the antecubital space of the arms, the top of the hand, and, in infants, the scalp.

18. What if I am unable to start a peripheral intravenous line in a child?

Pediatric lines are often difficult. If it is a critical situation, you may opt to start an intraosseous (IO) line. However, because this procedure is extremely painful, it should be used primarily in patients who are comatose. If an intraosseous line is not feasible and you only need to give medications, consider rectal or endotracheal administration.

19. What materials are needed to do an intraosseous infusion?

Basic Equipment for an Intraosseous Infusion

IO needle or Jamshidi-type bone aspiration needle

Isopropyl alcohol or povidone-iodine pads

Gauze sponges

Intravenous tubing

Intravenous fluid/medications

10-ml or 20-ml syringe with IV solution inside

Tape

20. What intraosseous sites can be used?
Some options include:
• The proximal tibia approximately 1–3 cm below the tibial tuberosity
• The distal tibia
• The distal femur

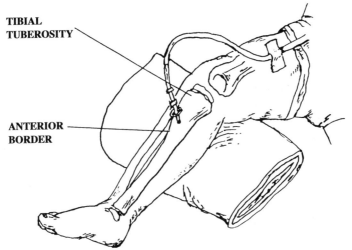

TIBIAL TUBEROSITY

ANTERIOR BORDER

Positioning of the leg, anatomic landmarks, and preferred site for an intraosseous line. (From Jaimovitch DG, Vidyasagar DV: Handbook of Pediatric and Neonatal Transport Medicine. Philadelphia, Hanley & Belfus, 1996, with permission.)

21. What are the steps in starting an IO line?
1. Identify the site and prep the skin.
2. Insert the needle parallel to the skin away from the epiphyseal plate using a boring, twisting motion until you feel a pop and decreased resistance.
3. Remove the stylette and try to aspirate bone marrow to confirm placement.
4. Attach intravenous tubing and infuse medications/fluid.
5. Secure the needle by taping with gauze sponges around it.
6. Tape down the tubing.

22. In addition to the characteristic pop and decrease in resistance that occur once the bone marrow cavity has been entered, what are some other signs that confirm needle placement?
• IV fluid and medication flow freely through the needle.
• There are no signs of infiltration or swelling.
• The needle can stand up by itself.
• Bone marrow can be aspirated. However, this is not completely reliable; you could have proper placement and still not be able to get any aspirate.

23. What kinds of fluids/medications can be put through the IO line?
Crystalloids, blood, atropine, epinephrine, lidocaine, calcium, dextrose (50% with water), dopamine. sodium bicarbonate, diazepam, and many others.

24. What are some complications associated with IO infusions?

Bone fracture	Fat embolism	Osteomyelitis
Compartment syndrome	Necrosis of skin	Subperiosteal infusion

Complications are rare, but they tend to be more serious than complications with peripheral IV placements.

25. Doesn't it take a long time for fluids and medications to reach the heart from an IO site?

No. In fact, circulation time from the IO site to the heart is generally less than 20 seconds. Therefore, rapid medication administration and effective volume resuscitation can be accomplished via an IO infusion.

26. When is central line placement indicated?

1. When access for a transvenous pacemaker is needed.
2. When central venous pressure and cardiac monitoring are indicated.
3. When more central drug delivery is needed.
4. When a peripheral IV site is not accessible.

27. What is the best location to start a central line?

Usually, the subclavian vein because it is easily identified by anatomic landmarks and it can be accessed quickly. Other options include the internal jugular vein and femoral vein, which may be used based on the practitioner's preference and training. Femoral veins are now used more frequently because no risk of pneumothorax exists, no neck manipulation is required, and no interruption of CPR is necessary.

28. Why are central lines usually not placed in the field?

Complications are more severe and more common than for peripheral IV placement. In addition, the procedure is technically more difficult and requires more training, time, and equipment.

Some Complications of Central Line Placement in the Field

Pneumothorax	Arterial puncture
Hemothorax	Infection
Tracheal perforation	Nerve injury
Intrathoracic catheter fragmentation	Cerebral infarct
Air embolus	

29. True or false? Central lines allow for more rapid fluid delivery than peripheral lines.

False. Poiseuille's law states that flow is proportional to the fourth power of the radius of the cannula and inversely related to its length. Therefore, short-length, large-bore intravenous catheters such as peripheral catheters will infuse the greatest amount of fluid in the shortest amount of time.

30. Can medications and fluids be given through indwelling lines?

Most indwelling lines can be used safely to give medications and fluids in the emergency setting (based on protocols). When questions arise, it is usually best to ask the patient or caretaker about the line since they will probably be able to provide information concerning its care and capabilities.

31. What is the correct anatomic name for the "intern's" vein, and where is it located?

The correct name is the superficial radial vein. It is a tributary of the cephalic vein and is located in the distal forearm.

BIBLIOGRAPHY

1. Bledsoe BE: Atlas of Paramedic Skills. Englewood Cliffs, NJ, Prentice-Hall, 1987.
2. Bledsoe BE, Porter RS, Shade BR: Paramedic Emergency Care, 2nd ed. Englewood Cliffs, NJ, Prentice-Hall, 1994.
3. Butman AM, Martin SW, Vomacka RW, McSwain NE Jr: Comprehensive Guide to Pre-Hospital Skills: A Skills Manual for EMT-Basic, EMT-Intermediate, EMT-Paramedic. Akron, OH, Emergency Training, 1995.

4. Campbell JE (ed): Basic Trauma Life Support for Paramedics and Advanced EMS Providers, 3rd ed. Englewood Cliffs, NJ, Prentice-Hall, 1995.
5. Chameides L, Hazinski MF (eds): Pediatric Advanced Life Support. Dallas, TX, American Heart Association, 1994.
6. Cummins RO (ed): Advanced Cardiac Life Support. Dallas, TX, American Heart Association, 1994.
7. Greenwald J: The Paramedic Manual. Englewood Cliffs, NJ, Prentice-Hall, 1988.
8. Roberts JR, Hedges JR: Clinical Procedures in Emergency Medicine, 2nd ed. Philadelphia, W.B. Saunders, 1991.
9. Sanders MJ: Mosby's Paramedic Textbook. St. Louis, Mosby, 1994.
10. Walraven G, Julihn M: Paramedic Review Guide: Case Studies and Self-Assessment Questions. Englewood Cliffs, NJ, Prentice-Hall, 1988.

62. PREHOSPITAL AIRWAY MANAGEMENT

Marilyn J. Gifford, M.D.

1. Is airway management essential for good patient care?

Airway is the "A" in ABC. It is not only essential but also the *first* thing that must be assessed and managed for any critical patient. It is also the "B" in ABC, since breathing is an integral part of airway management. In some patient transport situations, the prehospital care providers will spend the entire time and all their energy on addressing an airway problem; in those instances, their time will have been appropriately spent. There is never a fracture, wound, or injury more important than airway patency.

2. What is the best method of assessing an airway?

Look, listen, and feel.

Look at the airway. Is the face intact? Are teeth broken? Is there blood, vomit, or other material in the mouth? Nasal flaring? Then look at the patient's color. Look at the chest. Is it rising with inhalations? Is it symmetric? Is there evidence of respiratory *effort* (retractions)? What is the respiratory rate?

Listen to the airway. Does it sound like air is moving in and out? Any wheezes? Any gurgling, grunting, stridor, or other abnormal sounds that would indicate difficulty in moving air?

Feel the air exchange with your hand over the mouth and nose to determine respiratory rate and estimate tidal volume. Feel the chest wall to determine stability, crepitus, and symmetry of movement.

3. What are normal respiratory rates per minute?

Adults	12–20
School aged child	18–30
Preschooler	22–34
Toddler	24–40
Infant	30–60

4. When does an airway need intervention?

This is a tough question to answer. Any patient that is *not* alert, oriented, and breathing comfortably at a normal rate and volume has the potential to need intervention. If the patient can't maintain a clear airway on their own or needs help breathing, the airway needs to be managed. This can result from a huge number of medical illnesses and traumatic injuries.

5. What is the most common cause of airway obstruction in the unconscious patient?

The tongue. As it relaxes, it falls against the posterior pharynx.

6. What are other common causes of airway obstruction?

Food is the next most common cause. Hot dogs, candy, grapes, or nuts are common obstructive agents in children. Steak or other meat obstruction is common in intoxicated or elderly adults with inadequate chewing ability. Children additionally are at risk because toys, balloons, or small household objects may get lodged in their airways. Trauma patients further run the risk of teeth, vomit, or blood interfering with the airway.

7. What is the most effective way to remove an obstructing foreign body from an airway?

Although the Heimlich maneuver is the method of choice for laypersons, the most effective treatment by a paramedic is direct visualization with a laryngoscope and removal of the foreign body with forceps.

8. What are the first steps in establishing an airway for an unconscious patient?

First use personal precautions—gloves, glasses, and mask. Open the airway by using the head tilt/chin lift maneuver if possible, or open the airway by using the jaw thrust maneuver if neck injury is suspected.

9. When are oropharyngeal or nasopharyngeal airways necessary?

In the unconscious patient who is breathing spontaneously or in the patient who needs bag-valve-mask ventilation. The purpose is to maintain an open airway by keeping the tongue off the posterior pharynx.

10. What are the disadvantages of an oropharyngeal airway?

1. Cannot be used in a patient with an intact gag reflex.
2. If improperly inserted, can cause airway obstruction.
3. Easy to dislodge.
4. Cannot be inserted through clenched teeth.
5. Does not isolate or protect the trachea.

11. What are the advantages and disadvantages of a nasopharyngeal airway?

1. Better tolerated in a patient with the gag reflex but still can cause vomiting.
2. More difficult to dislodge than an oropharyngeal airway.
3. May cause nosebleed and increased risk of aspiration.
4. Cannot be used if midface trauma or chance of basilar skull fracture would allow its placement into the brain.
5. Does not isolate or protect the trachea.
6. If improper size (i.e., too long) is used, it may enter the esophagus.

12. What happened to the esophageal obturator airway (EOA)?

The EOA was developed as an airway device that could be inserted blindly by an individual lacking the level of training or skill required for intubation. The EOA had several complications, including esophageal rupture and death from anoxia secondary to incorrect placement. There are newer devices that are safer (e.g., the Combitube and the pharyngeal tracheal lumen [PTL] airway). There are currently no indications for the use of the EOA.

13. What are the indications for using the combitube or PTL airway?

In most systems, these are used as backup devices for the occasional patient who cannot be intubated—whether because of abnormal facial features, abnormal airway, or complicated trapped position that does not allow visualization of the trachea. There are some EMS systems that have approved training in the use of these devices for advanced EMTs (to be used instead of intubation).

14. Which patients need supplemental oxygen?

Any patient who looks ill and has any reason to be hypoxic. They may have one of the following.

1. Signs of respiratory distress, tachypnea, respiratory effort, noisy respirations, or cyanosis.
2. Abnormal vital signs—hypotension, tachycardia.
3. Altered level of consciousness.
4. Cardiac or respiratory arrest.

15. Which patients need ventilation?

Any patient who has an open airway and inadequate ventilation or no ventilation. Any patient (except one who is hypothermic) with a spontaneous respiratory rate < 10/min.

16. What is the approximate percentage of oxygen in various methods of delivery?

Inhalation Method	Flow Rate/Min	Oxygen in Inspired Air
Room air	0	21%
Nasal cannula	2	28%
	6	40%
Face mask	10	50–60%
Mask with reservoir	10	90%
Bag-valve-mask (BVM)	12	40%
BVM with reservoir	10–15	90%

17. What are the indications for intubation?

Oxygenation, ventilation, airway protection, or an alternate route for drug administration. Patients with increased intracranial pressure may also benefit from controlled hyperventilation, which would be impractical without intubation.

18. What size tube should I use?

Age	ET Tube (internal diameter in millimeters)
Preemie	2.5–3.0
Newborn	3.0–3.5
6 mo	3.5–4.0
1 yr	4.0–4.5
2 yr	4.5
4 yr	5.0
6 yr	5.5
8 yr	6.0
Adult female	7.0–8.0
Adult male	8.0–8.5

19. Is there any way to remember what size tube to use on a child?

One suggestion is to use a tube the size of the child's little finger; or, for children older than 1 year of age:

$$\text{Internal diameter (ID)} = \frac{16 + \text{patient's age in years}}{4}$$

Since tube sizes are always approximate, a tube 0.5 mm smaller than predicted size and one 0.5 mm larger should be available.

20. At what age should a cuffed endotracheal tube be used?

Age 6 is the youngest age to consider using a cuffed tube (size 5.5 mm ID).

21. When the tube is in the correct position in an adult, what will the depth marking read between the front teeth?

20–22 cm.

22. What are the two most commonly used laryngoscope blades?

Curved (MacIntosh) and straight (Miller, Wisconsin, and others).

23. What is the difference in the way the blades are used?

The tip of the curved blade is inserted into the vallecula, under the epiglottis. The tip of the straight blade slides *over* the epiglottis. Both will expose the glottic opening when traction is exerted upward on the handle of the laryngoscope.

24. **List the equipment that needs to be collected to be optimally prepared for intubation.**
  1. Laryngoscope with blades, fresh batteries, and fresh bulb.
  2. Suction.
  3. Oxygen.
  4. Bag-valve-mask.
  5. Endotracheal tube.
  6. 10-ml syringe for cuff inflation.
  7. Stylet.
  8. Tape/tube tie.
  9. Stethoscope.
  10. End-tidal CO_2 monitor.

25. **How can the tube position be confirmed after intubation?**
  1. Listen to the lungs on both sides.
  2. Listen over the epigastrium.
  3. Watch the chest rise.
  4. Check tube placement with laryngoscope.
  5. Check exhaled CO_2.
  The most important confirmation is watching the tube pass through the cords.

26. **Sometimes patients start to vomit during the intubation. Is there anything I can do to prevent this?**
  A technique known as Sellick's maneuver can sometimes be helpful. This maneuver involves pressure applied to the cricoid cartilage to occlude the proximal esophagus, minimizing gastric inflation and esophageal regurgitation, thus decreasing the risk of aspiration.

27. **What are the complications of intubation?**
  1. Right mainstem intubation with oxygenation of only the right lung.
  2. Inadvertent displacement to an esophageal location.
  3. Obstruction of the tube.
  4. Pneumothorax or tension pneumothorax.
  5. Esophageal intubation.

28. **When is nasal intubation preferable to oral intubation?**
  1. In a patient with clenched teeth or one who is unable to move the head or neck.
  2. In a patient who is breathing spontaneously.

29. **What are the complications of nasal intubation?**
  1. Epistaxis, which can also increase the risk of aspiration.
  2. Esophageal intubation.
  3. Intubation of the brain in the presence of cribiform plate fractures.
  4. Trauma (abrasions, bleeding, or perforation of upper airway).
  5. Infection.
  6. Intubation with a tube too small to ventilate adequately.

30. **Since there is a reflex increase in intracranial pressure with intubation, is there a way to decrease that response to prevent aggravating the intracranial pressure in the head-injured patient?**
  Administration of lidocaine, 1.5 mg/kg IV, approximately 60 seconds before intubation may prevent the increase in intracranial pressure.

CONTROVERSY

31. Is the ability to perform a prehospital cricothyrotomy a useful skill for a paramedic?

Pro. There will always be some patients who cannot be ventilated or intubated and are in urgent need of airway assistance. These patients may have their lives or brains saved by placement of an immediate surgical airway.

Con. There are some who argue that any technical skill taught will be used more often than necessary. There are few good models with which to teach or practice the skill. In addition, there are some patients whose injury invites disaster—for example, those with short swollen necks, bruises or tears in the upper airway, or large tracheal hematomas. Excessive time involved in creating a surgical airway can result in a patient whose life is saved at the expense of hypoxic encephalopathy and brain death.

BIBLIOGRAPHY

1. Abbott J, Gifford M: Prehospital Emergency Care: A Guide for Paramedics, 3rd ed. New York, The Parthenon Publishing Group, 1995.
2. Chameides L (ed): Textbook of Pediatric Advanced Life Support. Dallas, TX, American Heart Association, 1988.
3. Merrick C, Goldberg R (eds): Prehospital Trauma Life Support, 3rd ed. St. Louis, Mosby, 1994.
4. Cummins RO (ed): Textbook of Advanced Cardiac Life Support. Dallas, TX, American Heart Association, 1994.

63. M.A.S.T.

Robert E. Suter, D.O., and Robert M. Domeier, M.D.

1. What does MAST stand for?

The most common translation is *military anti-shock trousers*; another is *medical anti-shock trousers*. Most people use the term *MAST trousers*.

2. Aren't MAST trousers obsolete?

While some emergency medical services (EMS) systems have discarded their MAST trousers, there are still some recognized indications for their use. In addition, some systems use MAST as they always have.

3. What are some other names for MAST trousers?

Pneumatic counter-pressure device (PCPD) and pneumatic anti-shock garment (PASG).

4. What are MAST trousers?

A medical device that looks like a pair of pants when applied. They are held on the patient with Velcro closures. Inflatable air bladders in the legs and abdomen put pressure on the legs and abdomen.

5. What is the purpose of MAST trousers?

They are designed to raise blood pressure in patients who are in shock.

6. What are the effects of the application of MAST trousers?

MAST trousers have positive effects on blood pressure and cardiac output. These effects occur in patients with hypovolemia caused by hemorrhage or medical hypotension. The mechanism of this effect is still not fully understood. The increases in blood pressure and cardiac output in mild hypovolemia may be a reflex response to the positive pressure exerted on the lower extremities. In more severe hypovolemia, an increase in systemic vascular resistance occurs by compressing the veins in the legs and abdomen.

7. Why are MAST trousers controversial?

From the 1960s through most of the 1980s, MAST trousers were in widespread use in prehospital systems based upon a number of animal studies. A group of researchers then began to question whether MAST trousers actually helped to keep human trauma patients in shock from dying. In one of these studies, trauma patients in shock died more frequently when MAST trousers were applied than when MAST trousers were not used. This study, frequently referred to as the "911 Study," involved victims of penetrating trauma, including many chest injuries, a recognized contraindication to MAST use. Questions were raised as to the validity of the study's conclusions. However, many EMS systems adopted the findings and applied them to all groups of patients. This resulted in many people being completely against use of the MAST trousers in all circumstances.

8. Do MAST trousers really increase the blood pressure in shock patients?

Yes. A large number of studies have shown that blood pressure increases in patients with shock in whom MAST trousers have been applied.

9. How could something that raises blood pressure in shock patients be controversial?

In some patients increased blood pressure causes increased bleeding and worsened outcome. Any patient with uncontrolled bleeding could be harmed. Patients with penetrating chest injuries are an example; this scenario is comparable to the assumption that more water comes out of a faucet under higher pressure. Also, a number of animal studies have shown increased blood loss with MAST use in the setting of uncontrolled hemorrhage.

10. Differentiate controlled hemorrhage and uncontrolled hemorrhage.
Controlled hemorrhage occurs in a situation such as an extremity injury from which the patient has lost a significant amount of blood but which has been controlled through direct pressure or some other means. Internal injury such as when the patient may be bleeding into the abdomen or chest and has not undergone surgery is an example of potential uncontrolled hemorrhage.

11. It sounds like MAST trousers were developed about 30 years ago. Who invented them?
Actually, anti-shock garments have existed since 1903. George W. Crile invented a device he called the pneumatic rubber suit, noted that it increased blood pressure, and reported his work in an article entitled, "The Resuscitation of the Apparently Dead." It was not until the past 30 years that their use was described in emergency settings.

12. Is there a use for MAST trousers that everyone agrees is good for the patient?
Yes, there appears to be no real controversy over the use of MAST trousers in taking care of patients with hypotension due to pelvic fractures who have long transport times. This is essentially using MAST trousers as a compressive air-splint.

13. Can MAST trousers be used to treat ruptured abdominal aortic aneurysms (AAA)?
Yes, but surgery is the only real life-saving procedure. MAST trousers have been reported by a number of researchers to improve survival if surgery is not immediately available.

14. How would MAST trousers be helpful in a ruptured AAA?
By using MAST trousers to put direct pressure over the bleeding AAA, the bleeding theoretically is reduced, providing additional time to get the patient to surgery.

15. In what shock patients should MAST trousers be applied?
While system protocols may vary, the literature supports the use of the shock trousers in patients with severe hypotension who have lost blood but who have controllable sources of bleeding or have unstable posterior pelvic fractures.

16. Are there shock patients who should never have the MAST trouser applied?
Yes. Absolute contraindications to MAST trousers include pulmonary edema, penetrating chest injuries, and diaphragmatic rupture.

17. Are there other times that MAST trousers should not be used routinely?
Yes. Although MAST trousers have been widely used by EMS personnel to splint leg injuries and suspected pelvic fractures at accident scenes even when the patient is not in shock, they can cause complications such as compartment syndromes in the legs that make their use for these injuries questionable. Also, if there is an uncontrolled hemorrhage not directly compressed by the MAST trousers, increased hemorrhage may result and the MAST should not be used.

18. Is it acceptable to use MAST trousers to splint femur fractures even if the patient is stable?
Although many systems allow MAST trousers to be used as splints, femur fractures are better treated with traction splints. The traction splint provides good stabilization and decreases internal bleeding and pain without putting external pressure on the leg, which can cause compartment syndromes and skin damage. Lower leg injuries are well stabilized with blanket or pillow splints. To use MAST trousers as a routine lower extremity splint, one must make sure to inflate them with only enough air to provide support. Avoid placing too much pressure on the legs.

19. Why do you need to limit the amount of time that MAST trousers are left on?

The primary concern with prolonged MAST application is related to the pressure they place on the legs and abdomen. There have been a number of cases of compartment syndromes in the legs and pressure necrosis of the skin with prolonged MAST use.

20. How do you apply MAST trousers?

There are a number of "right" ways to put on MAST trousers. The classic way is to lay the garment out flat and open and log-roll the patient onto the trousers, fastening all of the Velcro straps and then inflating it one compartment at a time, starting with each leg, and ending with the abdomen. To help speed things up using this technique, many emergency medical technicians and paramedics have the MAST trousers laid out on a spine board in their rig so that they can place the trauma patient on the back board and the MAST trousers at the same time.

21. Are there quicker ways of applying MAST trousers?

Yes, in a patient in whom speed is of the essence and who would not appear to be at high risk for a lumbar spinal injury, the trousers may be applied in the same way in which one would dress a small child. With the Velcro straps loosely affixed, one would grab the patient's feet and have an assistant pull the MAST trousers onto the patient just like putting on a pair of pants. One would then inflate the trousers as before.

22. How much should each part of the MAST trousers be inflated?

When used to treat shock, inflate each segment until you hear the Velcro start to pop. Then recheck vital signs. The pressure in the MAST trousers at this point is about 100 mm Hg. Much lower pressure (well below systolic blood pressure) should be used if MAST trousers are being used to splint a leg in a stable patient.

23. How does one deal with MAST trousers that have gauges on them?

Many systems have taped over the gauges so that they cannot be read. However, many types of these MAST trousers are designed so that gauges cannot be removed. If the system insists attention be paid to the gauge pressures, the recommendation is 80–100 mm Hg.

24. Are any patients with trauma of the abdomen or chest helped by MAST trousers?

Maybe. The research is inconclusive, but even the "911 Study" seems to show that the patients with the lowest blood pressures, those with systolic blood pressure of 60 mm Hg or below, do improve with the MAST trousers and die less frequently then other patients. This finding was not the official finding of the study and is not universally accepted.

25. Should MAST trousers be used for cardiac arrests?

No, there has never been any proven benefit.

26. What should I remember about MAST trousers?

That they definitely improve blood pressure, but improving blood pressure in this way rather than treating the cause of the low blood pressure may not be in the best interest of the patient. If they increase respiratory distress, they should be removed.

BIBLIOGRAPHY

1. Aprahamian C, Gessert G, Bandyk DF, et al: MAST-associated compartment syndrome (MACS): A review. J Trauma 29:549–555, 1989.
2. Bass RR, Allison EJ Jr, Reines HD, et al: Thigh compartment syndrome without lower extremity trauma following application of pneumatic antishock trousers. Ann Emerg Med 12:382–384, 1983.
3. Batalden DJ, Wichstrom PH, Ruiz E, et al: Value of the G suit in patients with severe pelvic fracture. Controlling hemorrhagic shock. Arch Surg 109:326–328, 1974.
4. Burn N, Lewis DG, Mackenzie A, et al: The G-suit. Its use in emergency surgery for ruptured abdominal aortic aneurysm. Anaesthesia 27:423–428, 1972.

5. Cayten CG, Berendt BM, Byrne DW, et al: A study of pneumatic antishock garments in severely hypotensive trauma patients. J Trauma 34:728–735, 1993.
6. Clarke G, Mardel S: Use of MAST to control massive bleeding from pelvic injuries. Injury 24:628–629, 1993.
7. Crile GW: The resuscitation of the apparently dead and a demonstration of the pneumatic rubber suit as a means of controlling blood pressure. Trans S Surg Gyn Assoc 16:361–370, 1904.
8. Hagman J, Iguchi R, Kinsley J, et al: Diaphragmatic rupture following blunt trauma. Ann Emerg Med 13:49–52, 1984.
9. Mattox KL, Bickell W, Pepe PE, et al: Prospective MAST study in 911 patients. J Trauma 29:1104–1112, 1989.
10. McSwain NE: Pneumatic anti-shock garment: State of the art 1988. Ann Emerg Med 17:506–525, 1988.

64. NEEDLE DECOMPRESSION

John C. Riccio, M.D.

1. Why is it important to understand needle decompression?
It can save a life.

2. What is needle decompression?
Inserting a pointed instrument into a tension-filled chest. This vents the chest, converting a tension pneumothorax into an open pneumothorax, a less lethal entity. Though a relatively simple procedure, needle decompression can be the difference between life and death. Therefore, we must be proficient and knowledgeable about this procedure.

3. Name the *only* indication for needle decompression.
Tension pneumothorax.

4. What is a tension pneumothorax?
A one-way air leak from the lung or chest wall that causes air to enter but not exit the pleural space. Air enters the pleural space during inspiration but becomes trapped with expiration. The continued accumulation of air leads to a significant increase in intrathoracic pressure, which collapses the affected lung, displacing the mediastinum away from the tension pneumothorax, and thereby compressing the mediastinal structures, particularly the vena cava.

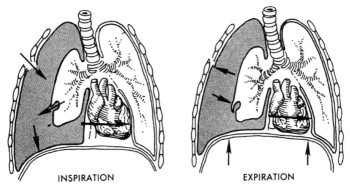

INSPIRATION   EXPIRATION

Tension pneumothorax. (From Vukich DJ, Markovchick VJ: Pulmonary and chest wall injuries. In Rosen P, et al (eds): Emergency Medicine: Concepts and Clinical Practice, 2nd ed. St. Louis, Mosby, 1988, with permission.)

5. What causes a tension pneumothorax?
The most common cause is iatrogenic barotrauma, which means that postintubation patients receiving positive pressure ventilation may develop a tension pneumothorax. Decreased lung compliance as evidenced by increased resistance to bag-valve ventilation and patients in cardiac arrest with pulseless electrical activity should immediately alert the caregiver to address the possibility of a tension pneumothorax.

Other causes include traumatic chest injuries where a lung leak fails to seal, a sucking chest wound that is improperly occluded (e.g., with a dressing taped on four sides versus three), and a spontaneous pneumothorax with a ruptured bullae that continues to leak.

6. How is a tension pneumothorax recognizable?

A tension pneumothorax is a clinical diagnosis characterized by respiratory distress, hypotension, tachycardia, unilateral absence of breath sounds, neck vein distention, and increasing difficulty in bagging. Late manifestations include subcutaneous emphysema, tracheal deviation, and cyanosis. It rapidly progresses to cardiac arrest, and delayed recognition can be fatal. Therefore, one should be vigilant in looking for a tension pneumothorax.

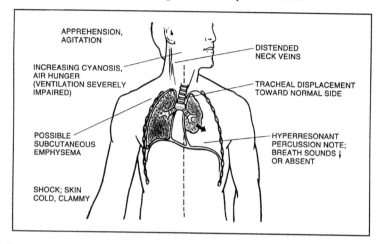

Physical findings of tension pneumothorax. (From Campbell JE (ed): Basic Trauma Life Support for Paramedics and Advanced Providers, 3rd ed. Englewood Cliffs, NJ, Prentice-Hall, 1995, with permission.)

7. Define Beck's triad.

Hypotension, jugular venous distension, and decreased heart sounds.

8. Is Beck's triad associated with tension pneumothorax?

No. It is associated with cardiac tamponade. They share the first two components of hypotension and elevated neck veins, but they are differentiated by diminished heart versus breath sounds. A tension pneumothorax has absent breath sounds with hyperresonant percussion on the affected side. These findings are not present with cardiac tamponade. Differentiating between these two life-threatening conditions is critical. A cardiac tamponade has similar symptomatology and initially can be confused with a tension pneumothorax. Patients with both conditions are in extremis with hypotension, tachycardia, and neck vein distension. Therefore, it is most important to determine if breath sounds are absent in the setting of hypotension, tachycardia, and neck vein distention.

9. People can survive with one lung. Why is a tension pneumothorax life-threatening?

People can survive with even less than one full lung. Therefore, something more must be compromising these patients. The displacement of the mediastinum depresses the vena cava, with loss of venous blood return to the heart. The heart does not fill, leading to inadequate cardiac output and eventually cardiac arrest.

10. Is a lot of advanced equipment needed to perform a needle decompression?

No. An antiseptic skin preparation solution such as povidine-iodine and a long 14-gauge catheter-over-needle device are the essential pieces of equipment. Follow your ABCs, provide supplemental oxygen, and wear gloves—universal precautions should always be observed.

11. Where is the needle inserted into the chest?

There are two approaches, anterior and lateral. The anterior approach is at the second intercostal space in the midclavicular line. The level of the second intercostal space can be rapidly identified by palpating the sternum for the angle of Louis, a prominence on the sternum about one quarter of the way down from the sternal notch. Do not insert the needle medial to the midclavicular line, because the internal mammary artery could be lacerated.

The lateral approach is at the fifth intercostal space in the midaxillary line. In men, the nipple is usually over the fifth rib, so it can be used as a quick reference point for the fifth intercostal space. When using the lateral approach, insert the needle during peak inspiration when the diaphragm is at its lowest in the thoracic cavity. If inserted during peak expiration, the needle could puncture the diaphragm, which may rise to the level of the fifth intercostal space during this phase of the respiratory cycle and, at the same time, lacerate the liver.

With either approach, the needle is inserted over the top of the rib to avoid the intercostal vessels and nerve.

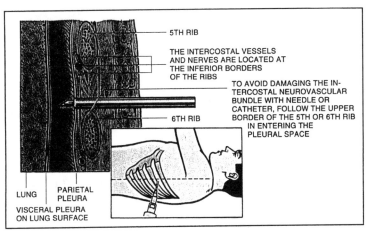

Needle decompression of a tension pneumothorax. (From Campbell JE (ed): Basic Trauma Life Support for Paramedics and Advanced Providers, 3rd ed. Englewood Cliffs, NJ, Prentice-Hall, 1995, with permission.)

12. What is the procedure for doing a needle decompression?

1. Confirm the diagnosis by physical findings (and obtain base station order if protocols mandate this).
2. Identify needle insertion site.
3. Prepare skin with antiseptic.
4. Insert the catheter-over-needle device.
5. Confirm placement by exit of air under pressure.
6. Remove the needle and leave the catheter in place.
7. Secure the catheter and attach a one-way valve if available.
8. Monitor the patient for improved clinical condition.
9. Transport to hospital for chest tube placement.

13. Can a tension pneumothorax recur after needle decompression?

Certainly. If a one-way valve is not used, in patients who are breathing spontaneously, air can be sucked back into the pleural space via the catheter, resulting in reaccumulation of intrathoracic pressure. The soft plastic catheter can also become kinked or occluded, preventing the escape of air from the tension pneumothorax. Needle decompression is only a temporizing measure, not definitive care. Therefore, the patient should be reassessed frequently for recurrence of tension pneumothorax following decompression. Repeat needle decompression may be necessary in these cases. In patients who are intubated and being bagged, there is no longer the possibility of air being sucked into the pleural space and it is acceptable to leave the catheter open or use a one-way valve.

14. Who can perform needle decompression?

A skilled health care provider trained and authorized in needle decompression, which includes physicians, paramedics, flight nurses, and mid-level providers with protocol approval.

15. If I believe a patient has a tension pneumothorax but the local protocols do not authorize me to perform needle decompression, what can I do?

- Establish an open airway
- Administer high flow oxygen
- Rapidly transport the patient to an appropriate facility
- Establish intravenous fluid resuscitation en route
- Provide ventilatory assistance as needed

16. What are the potential complications of a needle decompression?

- Hemothorax
- Lacerated lung
- Pneumothorax if tension pneumothorax was misdiagnosed
- Intercostal vessel or mammary artery puncture
- Pleural infection or empyema
- Cellulitis
- Hematoma
- Cardiac, liver, or diaphragmatic puncture.

BIBLIOGRAPHY

1. Campbell JE (ed): Basic Trauma Life Support for Paramedics and Advanced Providers, 3rd ed. Englewood Cliffs, NJ, Prentice-Hall, 1995.
2. Roberts JR, Hedges JR: Clinical Procedures in Emergency Medicine, 3rd ed. Philadelphia, W.B. Saunders, 1998.
3. Rosen P (ed): Emergency Medicine Concepts and Clinical Practice, 4th ed. St. Louis, Mosby, 1998.
4. Sanders MJ: Mosby's Paramedic Textbook. St. Louis, Mosby, 1994.

65. IMMOBILIZATION AND SPLINTING

Scott Branney, M.D.

1. What are the basic goals of splinting and immobilization?

The goal of splinting is to preserve function and ensure adequate blood flow as well as reducing the pain associated with musculoskeletal injuries. This is usually accomplished by splinting the affected body part from one joint above to one joint below the site of injury. The goals of immobilization are to protect the integrity of the spinal column, commonly through the use of cervical collars and spine boards.

2. What are the most important considerations in deciding when and how to apply splints?

When considering splinting a limb, however deformed or injured, you must remember the ABCs of trauma care. Establishment of an adequate airway, insurance of adequate breathing, assessment of circulatory status (including IV access), and protection of the spinal column all take precedence over the evaluation and treatment of injured extremities (except obviously exsanguinating wounds). Even totally ischemic limbs will remain viable for hours, and precedence must be given to intracranial, thoracic, and abdominal injuries.

3. How well do backboards and cervical collars work in immobilizing patients?

When only cervical collars are compared, it is found that Philadelphia collars permit less movement than either rigid plastic or soft foam collars. When combined with immobilization on a long backboard, however, rigid plastic collars provide greater immobilization than other types of collars. Typically, this results in approximately a 90% reduction in flexion, lateral motion, and rotation, with approximately 60% reduction in extension. Most patients whose head is directly on the backboard have their neck in slight extension. It has been suggested that 1 to 1.5 inches of padding between the head and backboard will put the neck in a more neutral position (and be more comfortable).

The opposite occurs with children. Since their head is relatively large compared to their body, placing their head flat on the board results in flexion of the neck. They benefit from 1 to 2 inches of padding under their body to bring the neck to a more neutral position.

4. What is the riskiest part of applying backboards or cervical collars?

Of those patients with neurologic deficits after spinal injuries, it is estimated that up to 25% develop the neurologic deficit after medical care has been initiated. Several studies have shown that logrolling patients onto backboards can result in significant movement of unstable thoracolumbar spinal segments, even when performed under ideal conditions by trained personnel. Thus, great care must be taken whenever a patient is being moved in order to immobilize the spine.

5. What about the use of towel rolls or sandbags?

Blocks of some kind are commonly placed along both sides of the head to provide additional stabilization. Sandbags and IV bags are not recommended. Both have enough mass to exert lateral pressure on the cervical spine if the patient must be rolled to the side (i.e., during vomiting) or if severe lateral G-forces are generated while in the ambulance. Rolled towels and commercial foam products both provide increased stability without significant weight.

6. What about strapping the patient to the backboard?

Strapping the patient to the backboard is commonly used to restrict lateral movement of the spine. Although many different styles of strapping and commercial products for this have been developed, only a few styles of strapping have been shown to reduce lateral motion. The efficiency of straps around the torso (at the armpits) and legs was shown to be greatly improved with the addition of a strap at the superior aspect of the pelvis. Strapping the arms to the chest as well as crossing straps over the chest offers no improvement in reducing lateral motion.

7. What about vacuum splints?

Vacuum splints are widely utilized in Europe as an alternative to traditional immobilization with cervical collars and backboards. Vacuum splints are, in effect, thin mattresses filled with small polystyrene balls. They may be easily molded to the body. When air is removed, they form a rigid splint that holds its shape. Vacuum splints with and without cervical collars have been shown to immobilize patients as well as backboards with cervical collars and are much more comfortable for the patient.

8. How well do the Kendrick extrication device and short boards work?

Both use of the Kendrick extrication device (KED) and strapping the patient to a short board have been shown to provide immobilization comparable to that of long boards for all planes of movement except lateral motion of the neck. Short-board immobilization can potentially make airway control more difficult because of its chin straps. There are no good controlled trials comparing extrication of the patient directly to a long board versus KED or short-board extrication.

9. How should you splint pelvic fractures?

Splinting pelvic fractures, particularly unstable ones, is the last good use for MAST pants. They provide excellent stabilization and may help to tamponade some of the bleeding associated with pelvic fractures. Contraindications to their use include pulmonary edema, suspected diaphragmatic rupture, and pregnancy.

10. What about inflatable extremity splints?

Inflatable extremity splints have several disadvantages. Although they are easy to apply, gauging their pressure with fingertip indentation of the splint or resistance to inflation by mouth commonly results in excessive pressure. Only mechanical pop-off valves have been shown to reliably control their inflation pressure. In addition, even with health volunteers, normal inflation pressures can cause oxygen tension in the limb to drop by two thirds. For patients with increased compartment pressure due to fractures, this can easily result in an ischemic limb when the splint is applied.

11. Besides commercial products, what else can be used to splint extremities?

Blood tubing boxes or newspaper sections make stiff yet light splints for forearm and wrist fractures, while pillow or blanket splints work very well for foot and ankle injuries.

12. What extremity injuries require special consideration when splinting?

Several orthopedic injuries cannot be easily reduced in the field or moved to neutral positions on a backboard. Hip fractures are best stabilized with a pillow or blankets between the patient's legs, with a supporting strap around the legs. Posterior hip dislocations (knee versus dashboard) can result in a hip that is flexed and internally rotated and should be supported in place until evaluated. Although uncommon, inferior shoulder dislocations (luxatio erecta) result in the arm being held straight up in the air, and any attempts to bring the arm to the patient's side are very painful.

13. What about open fractures or dislocations?

Most open fractures, particularly those contaminated with foreign material, should be splinted as they lie. This will prevent dragging foreign material back into the wound and increasing the chance of infection. Wounds should be covered with a sterile dressing, with pressure dependent on the degree of hemorrhage.

14. What should be done with avulsed or subluxed teeth?

Do not attempt to splint loose teeth or replace avulsed teeth in patients whose mental status is such that they might aspirate them. Aluminum foil, if available, can be folded around subluxed teeth to splint them to stable surrounding teeth, but only with caution. Avulsed teeth should be placed (by the patient) back into the sockets from which they were avulsed. If they cannot be replaced in their sockets, they are best transported in the patient's own saliva, either between cheek and gum or in a cup.

15. What should you do with impaled objects?

Whether we are talking splinters of wood or metal, nail gun injuries (fairly common), or pieces of fence or industrial equipment, impaled objects should not be removed. They should be stabilized as best they can, and the patient should be transported to the emergency department for their removal. Objects that may penetrate the eye should be stabilized and both eyes covered to prevent movement of the eyes. The dressing on the eye with the impaled object should not apply pressure to the eye (cups work well) to prevent extrusion of the contents of the globe.

CONTROVERSY

16. Should you reduce fracture-dislocations with distal ischemia in the field?

Pro. Reduction of fracture-dislocations will often immediately restore blood flow to the affected limb. This allows for transport and evaluation of the patient without the time pressure of having an ischemic limb. In addition, the patient may be much more comfortable after the dislocation has been reduced.

Con. Fracture-dislocations may not be that easily reduced. It is not uncommon for tendons or soft tissue to become trapped in the dislocation, requiring open reduction in the operating room. Since patients can tolerate an ischemic limb for hours, time spent on the scene attempting reductions may be better spent transporting the patient to the hospital for definitive treatment.

BIBLIOGRAPHY

1. Christensen KS, Trautner S, Stockel M, et al: Inflatable splints: Do they cause tissue ischemia? Injury 17:167, 1986.
2. Hamilton RS, Pons PT: The efficacy and comfort of full-body vacuum splints for cervical–spine immobilization. J Emerg Med 14:553, 1996.
3. Mazolewski P, Manix TH: The effectiveness of strapping techniques in spinal immobilization. Ann Emerg Med 23:1290, 1994.
4. McGuire RA, Neville S, Green BA, et al: Spinal instability and the log-rolling maneuver. J Trauma 27:525, 1987.
5. Schriger DL, Larmon B, Gasick T, et al: Spinal immobilization on a flat backboard: Does it result in neutral position of the cervical spine? Ann Emerg Med 20:878, 1991.

66. PREHOSPITAL NEUROMUSCULAR BLOCKADE

Preston Love, R.N., B.S.N., C.F.R.N., C.E.N., EMT-P

1. What are neuromuscular blocking drugs?
A group of drugs that work at the neuromuscular junction (where the nerve and muscle meet) to block or prohibit muscle contraction from taking place. These drugs effectively paralyze all skeletal muscles and the diaphragm. Throughout this chapter, remember that muscle contraction results from cell depolarization.

2. What do these drugs *not* do?
- They don't affect mentation or level of consciousness.
- They don't affect pain or sensation.
- They don't affect other senses.

3. How do neuromuscular blocking drugs work?
The body produces its own neurotransmitting substances, one of which is acetylcholine, which is released across the neuromuscular junction and is bound to a specific receptor site. This binding starts a chain reaction of other chemical reactions (involving sodium, potassium, calcium, and others), the end result of which is depolarization of muscle cells, which causes a muscle contraction.

4. How do the muscles relax?
At about the same time the acetylcholine is released, an enzyme called acetylcholinesterase is also released. Acetylcholinesterase breaks down the bond acetylcholine formed at its receptor site to then let the muscles relax.

5. What are paralytics?
Drugs that produce the same effect and are often referred to as muscle relaxants.

6. How are muscle relaxants used?
In the prehospital setting, they are used most frequently for rapid sequence intubation (RSI) and facilitation of mechanical ventilation. In rare circumstances, they are used for chemical restraint.

7. What is a rapid sequence intubation?
A technique for quickly securing an airway through endotracheal intubation. The technique calls for a smooth choreographed sequence of hyperoxygenation, cricoid pressure, drug administration, and intubation in the shortest time possible. Since patients in the prehospital setting are always assumed to have full stomachs, this method of intubation lessens the likelihood of aspiration of stomach contents. It also helps control intracranial pressure increases.

8. Which patients are candidates for RSI?
Some general guidelines include patients with:
Compromised or ineffective airways
Glasgow Coma Score of 8 or less
Signs/symptoms of increasing intracranial pressure
Airway burns

Severe maxiofacial trauma

Multisystems trauma involving any of the above

Additionally, these drugs are used to improve the response to mechanical ventilation by preventing the patient from "fighting" the ventilator.

9. Paralyzing agents can be divided into what categories?

Two broad categories known as depolarizing or nondepolarizing drugs based upon their action at the neuromuscular junction.

10. Explain the difference between depolarizing and nondepolarizing drugs.

Depolarizing drugs mimic the action of acetylcholine. They are called depolarizing because they work so well at fooling the body that muscle contractions actually take place.

Nondepolarizing drugs, on the other hand, use no deception. They will bind up to the site where acetylcholine wants to go and thus prevent acetylcholine from doing its job and, therefore, no muscle contraction can take place.

11. If a depolarizing drug actually causes the muscles to contract, how does it also make them relax?

Remember the second half of the normal muscle contraction/relaxation cycle, the part where acetylcholinesterase is released to "undo" the acetylcholine and let the muscle relax? The acetylcholinesterase does not work as well on the neuromuscular blocking drug. Because it takes the enzyme so long to dissolve the bond at the receptor site, a brief form of tetani ensues and the supplies of the other chemicals involved in the reaction are temporarily exhausted. At this point, the muscle has no choice but to relax and become flaccid.

12. Which drugs are the depolarizing agents?

Succinylcholine is the only depolarizing agent available in the United States.

13. What are the nondepolarizing drugs?

The nondepolarizing drugs most often used in prehospital care are vecuronium bromide (Norcuron), mivacurium (Mivacron), and a new drug: rocuronium bromide (Zemuron). Other drugs, which are not good choices for prehospital use, are atracurium (Tracrium), and pancuronium bromide (Pavulon).

14. What are some characteristics of a good prehospital drug?

Fast, predictable onset of action

Dose-dependent, reliable duration of action

Nondepolarizing

No side effects

Safe for all ages

15. Which drug is best?

This depends on several things. First, you need to determine how often you anticipate using these drugs and then look at what kind of patients you care for most often, transport times, and where the drugs will be stored (some of the drugs are sensitive to heat and cold).

16. Do some drugs have advantages over others?

Definitely. And all have disadvantages, too. The advantages include:

Succinylcholine. Oldest of all the drugs we use. Fastest onset of action of all neuromuscular blocking agents. Works in less than a minute and usually in 30–40 seconds when given intravenously. Can be taken intramuscularly, but takes a little longer to work. Duration of action is also very predictable at around 5–8 minutes. Inexpensive.

Vecuronium. Nondepolarizing. No intracranial pressure increase. No intragastric pressure increase. No intraocular pressure increase. No cardiovascular effects. Supplied as a powder, stable across a broad temperature range. May be reconstituted with and is compatible with most intravenous solutions. Dose-dependent onset and duration of action.

Rocuronium. Onset of 40–60 seconds; duration of action 20–30 minutes. No intracranial pressure increase. No intragastric pressure increase. No intraocular pressure increase. Dose-dependent onset and duration of action.

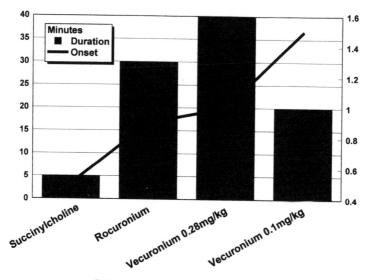

Prehospital neuromuscular blocking drugs.

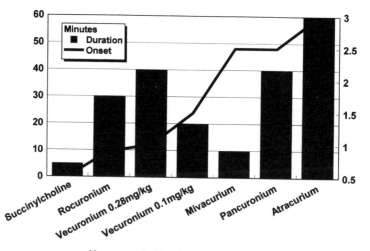

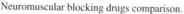

Neuromuscular blocking drugs comparison.

17. What are some of the disadvantages?

Succinylcholine. Because succinylcholine is a depolarizing agent, the simultaneous contraction of skeletal muscles causes an increase in intracranial, intragastric, and intraocular pressures. The debate still rages as to whether this is clinically significant. Not recommended for routine use in pediatrics; can cause intractable bradycardias. Causes serum potassium elevation of 0.5–1.0 mEq/dl and is therefore relatively contraindicated in burns and multisystem trauma greater than 24 hours old. Has been linked to malignant hyperthermia.

Vecuronium. Some believe the 45- to 90-second onset of action is too slow for RSI. Duration of action 30–40 minutes.

Rocuronium. Requires refrigeration for long-term storage. Duration of action, 20–30 minutes, may be too long for some services. Cost.

18. Can this knowledge improve my intubation skills?

No. You take your own skills and experience into every intubation you do. However, you will now be able to intubate patients that you could not have intubated before—not because you are necessarily better, but because the conditions are better. On the other hand, if you are unable to intubate the patient, you are going to have to bag-ventilate the patient until the drug wears off or someone else is able to place the endotracheal tube.

19. What steps are necessary in preparation for paralyzing someone?

All of the airway equipment necessary for the procedure should be immediately at hand next to the patient. Suction equipment should be on. High-flow supplemental oxygen should be given to maximize the amount of oxygen in the patient's blood and lungs since paralyzing them essentially causes a complete respiratory arrest.

20. Does anything else need to be done?

As mentioned earlier, the paralytic drugs cause muscle paralysis but do not affect the level of consciousness. Therefore, all patients who are awake but require paralysis for intubation should be given some sort of sedation as part of the intubation procedure. In addition, when the paralyzing agent is given, not only are skeletal muscles paralyzed, but all muscles are affected. This can include the esophageal-gastric sphincter, the paralysis of which would allow stomach contents to regurgitate. To minimize this, someone should assist you and put pressure on the trachea at the level of the cricoid cartilage to try to occlude the esophagus. This is also known as Sellick's maneuver.

BIBLIOGRAPHY

1. American Society of Hospital Pharmacists: Drug Information, AHFS. Bethesda, MD, ASHP, 1994.
2. Brown JA, et al: The literature and perspectives on muscle relaxants for rapid sequence induction. Nurse Anesthesia 2:72–88, 1991.
3. Capan LM: Trauma Anesthesia and Intensive Care. Philadelphia, J.B. Lippincott, 1991.
4. Davidson JE: Neuromuscular blockade. Focus Crit Care 18:512–520, 1991.
5. Ginsberg B, et al: Onset and duration of neuromuscular blockade following high-dose vecuronium administration. Anesthesiology 71:201–205, 1989.
6. Hedges JR, et al: Succinylcholine-assisted intubations in prehospital care. Ann Emerg Med 17:469–472, 1988.
7. Magorian T, et al: Comparison of rocuronium, succinylcholine, and vecuronium for rapid-sequence induction of anesthesia in adult patients. Anesthesiology 79:913–918, 1993.
8. Martyn JAJ, et al: Up-and-down regulation of skeletal muscle acetylcholine receptors. Anesthesiology 76:822–843, 1992.
9. Mehta MP, et al: Accelerated onset of non-depolarizing neuromuscular blocking drugs: Pancuronium, atracurium and vecuronium. A comparison with succinylcholine. Eur J Anesthesiol 5:15–20, 1988.
10. Miller RD: Anesthesia, 3rd ed. New York, Churchill Livingstone, 1990.
11. Syverud SA, et al: Prehospital use of neuromuscular blocking agents in a helicopter ambulance program. Ann Emerg Med 17:236–242, 1988.

XIV. Aeromedical Transport

67. AIR MEDICAL SYSTEM DESIGN AND CONFIGURATION

Michael W. Brunko, M.D.

1. Historically, where did modern air medical transport (AMT) get its start?

Airplanes were used for mass evacuations during World Wars I and II. Helicopters were used initially in Burma in 1944 and then on a larger scale during the Korean War with Sikorsky S-51 helicopters that were equipped with outboard stretchers, not allowing care in-flight. The larger, more powerful UH-1H ("HUEY") was used during the Vietnam War, allowing casualties to receive medical attention during transport. Almost 1 million wounded soldiers were transported during Operation Dustoff in Vietnam. The advances in AMT in wartime more than likely had an impact on morbidity statistics: per 100 casualties, there were 4.5 deaths during World War II, 2.5 deaths during the Korean War, and less than 1 death during the Vietnam War.

2. How did the military experience transition to the civilian application as we know it today?

Because of the helicopter's success in Vietnam, it gained attention after the war as a means of transport of civilians, especially for rural victims of trauma. (In the mid 1970s, 70% of trauma fatalities in the United States occurred in rural areas.) The military began to provide AMT to victims of rural traffic accidents through the Military Assistance to Safety and Transportation program, which gave rise to public programs such as the Maryland State Police and Los Angeles County Fire Department programs operating today. In 1972, the current-most representative model of rotor AMT began—the "hospital-based" helicopter. The initial program started at St. Anthony Hospital in Denver and primarily transported victims of trauma from the scene to the hospital. The number of hospital-based rotor-wing programs has steadily increased to nearly 200 in the United States, many of which have combined rotor/fixed wing transport capabilities.

3. What systems operate AMT today?

Most of the systems are hospital-based and combined rotor/fixed wing AMT service. More systems are beginning to merge regionally to form consortiums that are independent of a particular base. A minority of programs are private or public service programs, such as those operated by the Maryland State Police and the Los Angeles Fire Department.

4. How do you design an AMT program?

First a mission statement should be developed that encompasses the goals of the program. This usually involves assessing and evaluating the needs of a particular community and extending medical resources to that geographic area. Will the program extend to accident scenes (urban or rural), be restricted to interhospital transports, or accommodate both? You will need to evaluate how you can collaborate and interact with the current emergency medical services (EMS) systems without duplicating existing services. Of prime importance is the evaluation of how the program can attain maximal safety. Economics of developing the program also need to be studied. For instance, will your hospital, local government, citizens, or philanthropists undertake the start-up costs and how will they be maintained?

5. What types of aircraft can be used for AMT?

Rotor-wing (helicopters) and fixed-wing aircraft are currently used for AMT.

6. How do you select the best rotor-wing or fixed-wing aircraft?

The first decision is whether the program will purchase the aircraft or lease it from a vendor/operator who has experience in AMT. (Most programs lease their aircraft.) When choosing the ideal aircraft, you should consider altitude/pressurization limits, range, air speed and performance (especially at higher altitudes), space and configuration of the patient care area, loading door size and location, useful load capabilities, landing zone/runway needs, and capability for IFR (instrument flight rules) in addition to VFR (visual flight rules) flight. The ideal rotorcraft for AMT is economic, fast, agile, and has IFR capability; however, the actual usefulness of IFR helicopter flight depends on flying between instrument-approach–capable airports and being able to avoid icing conditions.

Helicopters are powered by single or twin engines. Twin engines generally are preferred because they provide more power and aid in the ability to transport a greater load. They also provide an additional safety measure in case one engine fails. However, twin-engine helicopters have a longer warm-up time—and thus a delayed ability to lift off promptly—and are more costly to operate than single-engine helicopters.

Fixed-wing aircraft used in AMT are generally turbine-powered, pressurized twin-engine aircraft. Jet aircraft are preferable for flights greater than 500 miles. Most fixed-wing aircraft used in AMT have IFR capability, cruise at 200–500 miles per hour, and have ranges of 1000–2500 miles.

7. What are the advantages of rotor-wing aircraft?

Helicopters can be based at a hospital or another location near your service area. Helicopters do not require a runway for takeoff and landing, are capable of landing in relatively small and secluded areas, and can usually be ready for takeoff in a matter of minutes.

8. What are the advantages of fixed-wing aircraft?

They have a much greater range than rotor-wing aircraft. Rotor-wing aircraft generally have a maximum range of about 350 miles, but fixed-wing aircraft can fly thousands of miles. Fixed-wing aircraft usually are able to transport a heavier load and are faster and more economical for most flight distances. Fixed-wing aircraft, which are pressurized, are preferable for the transport of patients in whom altitude changes could potentially worsen certain conditions.

9. What type of medical equipment should be carried on AMT aircraft?

- Oxygen supplies
- Cardiac monitors with defibrillator and external pacing capabilities
- Mechanical ventilators
- Infusion pumps
- Manual, Doppler, and automatic blood pressure-monitoring capabilities
- Pacemaker generators
- Pulse oximetry and capnography-monitoring capabilities
- Immobilization equipment

A program that does specialty transport needs equipment that is specific to the specialty, such as an incubator and neonatal ventilator for neonatal care.

All equipment should be lightweight, durable, compact, have extended battery capability, be easily secured, not interfere with aircraft avionics, and be able to withstand altitude, temperature, and gravitational changes without affecting performance. Equipment that relies on auscultation may be of limited use because of noise and vibrations that are common in most aircraft.

10. What types of crew configurations are used on AMT?

Most AMT programs use two medical crew members. Certain flight conditions (heat, humidity, altitude, multipatient transport) may necessitate flying with one crew member, as weight limitations are a larger factor in these circumstances.

In order of decreasing prevalence, AMT crews consist of nurse/paramedic, two nurses, nurse/physician, two paramedics, nurse/other (e.g., respiratory therapist), and one nurse only.

11. Is there an ideal crew configuration?

There is no proof that any one particular flight crew configuration is ideal. Logically, the ideal crew is adequately trained; if their experiences and backgrounds are different, they compliment each other in working well as a team. The mission statement and the types of transports the program provides may dictate the crew configuration.

12. What kind of training should the flight crew have?

The flight crew's training should be optimal for the majority of transports the program provides. In general, the training and experience of the flight crew should surpass what is available on local ground emergency medical services. Since most AMT programs transport critically ill or injured adults and children from health care facilities and accident scenes, the ideally trained individual should have experience in critical care medicine, pediatrics, and emergency medical services. Special training that is common to AMT but different from other patient care areas is knowledge of flight physiology, safety, communications, survival in case of a downed aircraft, and the uniqueness of delivering patient care in limited confines. The flight crew should have training in basic life support, PHTLS/basic trauma life support, pediatric life support, advanced cardiac life support, trauma, and neonatal resuscitation. They should be competent to perform all types of intubations, cricothyroidotomy, thoracostomy, peripheral and central venous line placement, pericardiocentesis, umbilical artery/vein catheterization, intraosseous insertion, ventilator and pacemaker management, and emergency vaginal deliveries.

13. Is it possible to train a flight crew to have expertise in all potential types of AMT?

Probably not. Most AMT services realize this and train their crews to be able to adequately care for and transport most patients. Many AMT services use on-call, possibly off-site specialty crews that can be available in a reasonably short time for flights requiring specialty services, such as neonatal services, high-risk obstetrics, and patients requiring intraaortic balloon pump devices.

14. When referring a patient from a hospital or emergency department for care elsewhere, how do you choose an AMT?

First and foremost, you must not decrease the level of care that the patient has already received. You must be aware of the types of AMT programs that are available and select the one that is most appropriate for the patient's injury or illness. If the patient requires specialty services such as tertiary pediatric, invasive respiratory, or cardiovascular care, it would be helpful to select a program that is experienced with these types of problems.

15. When should an AMT be used instead of ground transport?

The choice should be based on a variety of factors. In general, the **rule of Ts** should be considered.

- **Time** of transport is always a consideration, especially when considering the time it may take to transport a patient to a **trauma** or **tertiary** care center by air versus the time it would take to transport the same patient by ground to the local hospital. Time is especially crucial in the transport of a trauma patient in whom decreasing the time between the onset of injury and the receipt of definitive care is essential to increase the chances of survival.
- The geographic **terrain** is a consideration. The patient may be located in an isolated area that ground transport may not be able to reach.
- **Traffic** may dictate the use of AMT instead of ground transport.
- AMT may be useful when advanced life support ground units are unavailable because they are assisting other patients. Guidelines based on injuries or illnesses are available to aid in the decision to use an AMT.

Air Medical Transport Guidelines

Trauma Patients
- Lengthy extrication with severe injuries
- Motor vehicle accident (MVA) with ejection from vehicle
- MVA with death of same-car occupant
- MVA with pedestrian at > 20 mph
- Rollover MVA with unrestrained patient
- Motorcycle occupant thrown at > 20 mph
- Fall from heights greater than 20 feet
- MVA with front bumper displaced to rear by more than 30 inches
- MVA with front axle displaced to rear
- Penetrating injury from mid thigh to head
- Amputation or near amputation
- Severe hemorrhaging with systolic blood pressure < 90 mm Hg or requiring blood transfusion
- 15% or greater body surface area burns, burn of face, airway, perineum
- Glasgow Coma Scale ≤ 8
- Multiple trauma in pediatric patient
- Multiple trauma in patient > 55 years old
- Intubated patient

Medical/Surgical Patients
- Respiratory/cardiac arrest within last 12 hours
- Acute respiratory failure not responding to initial therapy
- Patient requiring continuous vasopressor, thrombolytic, or dysrhythmia medications
- Patients requiring pacemaker
- Invasive therapy for hypothermia
- Acute deterioration in mental status
- Patients with intra-aortic balloon pump
- Patients with arterial lines, pulmonary artery catheter, or ICP monitor
- Acidosis pH < 7.2
- Systolic blood pressure < 90 mm Hg or > 200 mm Hg
- Heart rate < 50 or > 150 beats per minute
- Glasgow Coma Scale < 8
- Patients with known or suspected acute aortic rupture/dissection
- Patient who required acute cardiac, neurosurgical, vascular or radiologic intervention available at referring facility
- Transport in critical care environment to a center that can perform organ transplant or procurement
- Patient with status epilepticus
- Patient with high-risk obstetrics condition not in active labor
- ICU or ICU transport when ground transport > 1 hour not requiring any of the above

Pediatric Patients
- Known or at risk for cardiac dysrhythmia or failure
- Known or at risk for respiratory arrest or failure
- Intubated patient
- Near drowning with signs of hypoxia or altered mental status
- Status epilepticus
- Acute bacterial meningitis
- Acute renal failure
- Unstable toxicologic syndrome
- Reye's syndrome
- Hypothermia requiring invasive therapy
- Systolic blood pressure
  - Neonatal < 60 mm Hg
  - Infant (< 2) < 65 mm Hg
  - Child (2–5) < 70 mm Hg
  - Child (6–12) < 80 mm Hg
- Respiratory rate < 10 or > 60 beats per minute

16. Can AMT integrate with ground EMS?

All AMT should maintain relationships with the EMS agencies within their geographic service area. The AMT program should take the initiative to educate the ground medics in the following areas:

- Appropriate triage criteria for requesting AMT.
- Locating, marking, and securing a safe landing zone for the aircraft that is used.
- Preparation of the patient for AMT.
- Safely approaching the aircraft to prevent injury.

An active education and feedback program must be in place so the ground agency can become an integrated part of the care and transport of the patient.

17. What does it cost to start up and operate a rotor-wing AMT program?

The average annual budget for a rotor AMT program is $2 million to $2.5 million, with approximately half of that amount dedicated to aviation costs. This amount considers the use and leasing of one or two aircraft. If the program were to purchase and operate its own helicopter, the initial cost could range from $1.5 million to $5 million per aircraft. The balance of the costs would be dedicated to personnel expenses and equipment and the amounts would depend on the types of staffing and equipment the program requires.

18. Who pays for the high cost of AMT?

Many AMT programs are subsidized by sponsoring hospitals. In recent years, many AMT programs have been forced to decrease their costs, which they primarily have done by merging programs into consortiums and sharing services within geographic areas. Some programs have developed "subscription services" in which a subscriber pays an annual membership to use the AMT service at a discount or free. Many air medical programs are able to continue operation despite the inability to recoup the cost of operation, because they receive strong local charitable donations and philanthropic contributions. A few AMT programs are subsidized by small fees that are included in a state's motor vehicle taxes.

19. How has managed care affected AMT?

It has forced the AMT industry to become more cost-effective and efficient in all aspects of its operation. Ongoing utilization management, including educating the users of AMT, has become very important in AMT administration. Many AMT programs are contracting with managed care insurers to transport the covered patients at set rates—using a multidimensional transport team of AMT, critical care ground transport, or advanced life support ground transport to match the most cost-effective means of transport with the patient's medical requirements.

20. Is there any proof that AMT is cost-effective?

Not when the bottom line is saving health care dollars. There is intuitive proof that providing a faster means of transport and decreasing the time until a patient receives specialized or definitive care, especially in regard to traumatic injury, decreases morbidity and mortality. Measuring the cost-effectiveness, especially in regard to risk/benefit analysis, is difficult because of the broad differences in patient presentations, injuries and illnesses, and the types of transports involved. Many multicenter studies are underway to study the cost/survival benefits of AMT.

21. Are there any types of patients who should not be transported by AMT?

Only patients who are provided a higher level of care should be transported by an AMT service. Patients who are pre-arrest or are in cardiac arrest should not be transported by AMT. Similarly, patients with serious medical conditions who have preexisting no resuscitative orders should probably not be transported by AMT. The combative patient who places at risk the safety of the air medical crew should not be transported. Such patients include violent prisoners, suicidal or homicidal patients, or intoxicated or head-injured patients who cannot safely be restrained. A woman who is in active labor or whose cervix is dilated 4 cm or more should not be transported by AMT.

22. How safe is AMT?

In the infancy of AMT, aviation accidents occurred two to three times more frequently than non-EMS accidents. These accidents were found to be three and one half times more likely to be fatal than non-EMS accidents. Since the late 1980s, safety has taken a priority with all AMT programs to decrease these disturbing statistics. Safety committees have been developing involving all members of the air medical crews. Access to the most up-to-date weather information and outfitting the aircraft with the best safety and survival gear has become standard. As a result, in 1987–1993 EMS rotor-wing aircraft crashed less often than other turbine helicopters. The fatal accident rate was three times less than in 1980–1986. However, the fatal accident rate for AMT is still higher than for every other category of aircraft based on the number of fatal accidents per flight hours.

Air medical programs should never accept a transport based on fear of losing that transport to a competing program or because they feel pressured by the referral hospital or agency. Crew safety should always be the top priority when considering transport of a patient.

23. Are guidelines available that ensure that certain standards for safety and care are met?

The primary agency responsible for the accreditation and maintenance of standards for AMT programs is the Commission on Accreditation of Air Medical Services (CAAMS). An AMT program can request that CAAMS review the program to meet the accreditation standards on a biannual basis. The Association of Air Medical Services (AAMS) also has standards, which are thought to be the minimum that should be met by AMT services. Some states may have particular air medical service guidelines in place.

24. Do medical directors of AMT programs have different qualifications than other EMS medical directors?

In some respects. The experience of most AMT medical directors originated from ground EMS medical direction. AMT medical directors must have knowledge in altitude physiology and aviation safety, the appropriate utilization of the AMT service, be active in educating the referral agencies in regard to the appropriate utilization of the service, and be actively involved in retrospective analysis of utilization of that service. One particular difference between ground EMS and AMT medical directors is that the AMT medical director must be actively involved in patient follow-up with referring agencies and physicians, because the referring parties geographically may be far away, making follow-up logistically difficult.

25. What is the medical director's primary function?

- The authorization, review, and updating of standing orders and protocols
- Medical training of the flight personnel, including the nurses and paramedics
- Active involvement in quality improvement and in maintaining an open line of communication to referral physicians and agencies in regard to follow-up.

Depending on the geographic location of the program, the medical director may be actively involved in outreach education to rural EMS agencies and hospitals that may need the services of the AMT program.

26. Are there any differences between the United States AMT design and the international AMT designs?

The primary difference is that the European systems extensively use physicians. Most of the programs in Australia and Europe use a physician in all transports, in particular for the resuscitation and stabilization of the patient either at the scene or referring institution prior to transport. Depending on the location, other members of the crew may have expertise in rescue and extrication. Other differences in transport relate to the repatriation of patients from Third World countries; a patient may require a higher level of care than what is available in his or her country or may need to be returned to his or her own country. These programs must deal not only with the lack of medical care available but also with governmental and bureaucratic rules that may be involved in crossing international borders.

27. What is the future of AMT?

"Matching" the patient with the proper level of health care resources via the most appropriate and cost-effective means of transportation will be essential. Critical care ground transport programs are being developed in conjunction with many AMT programs to provide a high level of critical care transport in situations where time of transport is not crucial. This will especially be useful as managed care penetrates more geographic areas and repatriation of patients to member hospitals becomes necessary.

BIBLIOGRAPHY

1. Association of Air Medical Services: Association of Air Medical Services Standards. Alexandria, VA, AAMS, 1992.
2. CAAMS: Accreditation Standards of Commission on Accreditation of Air Medical Services, 2nd ed. Anderson, SC, CAAMS, 1993.
3. Rodenberg H: Aeromedical transport and inflight medical emergencies. In Rosen P (ed): Emergency Medicine: Concepts and Clinical Practice, 3rd ed. St. Louis, Mosby, 1992, pp 229–253.
4. Rodenberg H, Blumen IJ (ed): Air Medical Physician Handbook. Salt Lake City, Air Medical Physician Association, 1994.

68. AEROMEDICAL TRANSPORTATION: PHYSIOLOGY OF ALTITUDE

Lee W. Shockley, M.D.

1. What happens physiologically when a person ascends to altitude?

Atmospheric pressure, of course, is a function of altitude; as one ascends, the atmospheric pressure decreases. For example, the atmospheric pressure on a standard day at sea level is 760 mm Hg; the pressure is roughly half of that at 18,000 feet and only a third of that at 28,000 feet. The effects of the decreasing atmospheric pressure with altitude are manifest in volume (Boyle's law), partial pressures of gases (Dalton's law), the solubility of gases (Henry's law), and temperature (Charles' law).

Effects of Decreasing Atmospheric Pressure

NAME	EQUATION	EFFECT OF ALTITUDE
Boyle's law	$P_1V_1 = P_2V_2$	Gases expand in volume
Dalton's law	$P_{total} = p_1 + p_2 + ...$	The partial pressure of a gas decreases with altitude
Henry's law	$Concentration_{dissolved\ gas} =$ constant x p_1	The amount of a gas that can be dissolved in solution decreases with altitude
Charles' law	$V = constant/T$	Temperature lapse rate of 2°C (3.5°F) per 1000 feet

P = pressure, V = volume, T = temperature

Physiologically, these laws indicate that, with increasing altitude (decreasing pressure), (1) gas-filled structures expand, (2) the partial pressure of gases (e.g., oxygen) drops, (3) dissolved gases (e.g., nitrogen) come out of solution, and (4) the ambient temperature drops.

2. Why is it important to understand the physiologic changes that occur with altitude?

A patient who is transported by air may be subjected to an environment with lower atmospheric pressure than he or she would be subjected to in a ground transport. Practically speaking, this means:

1. Trapped gases will expand in the relatively hypobaric atmosphere. A pneumothorax can increase in size or become a tension pneumothorax. Air splints or military anti-shock trousers (MAST) can get too tight and impair circulation. The patient with an ileus or intestinal obstruction can experience worsening symptoms (aerogastralgia) or even hollow viscus rupture. Air trapped in endotracheal tube cuffs and intravenous tubing will expand. Gases trapped in obstructed sinuses, ears, or abscesses will expand and can cause severe pain.

2. If the patient has a serious alveolar/arterial gradient problem (i.e., chronic obstructive pulmonary disease or pulmonary embolism) or an altered hemoglobin dissociation curve (i.e., carbon monoxide poisoning), it may be very difficult to adequately oxygenate him or her. Consider supplemental oxygen, pulse-oximetry monitoring, early intubation, or positive end expiratory pressure to maintain sufficient oxygenation. High-altitude diseases (high-altitude pulmonary edema, high-altitude cerebral edema, or acute mountain sickness) may be exacerbated by the transport at even higher altitudes.

3. Decompression sickness can worsen at altitude because more of the dissolved nitrogen comes out of solution as microbubbles. If these patients must be transported by air (such as to a

hyperbaric facility), they should be given 100% oxygen and transported at as low an altitude as possible.

4. The lower ambient temperature at altitude may worsen the condition of a hypothermic patient. Passive or active rewarming techniques may be necessary in-flight.

3. If the aircraft is pressurized, will ascent to altitude still affect patients?

It can. Although an aircraft is pressurized, it doesn't mean that the cabin altitude is sea level. Even commercial pressurized aircraft (such as the Boeing 737 and the McDonnell-Douglas DC-9) experience cabin altitudes of up to 8450 feet during cruise flight. Pressurization is a relative thing. The pilot of the aeromedical aircraft can tell you what the cabin altitude is.

4. Besides giving every patient supplemental oxygen, what should I do?

Pre-flight chest tubes and nasogastric tubes should be considered in patients at risk. In-flight, pay attention to expanding trapped gases in the medical equipment. This means continuous, careful monitoring and evaluation of patients and preparing to decompress the spaces in which trapped gas has expanded. Specifically, needle or chest tube thoracostomy for pneumothorax or nasogastric tube insertion for abdominal distention should be available during the transport and performed by appropriately trained personnel in the event of deterioration in the patient's condition.

BIBLIOGRAPHY

1. Benson NH, Low RB, Chisholm CD, et al: Air medical transport: An annotated bibliography of the recent literature. Am J Emerg Med 9:510–519, 1991.
2. Burney RE, Fischer RP: Ground versus air transport of trauma victims: Medical and logistical considerations. Ann Emerg Med 15:1491–1495, 1986.
3. Hansen PJ: Safe practice for our aeromedical evacuation patients. Mil Med 152:281–283, 1987.
4. Isaacs SM, Saunders CE, Dürrer B: Aeromedical transport. In Auerbach PS (ed): Wilderness Medicine: Management of Wilderness and Environmental Emergencies, 3rd ed. St. Louis, Mosby, 1995.

XV. Media and Public Relations

69. PUBLIC AND MEDIA RELATIONS

Mitchell E. Tilstra, EMD-P, EMD I/C

1. Should I wait for the media to call me for information on a story?

No! Prehospital personnel perform hundreds of thousands of life-saving acts every year. Unfortunately, most of the media coverage occurs when there is a perceived miscue or mistake. Emergency incidents strike interest in everyone. They are exciting, humanistic, and have a great impact on patient outcomes. When positive events occur, make sure the appropriate media are notified. It is essential that the public understand the caring and competency and readiness available within their communities.

2. Should everyone in the department be briefed about an incident so they all will communicate the information consistently?

Major or extraordinary incidents should be discussed with the appropriate people within the department or organization. It is ideal to have one person designated as the spokesperson for the media. The spokesperson must be available 24 hours a day for the initial break into media coverage. If the incident will be in the news longer than 4–5 days, departmental meetings should recur to brief staff members.

3. What are some tips for speaking with reporters?

It takes practice to conduct an interview that will satisfy you. Reporters are not trained in the practice of prehospital medicine just as you are not educated as a press secretary. Once the interview is over, you are at the mercy of the reporter and the editor. The important facts should be stated at the beginning of an interview because most editors will cut from the end of the story first. The usual interview will last about 5 minutes; a sit-down, scheduled interview as much as 20 minutes. However, only 15–30 seconds will be used and your statements will be sliced into "bites" with the reporter narrating between video and audio segues.

Reporters are trained to write stories that separate their angle from a competitor's. People who work in media tend to scan for sensational statements and will chose the "gem" statements to produce sound bites that contribute to the angle of their story. Do not make statements that have not been thoroughly thought out and discussed among your staff or superiors.

4. What are the advantages and disadvantages of having a public information officer?

Most police and fire departments and some hospitals have designated public information officers (PIOs) who are the only individuals that are permitted to address the media. Using the chief as the PIO initially demonstrates that the top person in the department is in touch with his or her organization and intends to handle the issue from the highest level. A PIO who serves as a relay between the department and the media may lose credibility if he or she does not have the operational knowledge or is not allowed to speak to nearly all matters for the department. If the PIO must constantly "track down that information and get back to you," aggressive reporters will find other sources to extract information that may not be the opinion of the department. Remember that, for the most part, the PIO has certain rules and restrictions but the reporter does not.

Conversely, consistently using a PIO always leaves the organization with a fallback position if the PIO misspeaks or represents the issues poorly. The chief or other high ranking official can correct statements made in poor judgment or haste.

5. What should I be aware of and always do in an interview?

1. Be aware of whether the interview is being conducted for radio, television, or print.

2. Be pleasant and positive. It's important to show human compassion and warmth in times of crisis.

3. Challenge misinformation. If a question is asked based on inaccurate information, do not answer the question. Correct the premise immediately without restating the question.

4. Slow down if you get angry. Take a deep breath and gather your thoughts.

5. End statements definitively. Reporters tend to keep the microphone aimed your way. This may cause you to make off-the-cuff or unprepared statements. This technique makes the interviewee feel as if there is something else he or she should say. The result of these spontaneous comments may end up as sound bites.

6. Speak plainly and direct your comments to the lay public. Avoid using industry jargon that the general public will not understand.

7. Tell the truth. Give accurate and factual information. If you are uncertain of the facts, say so.

8. Be candid and direct, especially on television. Deal with what's on peoples' minds, what frightens them. Sometimes there are no good answers.

9. Draw on your personal experiences to illustrate your point and use analogies to explain difficult technical situations.

10. Cite outside experts on prevailing industry standards or practices. Communities constantly compare themselves to one another.

6. What should I avoid doing during an interview?

Do not:

1. Be hostile, sarcastic, or confrontational.
2. Consider the interview a conversation. Everything is on the record.
3. Overload your message with complex or technical data.
4. Personally attack other organizations or competitors.
5. Answer a question with "no comment."
6. Attempt to cover up a mistake or mislead the media. Reporters are professionals who make their living extracting information and judging peoples' characters.
7. Theorize, speculate, hypothesize, or agree with a reporter who does so.
8. Interfere with any legitimate duties of the media.

7. What are some tips for videotaped interviews?

1. Be prepared and proactive. Communicate key messages.
2. Turn negatives into positives. This requires practice.
3. Think in terms of "sound bites." Try to deliver definitive answers lasting 7–10 seconds.
4. Let the microphone be the reporter's concern. Unusable audiotape is the reporter's or photographer's fault, not yours. It is the media's responsibility to assure proper sound levels are in place prior to the interview. Speak in your normal tone.
5. Always look directly at the reporter, not the camera. Watch others being interviewed and notice the difference between a well-seasoned interviewee and a novice.
6. Avoid being asked stupid questions. Use a handout or media kit. Fax it to the assignment editor the day before the interview. This may inspire the reporter to ask questions relative to the specific issues.

BIBLIOGRAPHY

1. Paine and Associates: Presented at The American Ambulance Association, Nashville, TN, November 1994.

XVI. *Emergency Vehicle Operation*

70. EMERGENCY VEHICLE OPERATION

Tom Tkach, NREMT-P

1. Isn't speed of the essence when responding on emergency medical calls?

EMS providers are constantly responding to life-and-death situations. Under such pressure, they can become obsessed with the need to travel at the utmost speed, disregarding their safety and the safety of other drivers. In reality, however, less than 10% of the calls turn out to be life-threatening cases. Emergency responses, therefore, usually turn out to be more dangerous to the responders than the nature of the emergency to the patient. In addition, recent research indicates that emergency responses save little time in the overall scheme of the emergency call, time easily recovered with good scene management skills.

2. Why is emergency vehicle operations (EVO) training necessary?

Most EMS providers believe that they face the greatest personal risk while dealing with calls such as shootings, stabbings, and gang fights. However, the greatest risk for injury actually comes from the potential for emergency vehicle accidents. More EMS providers are killed and injured in such accidents than in any other type of prehospital event. Appropriate EVO driver education can significantly decrease the risk of injury during EVO.

3. Besides decreasing the risk of injury, is there another reason to obtain bona fide EVO training?

With the increasingly litigious society in which EMS providers find themselves performing, there is an increased risk of personal liability if you're found responsible for an accident that occurs while you are operating an emergency vehicle. Substantial case law demonstrates that operators of emergency vehicles can be held liable for criminal and civil damages for their actions when judged responsible for an accident.

4. Why isn't a generic defensive driving class sufficient for emergency vehicle drivers?

The average defensive driving course is good for the average driver, but anyone who must navigate a five-ton emergency vehicle through heavy traffic at high speed must be a much more skillful driver. Emergency vehicle drivers must understand the physical dynamics of their vehicle, such as its tires and its load transfer properties. The emergency vehicle driver *must* know the limits of the vehicle. The average driving class is inadequate for teaching these crucial skills to the emergency driver.

5. What do EVO courses cover?

All emergency vehicle operators should enroll in a sanctioned emergency vehicle operations course (EVOC), which includes performance training and evaluation on a driving range. The best EVOC programs allow students to drive their emergency vehicles on a closed course at 100% capability to experience what the vehicle can and can't do on the street. Emergency vehicle drivers who learn the limits of both themselves and their vehicles in a controlled setting are much more conservative and therefore much safer drivers.

Reasons to Obtain Emergency Vehicle Driver Training

1. Reduce emergency vehicle accidents
2. Reduce risk of personal injury
3. Reduce liability
4. Increase level of attention
5. Create greater driver maturity
6. Create greater emotional control
7. Reduce stress level
8. Increase decision-making skill
9. Improve vehicle control skills for on-duty driving
10. Improve vehicle control skills for off-duty driving

6. What is one of the most frequent complaints made by the public to supervisors of EMS agencies?

That the emergency vehicle violated one or more traffic laws. The greatest number of citizen contacts with EMS occur while citizens are driving their own vehicle and are confronted by an emergency vehicle responding to an emergency call. Therefore, it is easy to understand why a significant number of complaints are related to driving. It is difficult for other drivers to understand the complexities of driving an emergency vehicle. Emergency vehicle operators must realize the great scrutiny they are under and always drive with due regard for the safety of all other drivers.

7. What are the psychological aspects related to driving an emergency vehicle?

Because of the great risk of accidents, a mature attitude, coupled with sound judgment and 100% concentration, are important psychological attributes of a good emergency vehicle operator.

8. What is an "on board computer" and how does it work?

Your brain functions like an on-board computer, receiving data in the form of visual, audio, and tactile sensations. This information is processed rapidly by your brain, and your driving actions and reactions are produced. Approximately 90% of the input your brain needs for driving comes from vision. Most of the remaining 10% comes from tactile senses, i.e., "feeling" the weight transfer of the vehicle. A small portion comes from auditory input.

9. What are the components of vision?

Visual acuity, focal vision, peripheral vision, and depth perception.

10. How does visual acuity affect driving ability?

Visual acuity is defined as the ability of either eye to differentiate small space intervals in the discrimination of form. Since most input from driving comes visually, high acuity is critical for safe emergency vehicle operations. Visual acuity can be affected by the amount of ambient light and age of the driver. Thus, driving at night impairs acuity and, as a driver ages, macular degeneration of the retinas is more pronounced, also impairing acuity.

11. What is focal vision?

Also referred to as central vision, focal vision is the portion of the visual field you are specifically looking at. The focal visual field accounts for only 3–5% of the total field of vision. Drivers who use only their focal vision to drive are using a limited amount of their available ability to see. Such drivers are referred to as having tunnel vision. An emergency vehicle driver must learn to use his or her total field of vision.

12. What is peripheral vision and why is it important?

Peripheral vision allows a person to perceive objects to either side of one's focal vision. Because the periphery of the retinas contain fewer nerve endings, images perceived through peripheral vision are not well defined. You can demonstrate this by holding your hands out to both sides while looking straight ahead. You can see your hands but cannot count your fingers. Peripheral vision is important to the emergency vehicle driver. If you learn to use your peripheral vision effectively, you gain valuable reaction time while clearing an intersection, for example, because you can perceive movement of approaching vehicles more quickly. You cannot tell what kind of vehicle it is until you look more directly at it, but you know a vehicle is approaching.

13. What is depth perception and why is it the most important component of vision for emergency vehicle driving?

When both eyes are open, the brain is able to compute the relative position of objects in the visual field. This ability to judge this "spatial depth" of objects is crucial for a driver. Depth perception allows the driver to determine if there is room to maneuver the vehicle through lanes and spaces as well as distance from objects. Emergency vehicle accident statistics show that a significant number of crashes are "vehicle dimension" incidents, in which the driver attempted to enter too small a space. Good depth perception requires good vision.

14. How can I improve my vision?

Visual improvement has been demonstrated through the use of a five-step method developed by three scientists. Practicing the components of this method, the Smith-Cummins-Sherman Visual Development System, allows a person to enhance his visual awareness and field of vision.

Smith-Cummins-Sherman Visual Development System

1. Aim high in steering: Keep your vehicle centered in your path by glancing well ahead at the roadway.
2. Get the big picture: Continually scan the unfolding traffic scene as you drive. Systematically scan all around your vehicle, especially your blind spots.
3. Keep your eyes moving: Never fix your focal vision on any one area.
4. Always have an escape: "Scan & Plan" to react to traffic changes.
5. Make sure they see you: Just because your emergency warning equipment is on doesn't mean other drivers know you're there. Always be alert for clues to wrong moves by other drivers.

15. What concerns do I need to have about night driving?

Most drivers believe that the only difference between day and night driving is that headlights are used at night. This misconception causes them to drive at night as they do in the daylight, a misconception that is all too often fatal. Visual difficulties begin at dusk as the eyes are forced to adapt to changing light levels, impaired color perception, deeper shadows, and headlights from approaching cars. With full darkness, normal driving cues are lost, acuity and depth perception are impaired, field of vision narrows, and sight distance decreases. All of these factors add up to an enormously increased risk during night driving.

16. How do I maximize my ability to drive safely at night?

Wear corrective lenses if you need them. Be as well rested as possible. Increase your cushion and reduce your speed. Know the range of your headlights so you don't overdrive your sight distance. Good vehicle prep is also crucial; clean all windows inside and out to reduce glare.

17. What is "load transfer"?

Also known as weight transfer, load transfer is a physical event that occurs in a vehicle whenever a "control action" is applied by the driver. This principle is best understood by imagining that the vehicle is balanced on a fulcrum placed under the center of the chassis. Whenever the driver applies a control action, i.e., turning the steering wheel, applying the brakes, or stepping on the accelerator, the weight of the vehicle shifts on this fulcrum, transferring the load around to different wheels. Anyone who has ever ridden in the back compartment of an ambulance is well acquainted with load transfer.

18. What does load transfer have to do with driving?

It is not so much the actual transfer of weight that affects driving dynamics but the fact that load transfer affects the size of the contact patch of the tires on the vehicle. As the weight of the vehicle transfers toward one of its corners or sides, the amount of weight on the corresponding tire(s) increases. As a result, the tire's area of contact with the road surface gets larger while the contact patches of the tires on the other side of the vehicle get smaller. These changes in contact patch size can affect handling and control of the vehicle. Proper load transfer management maintains maximum contact patch size, allowing the greatest control. A good driver must learn to minimize load transfer if optimal vehicle control is to be maintained.

19. Why does an emergency vehicle have greater amounts of load transfer than the average passenger car?

An ambulance or rescue vehicle is much heavier and has a higher center of gravity than the average vehicle. These design characteristics add to the magnitude of the load transfer that occurs under maneuvering, which increases the chance of losing control. Excessive load transfer causes tires to lock up more easily under braking and lose traction while cornering, causing a loss of vehicle control.

20. How can load transfer be controlled?

Smooth and gentle control actions will minimize load transfer and allow optimal control of the vehicle. Most new emergency vehicles are equipped with diesel engines that have an incredible amount of compression. Suddenly taking your foot off the accelerator of this engine simulates a tap on the brakes, creating increased load transfer. Sudden turns cause tremendous load transfer and should be avoided. One maneuver in particular to avoid is braking and cornering simultaneously. Braking should be done "in-line" before entering any curves or corners. The old adage of "brake and accelerate as if there was an eggshell between your foot and pedal" has real merit. Remember that when you are driving to the limit of adhesion of the tires, any increase in load transfer is an invitation to disaster. Gentle control actions on the steering wheel, accelerator, and brake pedal will allow the greatest control.

21. Are there other design characteristics of the typical emergency vehicle that can create handling problems?

Any vehicle that has dual rear wheels has twice as many tires in back as in front, giving twice as much traction to the rear of the vehicle than the front. This creates a distinct handling problem called understeer. In an understeering vehicle attempting to negotiate a corner or curve, the front tires lose traction with the road surface before the rear tires, forcing the front end of the vehicle to "push" out in the opposite direction the vehicle is attempting to travel. Understeer is controlled by good throttle control. Slightly lifting off the accelerator will scrub some speed off the vehicle and allow the front tires to regain traction and track around the turn.

22. Which is more dangerous, emergency driving in an urban or a rural area?

Each setting has its own unique dangers. Urban areas have higher traffic volumes, more pedestrians, and higher call volumes. Rural emergency responses expose the driver to large animals in the roadway, less light, and less adequate road conditions. Rural and urban responders must be just as vigilant as the other.

23. What weather conditions increase the risk for an emergency vehicle?

Rain, snow, and ice have the result of reducing a driver's vision, reducing control, and increasing stopping distance. These impairments are magnified for the emergency driver because the vehicle is heavier and more difficult to control in normal driving conditions. One must be even more conservative when driving in adverse conditions.

24. What are the secrets to driving in rain?

Driving conditions are always worst during the initial minutes of a rainstorm as the road grime floats on the water in the roadway. Brakes get wet, impairing stopping ability, and heavy rain impairs visibility. Reduce your speed and increase the cushion between other drivers. Be wary of hydroplaning, which can occur in an emergency vehicle just as with any other vehicle. Be prepared to react to the subsequent control loss by reducing speed.

25. How do I know when there is enough water on the road to create hydroplaning?

It takes as little as $1/16''$ of water on the roadway to cause hydroplaning, reducing your ability to steer and stop. With that amount of water, reflections from other vehicles' brakelights and headlights are visible on the road and tires will leave a visible wake.

26. What are some secrets to driving on snow and ice?

In winter conditions, bridges and shaded areas freeze first and melt last. Since any sudden control actions can cause you to lose control due to the increased load transfer of the emergency vehicle, speed reduction and gentle control input is essential. Increase the following distance from other vehicles. One extremely helpful tip when attempting to stop on icy roads is to slip the transmission into neutral, removing the engine compression from the load transfer equation.

27. What is the most common mistake made by both civilian and emergency vehicle drivers that creates an accident?

When a driver, including the emergency vehicle driver, gets in a bad situation, the most common mistake is to lock up the brakes of the vehicle. Once the brakes are locked, tiny balls of rubber tear loose from the tires. Essentially the vehicle "floats" on these rubber marbles, causing it to travel in the direction it was headed at the instant the brakes locked up. The resultant loss of directional control often causes the vehicle to strike whatever the driver was attempting to avoid. One of the fundamental driving skills taught in EVOC is appropriate use of emergency braking techniques. A properly trained emergency vehicle driver can evade almost all impending collisions because this panic braking and control loss will not occur.

28. Can a vehicle with an antilock braking system (ABS) stop in a shorter distance than a vehicle with standard brakes?

No. The only road surface on which ABS brakes can stop the vehicle more quickly is on gravel. The advantage of ABS brakes is that they will not lock up under maximum braking input, allowing the tires to maintain rolling friction and enabling the driver to still maneuver the vehicle. On an emergency vehicle with a standard braking system, a driver can simulate ABS brakes with use of a technique called threshold braking.

29. What is threshold braking?

Application of the maximum braking input while still allowing the tires to keep rolling, thereby maintaining vehicle control. It requires lots of practice and a skillful driver who can feel load transfer and listen for the characteristic sound made by tires at the limit of their adhesion. During an emergency stop, the driver applies maximum pressure to the brake pedal. Just before a tire loses traction, i.e., its "point of incipient skid," a high-pitched whining sound is produced. When that sound is heard, the driver must "flare" his toes on the brake pedal, bleeding a small amount of hydraulic pressure off the brakes, thereby allowing the tires to keep rolling. This technique allows maximum braking ability while preserving steering control.

30. What is brake fade?

Build-up of heat in the braking system impairs braking ability and can dramatically increase pedal force requirements. During responses, heat is generated by the heavy use of brakes and can affect the composition of the brake component material. In a vehicle with drum brakes, this can cause formation of a layer of superheated gas molecules to build up between the brake drum and brake shoes, preventing contact. The brake pedal gets soft and stopping ability is impaired. In extreme cases, the brakes can simply disappear. In a vehicle with disc brakes, excessive heat can be generated in the brake pads, which then transfers into the brake fluid through the calipers. The brake fluid can actually boil, at which time all braking is lost.

31. What should I do if brake fade occurs?

If the brakes fade while en route to a call, minimize your speed and use of brakes. If the brakes are lost completely, the only option is to terminate your response. Assuming you arrive at the scene and the brake fade is due to excessive drum and shoe heat, cooling will occur while you are attending to the call. Once you load the patient to begin transport, the brakes should be functional again, but the vehicle should be serviced as soon as possible. If brake fade is due to boiling of the brake fluid, steam will be generated in the brake lines and it's unlikely that the brakes will recover with cooling. The vehicle should be removed from service immediately.

32. Are turns and curves of concern?

Remember that the laws of physics impose limits on your cornering ability. Centrifugal force quadruples as speed doubles; therefore, there is a maximum speed for each curve. The tighter the curve, the slower the speed must be. In addition, the design characteristics of a heavy emergency vehicle increase the amount of load transfer that occurs while maneuvering. A good emergency driver must know the limit of the vehicle, especially as it relates to cornering speed.

33. How should I negotiate turns and curves?

First, brake to the proper speed before entering the turn. Because braking distance quadruples as speed doubles, any hard braking at high speed should be done "in-line," with the vehicle traveling in a straight line. This will minimize lateral load transfer. Then position the vehicle for entry as far outside the lane as you can, using as much road as possible. By noting the inside point of the road edge, establish an apex (the lowest point of the turn), driving low across it while maintaining your speed. Now exit high from the curve, again using as much road as possible. This is called high-low-high cornering and it allows you to maintain a higher speed through the corner with less load transfer. Finally, as you reach the apex of the turn, accelerate gently, transferring some of the load off the front tires, allowing them to track more efficiently around the turn.

34. What are the types of skids and how do I recover from them?

Three types of skids are involved with driving: the braking skid, the cornering skid, and the power skid. The power skid can't occur in a heavy emergency vehicle because the engine can't produce enough power to spin the tires. Braking skids, however, are common because of the panic braking applied by many emergency vehicle drivers. Recovery from a braking skid is easy—get off the brakes, thereby recovering rolling friction and regaining control. A cornering skid occurs when too much speed is carried into a turn. Usually the front tires will lose traction first, creating an understeer situation. Applying the brakes makes a cornering skid worse due to increased load transfer. Recovery is accomplished by easing off the accelerator and avoiding braking.

35. What are some of the most dangerous situations for an emergency vehicle?

Intersections account for more than half of the accidents involving emergency vehicles. Blind intersections are the worst because oncoming lateral traffic cannot be seen. The most perilous situation occurs when an emergency vehicle is attempting to negotiate a red light at an intersection of multilane roads. "Green" traffic in some of the lanes crossing your path will stop, leaving an "open lane" with a green light for opposing traffic. This is a setup for disaster: a driver in the gridlocked cars behind the stopped "green" traffic will not see or hear your emergency equipment, become frustrated by the stopped cars on a green light, and blast through the open lane. Maneuvering near large trucks and buses is risky since it is practically impossible for them to stop or turn suddenly. You must develop respect for them since they physically cannot pull over and yield like other cars.

36. What is the "warning process"?

The process by which other drivers become aware of and respond to an emergency vehicle. The three components of the process are detection, recognition, and response, and they are integral to one another. The better the emergency equipment is and the better it is maintained, the sooner the vehicle is detected by other drivers, giving them maximum time to recognize the vehicle and respond appropriately.

37. What color of emergency lights should an emergency vehicle have?

Most sources recommend red and blue lights since red is more readily detected in daylight and blue is more readily detected at night. Many agencies also use white. The real key to visibility is to have very bright lights of different colors and lots of patterns of light.

38. What kind of audible warning devices should the vehicle have?

The average sound level of normal street traffic is 90 decibels. The siren should generate at least 120 decibels to be heard over normal street traffic, but that alone isn't enough to be heard by all drivers. Since human hearing is quite effective in identifying changes in pitch and tone, the key to being heard is to continually vary the siren settings while responding.

39. Where can I learn more about emergency driving classes?

Contact your state EMS office for listings of EVOC courses. Most local police agencies will have listings of available programs. The National Safety Council also has developed an EVOC program.

BIBLIOGRAPHY

1. Abbott T: Training Program for Driving Instructors. Colorado Springs, CO, Paragon School of Driving.
2. Bondurant B, Blakemore J: Bob Bondurant on High Performance Driving. Motorbooks International Publishers & Wholesalers, 1993.
3. Federal Emergency Management Agency: United States Fire Administration Emergency Driver Training Manual.
4. Greenwald J: Driving Yourself Sane. Health 4:88–89, 1994.
5. International Association of Directors of Law Enforcement Standards and Training.
6. Rice B, Coxon K, Carle L, et al: DHHPD Driving Performance Standards, Policies, and Procedures. Denver, DHPD, 1981–1997.

INDEX

Page numbers in **boldface type** indicate complete chapters.